PRESTON'S ROYAL INFIRMARY

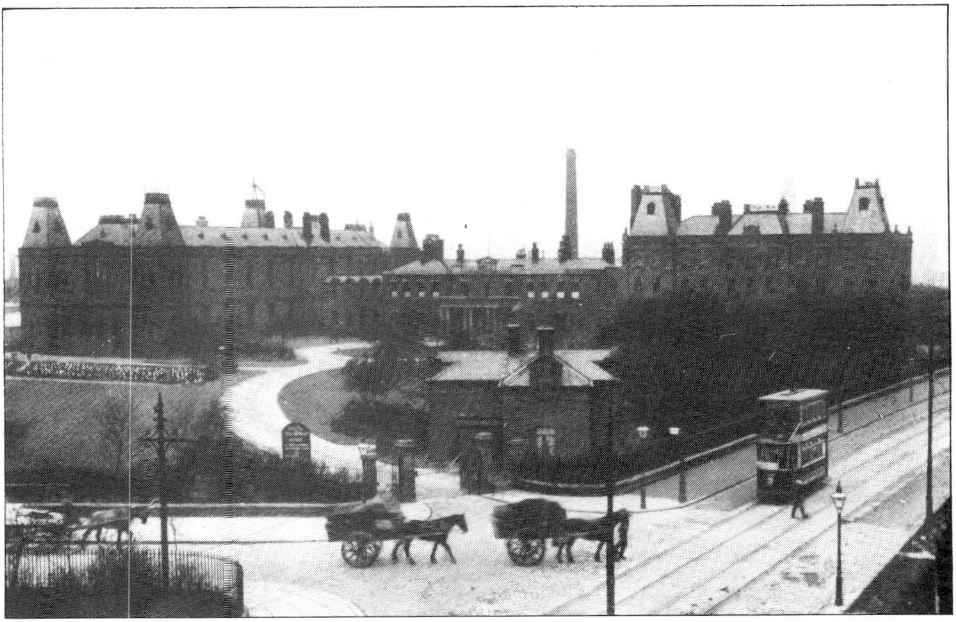

A History of Health Care in Preston 1809-1986

John Wilkinson

Carnegie Press, 1987

Preston's Royal Infirmary:
A History of Health Care in Preston, 1809 - 1986.
by John Wilkinson

Published by Carnegie Press,
125 Woodplumpton Road, Cadley, Preston
Tel (0772) 728868

Printed by T. Snape & Co. Ltd., Bolton's Court, Preston.

Hardback ISBN 0 948789 14 X
Softback ISBN 0 948789 15 8

The publishers wish to acknowledge the help, encouragement and support of the Preston District Health Authority, at all levels, in the publication of this book. Without their co-operation, particularly over the subscription appeal, it may never have appeared in print.

FIRST

ANNUAL REPORT

OF THE

PRESTON & COUNTY OF LANCASTER

ROYAL INFIRMARY.

FOR THE YEAR 1870.

PRESTON:
Printed by T. Snape & Co., 141, Church Street, & 11, Bolton's Court.
1871.

This book is dedicated to all those who, over the years, have in any way contributed to the care of sick people in Preston.

Contents

List of Subscribers

The following have kindly lent their support to the publication of this book.

Addison, Mrs. M. C., Fulwood, Preston
Afrin, Councillor V. M., Preston
Ahamed, Marie, Euxton, Chorley, Lancashire
Ainsworth, Heather, Longton, Preston
Allen, A. B., Walton-le-Dale, Preston
Allen, Mrs. A. H., Broughton, Preston
Allen, Myra, Penwortham, Preston
Allen, Mrs. M. M., Leyland, Lancashire
Allen, Peter John, Clayton-le-Woods, Lancashire
Allen, Vernon, Freckleton, Preston
Anderson, Mrs. P., Corsebar, Paisley, Scotland
Anderton, Malcolm, Fulwood, Preston
Andrews, Mrs. Barbara, Ribbleton, Preston
Antcliffe Mrs. M. T., Preston
Armstrong, G., Feniscliffe, Blackburn, Lancashire
Arnott, George Mair, Victoria, British Columbia Canada
Ashcroft, Mrs. Dorothy, Sassafras, Victoria, Australia
Ashcroft, S. J., Longton, Preston
Ashman, Chris, Leyland, Lancashire
Ashton, Mrs. B. C. Ribbleton, Preston
Ashton, John Barry, Penwortham, Preston
Askew, Miss A. E., Fulwood, Preston
Atherton, Mrs. Jean, Ashton, Preston
Axcell, Mrs. S. M., Leyland, Lancashire
Bailey, Mrs. A. E., Goosnargh, Preston
Bailey, Mrs. Julia, (née O'Connell), Ashton, Preston
Bailey, Mrs. Susan, Goosnargh, Preston
Baines, Mrs. A., Whittingham, Preston
Baldwin, Margaret, Broughton, Preston
Baldwin, Mrs. Mary P., Penwortham, Preston
Balshaw, Mrs. J. E., Ashton, Preston
Bamber, Mrs. M. Ashton, Preston
Baniabassian, Mrs. C. S., Bamber Bridge, Preston
Banik, Dr. J. L., Fulwood, Preston
Banister, Eileen E., Brindle, Chorley, Lancashire
Bannister, Councillor, A. F., Penwortham, Preston
Bannister, Kathryn A., Lea, Preston
Barker, Dr. Clive, Clayton Brook, Preston
Barker, Mrs. Marie, Oak Ridge, Tennessee, U.S.A.
Barnes, Mrs. C., Fulwood, Preston
Barnes, Susan, Walton-le-Dale, Preston
Barnett, Mr. & Mrs. S., Nelson, Lancashire
Baron, Paul, Ashton, Preston
Bates, Mr. T., Fulwood, Preston
Batty, Ellen R., Dronfield Woodhouse
Bayman, Joan, Bamber Bridge, Preston
The Beardsworth Family, Bamber Bridge, Preston
Beare, Mr. & Mrs., Fulwood, Preston
Bell, M. A., Fulwood, Preston
Bennett, Mrs. A., Ashton, Preston
Bentley, Patricia A., Hutton, Preston
Bickley, A. G., Deepdale, Preston
Biggins, Elizabeth, Penwortham, Preston
Billet, Mrs. A., Penwortham, Preston
Billington, Mr. & Mrs. J., Leyland, Preston
Billington, J. & W., Grimsargh, Preston

Billington, Mr. & Mrs. N., Brookfield, Preston
Binns, Mrs. F. M., Newport, Gwent
Birkenhead, Mr. R., Fulwood, Preston
Black, Mrs. I. S. B., Compton, Winchester, Hants
Black, Mrs. M. M., Fulwood, Preston
Blackburn, J. R., Ashton, Preston
Blackburn, Margaret M. & Bob, Fulwood, Preston
Blackley, Mrs. Annes, Upton, Wirral, Merseyside
Blakeman, Valerie, Blackpool, Lancashire
Blau, Ronald & Sheila, Fuengirola, Malaga, Spain
Blundell, Tom, Goosnargh, Preston
Bolas, Marie, Chorley, Lancashire
Bolton, Alec & Jayne, Bilsborrow, Preston
Bolton, Janet, Brock, Preston
Bolton, Miss M., Woodplumpton, Preston
Booth, Mrs. D., Little Bispham, Blackpool, Lancashire
Booth, Ivy, Penwortham, Preston
Boreham, L. J., Ingol, Preston
Bowcock, Mrs. M., Penselwood, Wincanton, Somerset
Bradbury, Mrs. Joan, (née Horn), St. Helens, Merseyside
Brady, Sylvia, Barton, Preston
Brailsford, Mr. W. W. & Mrs. C. J., Longton, Preston
Breakell, Margaret, New Longton, Preston
Brearley, Dr. B. F., Scorton, Preston
Bridge, Audrey, (née Mason), Whiting Bay, Isle of Arran, Scotland
Bright, C. M., Gosfield, Halstead, Essex
Brindle, Maureen, Fulwood, Preston
Brogden, Mrs. A. M., Much Hoole, Preston
Brooks, Mr. & Mrs. James, Ingol, Preston
Brooks, Mrs. J. A., Fulwood, Preston
Brooks, Ray, Hove, Sussex
Broughall, F. M., Penwortham, Preston
Brown, Mrs. B., Fulwood, Preston
Brown, Mrs. Elsie, (née Wharton), Fulwood, Preston
Brown, Susan, Ingol, Preston
Bryan, Mrs. B., Fulwood, Preston
Buckles, Ethel, Hutton, Preston
Buckley, Mrs. C., Fulwood, Preston
Buckley, Mrs. J., Ingol, Preston
Burland, Mrs. B. A., South Uist, Scotland
Burnett, M., Penwortham, Preston
Burns, Rev. Canon E. J. & Mrs., Fulwood, Preston
Burns, Mrs. Rita, Fulwood, Preston
Burns, Mrs. Sandra, Walton-le-Dale, Preston
Burton, Mrs. E., Fulwood, Preston
Burton, Stella, Great Harwood, Lancashire
Butler, M. J., Fulwood, Preston
Button, Dr. R. I., Walton-le-Dale, Preston
Byrne, Mrs. Ann M., Roosevelt Park, Johannesburg, South Africa
Byrom, Miss Diane M., Kirkham, Preston
Caffrey, Linda, Lea, Preston
Cairns, Miss Sheila, Penwortham, Preston
Calderbank, J. F., Fulwood, Preston
Campbell, Dr. A. N., R.P.H., Preston
Camps, Mrs. M., Fulwood, Preston
Caplin, Dr. George, Fulwood, Preston
Capper, Joan, SRN, SCM, Marshside, Southport, Lancashire
Carr, Elaine, Lostock Hall, Preston
Carsley, Mrs. Linda, Preston
Carter, Mrs. G. R., Fulwood, Preston
Carter, Mrs. Pauline M., Poulton-le-Fylde, Lancashire
Case, D. B., Penwortham, Preston
Cassie, Mr. & Mrs. A. M., Fulwood, Preston
Catterall, J., Fulwood, Preston
Catterall, P. G., Fulwood, Preston

Chaloner, Mrs. D. E. Fulwood, Preston
Chambers, Joan A., (née Craig), St. Annes-on-Sea, Lancashire
Charnley, Mrs. Barbara, Penwortham, Preston
Chatterjee, Mr. A. K., Fulwood, Preston
Chessell, Joyce, Grimsargh, Preston
Childs, Mr. F. A., Higher Walton. Preston
Clare, Barry, Anderton, Chorley, Lancashire
Clarke, J. F. B., Euxton, Chorley, Lancashire
Clarkson, R. H., Walton-le-Dale, Preston
Clegg, Mrs. Elsie, Whitehall, Darwen, Lancashire
Cleminson, Mrs. Kate, Penwortham, Preston
Cliff, Mr. & Mrs. G., Fulwood, Preston
Clifford, C. M., Newport, Gwent
Clucas, D. B., R.P.H., Preston
Clulow, Jean, Penwortham, Preston
Coaker, Melanie Jane, Fulwood, Preston
Cocks, Yvonne M., Penwortham, Preston
Colgan, Nell, Penwortham, Preston
Collinson, Mr. H., Preston
Collinson, Mrs. M. P., Fulwood, Preston
Consiglio, Dr. R. V. A., Bilsborrow, Preston
Conway, Henry, Ashton, Preston
Cook, Mrs. K. M., Longridge, Preston
Coombes, Mrs. M. A., Ashton, Preston
Cooper, Dr. W. A. Bruce, Fulwood, Preston
Corbin, Mary I., Fulwood, Preston
Corcoran, Mrs. Joan G., Lea Town, Preston
Cornwell, Mr. P., Walton-le-Dale, Preston
Cosgrove, Mr. N. W , Fulwood, Preston
Costello, Edith A., Fulwood, Preston
Costello, M. C., Newark, Notts
Cottam, Mrs. Irene, Fulwood, Preston
Cottier, F. M. & G., Whitestake, Preston
Counsell, P. A., Penwortham, Preston
Covell, N. A. G., Lytham, Lancashire
Coward, Dr. R. A., Lostock, Bolton, Greater Manchester
Cowell, Mrs. J., Grimsargh, Preston
Cowie, Mrs. Rosemary, Ickleford, Hitchin, Herts
Craven, Mrs. J., Fulwood, Preston
Croasdale, J. & M. E., Ulnes Walton, Preston
Croft, G. Marjorie, Longridge, Preston
Cronkshaw, Pauline G., Fulwood, Preston
Cronshaw, E., Penwortham, Preston
Crook, Angela, Fulwood, Preston
Crook, Miss Joan, Preston
Crook, Mrs. Mary, Preston
Crook, Miss Sheila, Fulwood, Preston
Crook, Mr. Stephen, Preston
Crook, Mrs. Susan, Fulwood, Preston
Cross, Janet A., Kingsbridge, South Devon
Cross, Jim, Leyland, Preston
Cross, Mrs. M. A., Garstang, Preston
Crowther, G. J., Samlesbury, Preston
Cunliffe, A. W., Wrea Green, Preston
Dagger, Freda, (née Cooper), Fulwood, Preston
Darby, Mrs. B. A., Shipton Gorge, Bridport, Dorset
Davies, Mrs. Beryl, Walton-le-Dale, Preston
Davies, Dr. Dilys & Dr. Tudor, Penwortham, Preston
Davies, Dr. D. J., Penwortham, Preston
Davies, Edith, SRN, Fulwood, Preston
Davies, Gloria, Lostock Hall, Preston

Davies, Stephen, Ashton, Preston
Davis, Mr. H. B., Preston
Dawoud, Dr. E. S. M., Clayton-le-Woods, Lancashire
Daws, Mr. R. A., FRCS, Ashton, Preston
Dean, A. R., Broughton, Preston
Delaney, Mrs. Jean, A., Hoghton, Preston
Dempsey, J. P., P.H.A., Preston
Dempsey, Michael, C., Fulwood, Preston
Desanti, Mrs. M. J., Penwortham, Preston
Desmond, S. R., Cabus, Garstang, Preston
Diamond, Mrs. Patricia, JP, Penwortham, Preston
Dickinson, Mrs. Ann, Hoghton, Preston
Dilworth, Mrs. Joyce, Higher Walton, Preston
Dimmock, Mrs. Jill E., Higher Walton, Preston
Dixon, Mrs. H. G., Preston
Dixon, Miss Janet, Fulwood, Preston
Dobson, A. J., Fulwood, Preston
Dodgeon, Ekaterine, Fulwood, Preston
Donald, Dr. C., Hoghton, Preston
Done, H. J., Broughton, Preston
Donnelly, Mrs. D., Croston, Preston
Donnelly, Mrs. M., Preston
Downward, Mrs. Hannah, New Longton, Preston
Drain, Geoffrey, CBE, Swiss Cottage, London
Duck, George, Fulwood, Preston
Duff, Mr. & Mrs. T. B., Grimsargh, Preston
Dunn, D., Walton-le-Dale, Preston
Dunsmore, Mrs. J., Fulwood, Preston
Dyer, Mrs. Barbara, Fulwood, Preston
Dyer, Jean A., Fulwood, Preston
Eagle, Miss I. M., Higher Bartle, Preston
Eastham, Mrs. Ann, (née Edwards), Garstang, Preston
Eastham, Mrs. S., Higher Walton, Preston
Eaves, Evelyn, Fulwood, Preston
Eddershaw, M., Chipping Norton, Oxon
Edmondson, Mrs. A., Lostock Hall, Preston
Edmondson, R., Penwortham, Preston
Edwards, Mrs. Joan, Goosnargh, Preston
Eland, Christine Anne, Ribbleton, Preston
Ellis, Mr. F., Penwortham, Preston
Emmett, Mr. Neil, Walton-le-Dale, Preston
Evans, Mr. John, Penwortham, Preston
Evans, Mrs. K., Cwmfelin, Maesteg, Mid Glamorgan
Eves, Dr. Michael J., Preston
Ezard, Mrs. Christine, Porthcawl, Mid Glamorgan
Fairburn, Mrs. Eveline, Exmouth, Devon
Fairclough, Dr. M., Fulwood, Preston
Fairhurst, Miss A., Westhoughton, Greater Manchester
Fallows, Mr. Arthur, Eccleston, Chorley, Lancashire
Farrell-Roberts, Jean, Ingol, Preston
Field, Mrs. C. A., Whittle-le-Woods, Chorley, Lancashire
Finch, S. V., Ashton, Preston
Fisher, Norma A., Ribbleton, Preston
Fitzsimons, Mrs. K., Sale, Cheshire
Flaherty, T., R.P.H., Preston
Flannery, C., Ashton, Preston
Flannery, Mrs. C., Cottam, Preston
Fletcher, Miss Dorothy, Preston
Fletcher, Ian, Preston
Fletcher, Mrs. J. A., Penwortham, Preston
Fletcher, John & Margaret, Bolton, Greater Manchester
Flintoff, Thomas, R., MBE, JP, Garstang, Preston
Flynn, Judith M., Fulwood, Preston
Ford, Mr. Joseph, Lostock Hall, Preston
Fordham, I. J., Carnforth, Lancashire

Foster, Peter S. G., Lytham St. Annes, Lancashire
Fowler, Mrs. Alice, Deepdale, Preston
Fox, Brenda M., Garstang, Preston
Fryer, Dr. J. M., Goosnargh, Preston
Gallagher, K. T., Fulwood, Preston
Gardener, Mrs. R., Norwich, Norfolk
Gardner, D. T., Chorley, Lancashire
Garstang, Mrs. Vivienne, Grimsargh, Preston
Garth, Darren R., Fulwood, Preston
Garth, Patricia & Malcolm, Fulwood, Preston
Gates, E. P., Goosnargh, Preston
Gatt, J. A., P.R.I., Preston
Gaul, Mrs. K. A., Tewkesbury, Glos.
Geake, Dr. M. R., St. Minver, Wadebridge
Ghosh, Mrs. J. M., Penwortham, Preston
Gibb, Dr. Robert, Kirkby Stephen, Cumbria
Gibbons, Mrs. G. S., Harlestone, Northampton
Gibbs, D. J., Ribbleton, Preston
Gibson, Miss H. J., Walton-le-Dale, Preston
Giddins, Mrs. E. G., Ribbleton, Preston
Gifford, Mrs. A. M., Ribbleton, Preston
Gill, Mrs. N., Fulwood, Preston
Gillison, Mrs. Joan, Whitestake, Preston
Gleeson, Mrs. Barbara, SRN, QN, Chadderton, Oldham
Goddard, D. L. E., Goosnargh, Preston
Goddard, H. A. & A. G., Fulwood, Preston
Golding, D. Fulwood, Preston
Goode, Mrs. S., Ashton, Preston
Goodier, Mrs. E. Dunnington, York
Gould, Mrs. D. M., Fulwood, Preston
Gowers, Elizabeth Ann, Patcham, Brighton, Sussex
Graham, C., Preston
Gratrix, Amy, Penwortham, Preston
Gray, A. J., Longridge, Preston
Green, Joan E., Chorlton, Manchester
Greenhalgh, Mrs. V. J., Leyland, Preston
Greenwood, Eleanor, Preston
Gregson, G. A., Lytham, Lancashire
Griffith, Mrs. J., Shaftesbury, Dorset
Griffiths, J., Walton-le-Dale, Preston
Grimley, Ann, R.P.H., Preston
Grimshaw, Alec, Longridge, Preston
Grimshaw, Audrey, Erin, Ontario, Nobito, Canada
Grimshaw, Joan, (née Neilson), New Longton, Preston
Grisdale, Jean M., Fulwood, Preston
Gulati, Dr. R. K., Tarleton, Preston
Guy, Mr. Michael, Heysham, Lancashire
Haigh, T. J., Fulwood, Preston
Haire, Mrs. Anne, Pilling, Preston
Haldon, Mrs. Susan, Lea, Preston
Hall, Mrs. E., Preston
Hall, F. M., Penwortham, Preston
Hall, Mrs. Mary Eileen, Kirkham, Preston
Hall, Ruth, Ribbleton, Preston
Hall, Susan, Blackburn, Lancashire
Halliwell, Mrs. Olive, Fulwood, Preston
Halsall, Christine M., Fulwood, Preston
Halsall, Walter W., Fulwood, Preston
Hamer, Mrs. Dorothy, Fulwood, Preston
Hammond, Mrs. M. M., Fulwood, Preston
Hampson, Mrs. M. M., Fulwood, Preston
Hanby, Miss Caroline Patricia, Fulwood, Preston
Hanley, Mrs. I., Chipping, Preston
Hardman, Karen A., Fulwood, Preston
Hardwick, Mrs. J. F., Brookfield, Preston

Hargreaves, Mrs. M. H., Cottam, Preston
Harris, Mrs. M., Fulwood, Preston
Harris, Miss May, Preston
Harris, Pauline, Goosnargh, Preston
Harrison, J. P., Preston
Harrison, Teresa, Fulwood, Preston
Hart, E. Janet, New Longton, Preston
Harvey, Mrs. W. J., Horsell, Woking, Surrey
Haughie, Dr. T. M., Broughton, Preston
Hawkins, Patricia, (née Yates), Southport, Merseyside
Haxby, K. F., (née Brindle), Park Green, Edinburgh
Hayes, Mrs. B. A., Preston
Hayhurst, Julie, Longridge, Preston
Hayhurst, Mrs. T., Preston
Hayton, Dylis, B., Penwortham, Preston
Heaps, Theresa M., Fulwood, Preston
Hearn, A. R., Fulwood, Preston
Heaton, Judith M., (née Wormleighton), SRN, Whalley, Blackburn, Lancashire
Heffernan, Dr. C. K., Blackburn, Lancashire
Herron, S. C., Whitley Bay, Tyne & Wear
Heywood, Mrs. T., (née Spencer), Alderley Edge, Cheshire
Hickson, Bob, Tunbridge Wells, Kent
Higgins, Mrs. B. I., Shevington, Wigan, Lancashire
Higham, Lynne M., Walton-le-Dale, Preston
Hill, H., Fulwood, Preston
Hill, Norman, Hollinwood, Oldham
Hills, Mrs. T., Fulwood, Preston
Hindle, Mr. J. R., Brock, Preston
Hitchen, Dr. B. P. L., Fulwood, Preston
Hitchen, Mrs. H. M., Fulwood, Preston
Hitchin, Violet, M., Grimsargh, Preston
Hodd R. E., CBE, Blackpool, Lancashire
Hodgson, Stephen F., Blackpool, Lancashire
Hogarth, John, Preston
Holden, Dora, Altrincham, Cheshire
Holden, Francis A., Fulwood, Preston
Holden, Mrs. Isabel, Ribchester, Preston
Holderness, R., Fulwood, Preston
Holland, Miriam, (née Harrington), Wimborne, Dorset
Holman, Mr. K. R., Bolton, Greater Manchester
Holman, Mr & Mrs. P. D., Teddington, Middlesex
Holman, Mr. & Mrs. R., Penwortham, Preston
Holroyd, Shirley, Whitestake, Preston
Holt, Miss A. Velvia, Blackburn, Lancashire
Hopkin, P. M., Penwortham, Preston
Hopkinson, Michael Peter, Penwortham, Preston
Horan, Dorothea, Davyhulme, Manchester
Horner, Dr. J. S., Goosnargh, Preston
Hoskins, Mrs. Pat, Walton-le-Dale, Preston
Houghton, Mrs. Enid, M., Grimsargh, Preston
Houghton, Mrs. S., Ashton, Preston
Howard, Mrs. C., Penwortham, Preston
Howarth, Mrs. A., Chorley, Lancashire
Howarth, David Andrew, Fulwood, Preston
Howarth, Mrs. N. P., Whittle-le-Woods, Chorley, Lancashire
Howe, A., Penwortham, Preston
Howe, Mrs. Ruth, Brampton, Cumbria
Howitt, Florence M., Kingston, Ontario, Canada
Hunter, Mrs. D., Goosnargh, Preston
Hunter, Mrs. P., Lancaster, Lancashire
Hurst, Mrs. J., Preston
Hurst, Norman & Edna, Lea, Preston
Hutchinson, Dr. D. N., Blackburn, Lancashire
Ince, Mr. J. B., Hutton, Preston
Irwin, Dr. D. T., Ribbleton, Preston

Isherwood, J. K., Bamber Bridge, Preston
Jackson, Mr. D., Fulwood, Preston
Jackson, Mr. G. P., Higher Walton, Preston
Jackson, H. W., Penwortham, Preston
Jackson, Patricia, Whittingham Hospital, Preston
Jama, Ahmed A., Walton-le-Dale, Preston
James, Miss J. W., Ingol, Preston
Jameson, Mrs. A., Penwortham, Preston
Jeffrey, Francis, Preston
Jeory, Mrs. J., Ashton, Preston
Jewell, Councillor Mrs. Edna, Lea, Preston
Johnson, K. & M., Ingol, Preston
Johnson, Mr. Michael, Preston
Johnston, Mrs. M. L., Hincaster, Milnthorpe, Cumbria
Jolly, A. J., Penwortham, Preston
Jolly, Mrs. Mary, Walton-le-Dale, Preston
Jones, Mrs. Catherine F., Penwortham, Preston
Jones, Clare, Barton, Preston
Jones, Dr. G. N. Cheadle Hulme, Cheshire
Jones, Ken, Blackpool, Lancashire
Jones, Mrs. Mary, Keighley, West Yorkshire
Jordan, Jacqueline, (née Fann), Bongate, Appleby, Cumbria
Joyce, Nuala, (née Cullen), Hoghton, Preston
Kay, Mrs. A. L., Leyland, Preston
Kealey, Teresa M., Leyland, Preston
Kelly, Mr. Thomas, Hoghton, Preston
Kempster, Mrs. E. M., Fulwood, Preston
Kidd, Miss Grace, Blackburn, Lancashire
Kilshaw, Peter James, R.P.H., Preston
King, Mrs. Anne, Sherwood, Preston
King, Mrs. June, Freckleton, Preston
Kington, Mrs. P. M., Ribbleton, Preston
Kinrade, Norman, Maghull, Merseyside
KIrby, Mr. Henry L., Ribbleton, Preston
Kirby, Miss J. M., Fulwood, Preston
Kitching, Mrs. M. L., Goosnargh, Preston
Knapton, Marie, (née Raby), Brecon, Powys
Knight, Patricia A., Freckleton, Preston
Knight, Miss Sarah L., Longridge, Preston
Knipe, Miss J. M., Grange-over-Sands, Cumbria
Krypczyk, A. M., Blackpool, Lancashire
Kurvers, Mrs. C., (née Van Maarsen), Soest, Holland
Kulbacki, Lesley, Hoghton, Preston
Lake, J., Hutton, Preston
Lake, Mrs. M. J., Hutton, Preston
Lamont, C. M., Fulwood, Preston
Lancashire Polytechnic, Preston
Lancaster, Mrs. J., Walton-le-Dale, Preston
Law, Mrs. Mary, Heysham, Morecambe, Lancashire
Lang, Robert L., Ribbleton, Preston
Laraway, Margaret, Camberley, Surrey
Lawler, Mrs. B., Northwood, Middlesex
Lawrence, Pauline B., Penwortham, Preston
Lawrenson, Dr. G. A., OBE, Lytham St. Annes, Lancashire
Lawrenson, Joyce, Fulwood, Preston
Lawson, J. W., Euxton, Chorley, Lancashire
Lea, Mrs., (née Brassington), Haverbreaks, Lancaster, Lancashire
Leadbetter, Mrs. A., Ashton, Preston
Leadbitter, Janine, Whittingham, Preston
Leahy, Norma, (née Taylor), Thompson, Manitoba, Canada
Leck, Mr. J. A., R.P.H., Preston
Lee, Austin, Frenchwood, Preston
Lee, Nancy-Jane, Cockerham, Lancaster, Lancashire
Lee-Watkinson, Veronica, Fulwood, Preston

Leigh, Mrs. W. E., (née Fleming), Fulwood, Preston
Leigh, N. F., Fulwood, Preston
Leitch, Mrs. N. M., Walmer Bridge, Preston
Lester, Mrs. D. A., New Longton, Preston
Lewington, Mrs. E. J., Northampton
Lewis, Mrs. J., Fulwood, Preston
Leyland, Gweneth, Southport, Lancashire
Livesey, D., Bamber Bridge, Preston
Livesey, E., Ashton, Preston
Livesey, Kathleen Isobel, Broadgate, Preston
Livesey, T. D., Lea, Preston
Lisle, Miss V. M., Walney Island, Barrow-in-Furness, Cumbria
Lloyd, Mr. G., Fulwood, Preston
Lockhart, Mr. T., Fulwood, Preston
Logan-Smith, Mrs. Jean, Lytham, Lancashire
Love, Mr. & Mrs. E. B., Mayals, Swansea
Lucas, Miss D., Thornbank, Bolton, Greater Manchester
Lumb, Mrs. D. M., Preston
Lynch, Dr. P. G., St. Annes, Lancashire
Lythgoe, J. P., Fulwood, Preston
McAiney, J. D., Ingol, Preston
McCandlish, Frank, Ashton, Preston
McCann, Mrs. Carole, Fulwood, Preston
McDade, Mrs. Brenda, Preston
McDowell, Dr. C. & Mrs. E. M., Leyland, Lancashire
McEvoy, Mr. & Mrs., Hutton, Preston
McFee, Mrs. M., Stanwix, Carlisle, Cumbria
McGarry, Mrs. Rita, Grimsargh, Preston
McGowan, Mrs. M. B., Longridge, Preston
McIlwaine, Dr. Eileen, Ashton, Preston
MacKelvie, Mary, Derwen Fawr, Swansea
Mackie, Coughlin & Barnes, Drs., Gt. Eccleston, Preston
McLaren, Mrs. Eva, Fulwood, Preston
McMellon, Mrs. D., Walton-le-Dale, Preston
McMullen, Dorothy E., Preston
McNamara, M., Dalkey, Co. Dublin, Ireland
Maddocks, D. H, Goosnargh, Preston
Malone, Miss M., Oswaldtwistle, Lancashire
Manley, Mr. David J., P.H.A., Preston
Manson, W., Hurst Green, Blackburn, Lancashire
Marginson, Miss J. E., New Longton, Preston
Marle, Mrs. M., Penwortham, Preston
Marquis, Mrs. Shirley, Blackpool, Lancashire
Marsden, Ann, Eccleston, Chorley, Lancashire
Marsden, Mrs. M., Longridge, Preston
Masheter, Mr. F. J. & Mrs. E., Preston
Mason, Anne, (née Dalton), Croston, Preston
Mason, Mrs. E. A., Craig-y-Don, Llandudno, North Wales
Mason, Edna M., Hoghton, Preston
Massey, Miss Doris, Barton, Preston
May, M. A., M.R.I.P.H.H., Preston
Mercer, Miss Lorna K., Preston
Mercer, T. Joyce, Lea, Preston
Merrifield, Miss Ingrid, Preston
Midwifery School, S.G.H., Preston
Millen, Elayne, Kennington, Ashford, Kent
Millns, Dr. D., Fulwood, Preston
Milton, John, Fulwood, Preston
Mitchell, Dr. J. D., Fulwood, Preston
Moir, Dr. C. C., Fulwood, Preston
Moir, Miss C. M., Fulwood, Preston
Molander, Elizabeth G., Gt. Bookham, Leatherhead, Surrey
Molyneux, Mrs. S., Garstang, Preston
Monk, Arnold, Clayton-le-Woods, Chorley, Lancashire
Montgomery, Cllr. Mrs. E., JP, Euxton, Chorley, Lancashire

Moon, Mrs. Janet M., Chorley, Lancashire
Moon, Mrs. Ursula, Preston
Moore, Mrs. Anne M., Clayton-le-Moors, Accrington, Lancashire
Moores, Miss M. E., Ashton, Preston
Morgan, Barbara, Fulwood, Preston
Morgan, Mrs. E. G., Ribbleton, Preston
Morgan-Capner, Dr. P., Melling-via-Carnforth, Lancashire
Morris, Mr. J. M., Blackburn, Lancashire
Morton, Mrs. R., Penwortham, Preston
Moss, Christine, A. Croston, Preston
Moss, Mrs. Maureen, Preston
Murray, Elizabeth Alice, (née Carter), Fulwood, Preston
Murray, Jeanne, Fulwood, Preston
Murray, Stephanie, Hoghton, Preston
Myerscough, Mr. F. L., Woodplumpton, Preston
NALGO (Preston Health Branch), R.P.H., Preston
Naylor, Carole, Lostock Hall, Preston
Nayman, Mrs. J., Morecambe, Lancashire
Nelson, Lavinia, M., Edinburgh, Scotland
Nesom, Anne, North Battleford, Sask., Canada
Newton, Mr. P. C., Goosnargh, Preston
Nickson, Mrs. F. M., Lancaster, Lancashire
Nicholls, Mr. R., Kendal, Cimbria
Nicholson, Dr. C. M , Longridge, Preston
Nicholson, Dorothy, Manly, New South Wales, Australia
Noble, Dr. W. A. & Mrs. J., (née Burrow), Broughton, Preston
Noblett, Ann P., Hoghton, Preston
Noblett, Dr. R. W., Ingol, Preston
Nooriafshar, Judith, (née Bunce), Maryland, New South Wales, Australia
Norburn, L. M., Leyland, Preston
Norcross, Jean, Penwortham, Preston
Norman, Christine, Leyland, Preston
Nowell, Miss Myra, Silverdale, Carnforth, Lancashire
Nutley, Marion, (née Norris), Deepdale, Preston
Nuttall, Mr. J. I., Chorley, Lancashire
N.W.R.H.A., Piccadilly South, Manchester
Oakes, Julie, Higher Bartle, Preston
Oakley, Marjorie, Walton-le-Dale, Preston
Oatridge, E. J., Broughton, Preston
O'Connor, Mrs. G., Fulwood, Preston
Oddy, Mrs. J. H., Brinscall, Chorley, Lancashire
O'Donnell, E., Fulwood, Preston
Ogden, Maureen, Fulwood, Preston
Ogleby, B. H., Penwortham, Preston
O'Herlihy, Mrs. Hazel, (née Horsfield), Leyland, Preston
Oldham, Christine E., Fulwood, Preston
Ollerenshaw, Dr. A. F., Preston
O'Neill, Evelyn, Leyland, Preston
Openshaw, Mrs. A. B., Penwortham, Preston
"Our. P.T.S., JANUARY 1942"
Owen, Dr. W. G., Walton-le-Dale, Preston
Packham, Mrs. P., Kendal, Cumbria
Paget, R. J. & M., Fulwood, Preston
Palmer, Mrs. V., Denton, Norfolk
Parish, Mrs. Dorothy M., Poole, Dorset
Parker, Mr. & Mrs. D., Fulwood, Preston
Parker, Mrs. E. M., Grimsargh, Preston
Parkes, Miss S. J., Penwortham, Preston
Parkinson, Mrs. D. M., Whittle-le-Woods, Chorley, Lancashire
Parkinson, Miss V. M., Apsull, Wigan, Lancashire
Parry, Linda, Newton-with-Scales, Preston
Parry, Dr. R. T., Fulwood, Preston
Payne, Caroline, District Lab., Preston

Payne, Mrs. M. A., Patney-Devizes, Wiltshire
Philipson, Mrs. C. M., Fulwood, Preston
Phillips, Katie, Preston
Pickles, Audrey, Dowbridge, Kirkham, Preston
Pickstone, Mrs. A., Penwortham, Preston
Platt, Bernice, Fulwood, Preston
Pluck, Dr. Derek J., Fulwood, Preston
Pooley, Ada, Longridge, Preston
Pope, Mrs. C., (née Shuttleworth), Fulwood, Preston
Potts, Mr. Gary, Ribbleton, Preston
Powell, David, Plungington, Preston
Powley, Mrs. J., Low Hesket, Carlisle, Cumbria
Pownall, Councillor Joseph & Mrs. Vera, Frenchwood, Preston
Preston Royal Infirmary Nurses League, Fulwood, Preston
Pritchett, Dr. A., Fulwood, Preston
Prosper-Hospital, The Staff of, Recklinghaüsen
Pugh, Mr. & Mrs. R. G., Fulwood, Preston
Pye, Mr. Harold, Ashton, Preston
Rae, Mrs. Joyce E., Fulwood, Preston
Rainford, J., Longridge, Preston
Rainford, Mrs. Janet C., Ashton, Preston
Rainton, Colin D., Leyland, Preston
Ramsden, F. & G., Fulwood, Preston
Rankin, W. R., Watford
Rath, Mrs. Joan, Fulwood, Preston
Rawling, Pauline, Lea, Preston
Rawlinson, Mr. Sydney, Ashton, Preston
Ray, Mrs. Alice, (née Pearson), Bare, Morecambe, Lancashire
Reader, John, Lea, Preston
Real, Mr. W. E. C., Fulwood, Preston
Reaney, Mr. & Mrs. T., St. Annes-on-Sea, Lancashire
Reeves, Winifred, Preston
Regan, Anne T., Fulwood, Preston
Regan, J. A., Ribchester, Lancashire
Reid, Mrs. C. M., Whittle-le-Woods, Chorley, Lancashire
Reid, Dr. Judith A., Fulwood, Preston
Rice, Elizabeth, (née Palmer), Avon, Mass., U.S.A.
Richards, Susan M., Longridge, Preston
Rigby, Hannah, Southport, Merseyside
Riley, Mr. T. E., Walton-le-Dale, Preston
Rimmer, Miss M., Eccleston Park, Prescot, Merseyside
Roberts, Mrs. M., Fulwood, Preston
Robertson, Mr. I. G., Fulwood, Preston
Robertson, L., Freckleton, Preston
Robinson, Mrs. J. M., Fulwood, Preston
Robson, W. A., Longridge, Preston
Roddie, Mrs. R., Walney Island, Barrow-in-Furness, Cumbria
Ronksley, Mrs. M., Clifton, Preston
Rooke, Mrs. E., Ribbleton, Preston
Rooke, Mrs. Irene, Southport, Merseyside
Rooney, Mrs. Irene M., Fulwood, Preston
Roscoe, Emma Louise, Penwortham, Preston
Roscoe, Lisa Jane, Penwortham, Preston
Roscow, Joan, Wheelton, Lancashire
Ross, Dr. Esther, Whittingham Hospital, Preston
Rounding, George, R. J., Hoghton, Preston
Routledge, Mrs. E. T., Broughton, Preston
Russell, J. Y. W. Broughton, Preston
Saikia, N. K., R.P.H., Preston
Salpekar, Dr. P. D., Clayton-le-Woods, Chorley, Lancashire
Sams, Mrs. Marie, Leyland, Preston
Sandham, I., Fulwood, Preston
Saunders, Mrs. Olive A., Fulwood, Preston
Saxon, Stanley, Fulwood, Preston

Sayers, Gloria, Preston
Sayner, Mrs. J. S., Ashton, Preston
Scott, Ann Maria, Penwortham, Preston
Scott, Cottier, Ball, Inglis & Brearley, Drs., Bamber Bridge, Preston
Sedgwick, Janet, Billington, Blackburn, Lancashire
Sephton, Dawn, Hesketh Bank, Preston
Sergeant, Mr. D. E., Astley Village, Chorley, Lancashire
Sharples, Miss R., Ingol, Preston
Shaw, Mrs. Margaret, Fulwood, Preston
Shergold Mrs. J., Fernhill Heath, Worcester
Sherlock, Mrs. Sylvia, Fulwood, Preston
Shelvin, M. T. F., Ashton, Preston
Shorrock, Mrs. M., Preston
Sim, Mrs. E., Garstang, Preston
Simmons, Mrs. A. Penwortham, Preston
Simmons, Mrs. S., Lea, Preston
Simons, Mr. Cyril, Penwortham, Preston
Simpson, Miss Jean D., Kendal, Cumbria
Simpson, Dr. W. A., Hoghton, Preston
Slater, Dr. A. & E. V., Broughton, Preston
Slater, E. E., (née Carver), Hayle, Cornwall
Slater, Jeanette L., Fulwood, Preston
Slater, Mrs. Lynn, Freckleton, Preston
Slater, Mr. M., Fulwood, Preston
Smail, Mr. R., Inskip, Preston
Small, Mrs. M. Goosnargh, Preston
Smirk, Mrs. J. M., (née Lockwood), Fulwood, Preston
Smith, Andrea, Adlington, Lancashire
Smith, Mr. Carl, Farington Moss, Preston
Smith, Florence M., Longridge, Preston
Smith, Harold & Kathleen, Penwortham, Preston
Smith, Dr. R. Ian, Ribbleton, Preston
Smith, Janice, Penwortham, Preston
Smith, Mrs. L., Deepdale, Preston
Smith, Mrs. M. P., Fulwood, Preston
Smith, Ron & Freda, Fulwood, Preston
Smith, Mrs. Valerie, Bury, Greater Manchester
Smith, Mrs. W., Ribbleton, Preston
Smythe, R. & M., Fulwood, Preston
Snalam, Christine M., Inskip, Preston
Sotheran, Mrs. H. M., Garstang, Preston
Southworth, F. G., Southport, Merseyside
Spriggs, Mrs. A. P., (née Heaps), Penwortham, Preston
Springate, Betty, (née Tindall), London
Steele, Mrs. Catherine, M., (née Wilson), Kilmarnock, Ayrshire, Scotland
Stephenson, Mr. G. W., Ribbleton, Preston
Stewart, Douglas, Fulwood, Preston
Stirzaker, Miss L. E., Deepdale, Preston
Stockton, Marilyn, Fulwood, Preston
Stones, Frances, Ashton, Preston
Strong, Mrs. Margaret, Lytham St. Annes, Lancashire
Stuart, Sheila M., Ribbleton, Preston
Stutter, Mrs. C. A., Ingol, Preston
Suddick, Dr. E. M., Fulwood, Preston
Sullivan, Dr. and Mrs. G., Penwortham, Preston
Sumner, B. M., Guilden Sutton, Chester, Cheshire
Sumner, Josephine, Preston
Sumner, Mrs. Joyce, Moulton, Northwich, Cheshire
Sumner, Valerie, Fulwood, Preston
Sutcliffe, Harold, Fulwood, Preston
Sutcliffe, Mr. N., Garstang, Preston
Sutcliffe, Pavella D., Deepdale, Preston
Swarbrick, Miss Linda J., Penwortham, Preston
Swarbrick, R., Bracknell, Berkshire

Swinburn, W. R., Cheadle Hulme, Cheshire
Swindlehurst, Elsie, Fulwood, Preston
Tallon, Roy, Ranskill, Retford, Notts.
Tapley, G. A., Tarleton, Preston
Tapp, Dr. E., Lostock, Bolton, Greater Manchester
Tarrant, Miss E., Ashton, Preston
Taylor, Mrs. C., Ribbleton, Preston
Taylor, E. G., Ingol, Preston
Taylor, P., Lytham, Lancashire
Taylor, Dr. Ken, Ashton, Preston
Taylor, W. & J., Fulwood, Preston
Telfer, Mr. & Mrs. G., Walton-le-Dale, Preston
Temperley, J. M., R.P.H., Preston
Thomas, Barbara A., Fulwood, Preston
Thomas, Mrs. Sylvia, Fulwood, Preston
Thompson, Marlene A., Fulwood, Preston
Thompson, Mr. Michael A., Longridge, Preston
Thomson, Catherine, Los Angeles, California, U.S.A.
Thomson, Richard David, Fulwood, Preston
Thomson, R. G., Fulwood, Preston
Thornton, Mrs. L., Ribbleton, Preston
Thornton, Miss. Margaret, Deepdale, Preston
Thornton, P., Hoghton, Preston
Threlfall, Mrs. Hilda, Chorley, Lancashire
Threlfall, Mrs. J., Fulwood, Preston
Thurnhill, Mrs. Lucy, Penwortham, Preston
Tilburn, Mrs. Ethel May, (née Harper), Barrow, Cumbria
Tiley, D. E., Fulwood, Preston
Tilley, Mr. L. H., Ribbleton, Preston
Timbrell, Rev. K. S., Whittingham, Preston
Timms, D. J., R.P.H., Preston
Tod, W. H., MD, FRCOG, Fulwood, Preston
Todd Mrs. Ellen, (née Cuerden), Ribbleton, Preston
Todd, Mrs. Sylvia, (née Chambers), Fulwood, Preston
Tomlinson, Jean, M., Clayton-le-Woods, Chorley, Lancashire
Topham, Miss J., Deepdale, Preston
Towers, Eileen, Nether Kellet, Carnforth
Townley, Mrs. H., Cockerham, Lancaster, Lancashire
Travis, Mrs. B., Stoneleigh, Epsom, Surrey
Trenouth, Dr. M. J., Fulwood, Preston
Turner, B., (née Preston), Fulwood, Preston
Turner, Betty, Cadley, Preston
Turner, G. & D. M., Longton, Preston
Turner, Mrs. J., Hoghton, Preston
Turner, Mrs. Jean, Cranwell, Sleaford, Lincolnshire
Turner, Margaret, NNEB, Preston
Turner, Sheena M., Grimsargh, Preston
Turner-Bishop, Mr. Aidan, Frenchwood, Preston
Tutton, G. K., Hoghton, Preston
Vernon, Miss Joan, Ingol, Preston
Vero, Mr. D., Fulwood, Preston
Vicary, Beverley P., Fulwood, Preston
Wade, Mrs. Claire M., Fulwood, Preston
Walker, Alma, Leyland, Preston
Walker, Mrs. D., New Longton, Preston
Walker, Susan, SRN, SCM, Leyland, Preston
Walmsley, Anne, Fulwood, Preston
Walmsley, Mary, Rishton, Blackburn, Lancashire
Walmsley, Mrs. S. D., Newton-with-Scales, Preston
Walsh, Mrs. Eva, Preston
Walsh, Stephen, Clayton-le-Moors, Lancashire
Walsh, W. Maurice, MD, Dph, Penwortham, Preston
Wane, Miss S. M., Longton, Preston
Ward, Andrew, Fulwood, Preston
Ward, Des & Maura, Walmer Bridge, Preston
Ward, Mr. J., Fulwood, Preston
Ward, Dr. J. C., Goosnargh, Preston

Ward, Rev. Thomas C., Ribbleton, Preston
Waring, Mrs. M., Bournemouth
Watkinson, Mrs. Carol, Ribbleton, Preston
Watson, L. A., Lostock Hall, Preston
Watt, Dr. D. A. L., Grimsargh, Preston
Watts, Mrs. A. V., Astley Park, Chorley, Lancashire
Watts, Iris, (née Woodacre), Southport, Merseyside
Watts, J., R.D.&.E.H., Wonford, Exeter
Webster, Mr. & Mrs. M., Croston, Preston
Wellcome Unit For The History Of Medicine, The University, Manchester
Welsby, Mrs. Elaine, Fulwood, Preston
Weston, Mrs. W., Lydiate, Merseyside
Whalley, J., Garstang, Preston
Whalley, Mr. W., Higher Walton, Preston
Wharton, M. R., R.P.H., Preston
Wheatland, Mrs. V. M.M Fulwood, Preston
Whitehead, Mrs. D. E., Southport, Merseyside
Whitehead, Mrs. J., Newton, Mearns, Glasgow
Whitewright, Dr. & Mrs. A., Bromley Cross, Bolton, Great Manchester
Whittaker, J., Penwortham, Preston
Whittle, Mrs. M., Penwortham, Preston
Wibberley, Jill, Littlemore, Oxford
Wickham, H. Fulwood, Preston
Wilcock, Mrs. Teresa, Longridge, Preston
Wilkes, Chevalier Ronald, KtT, PCM, KPR,& Dame V. El-Ramly, DT, Catforth, Preston
Wilkinson, David John, Coppull, Chorley, Lancashire
Wilkinson, Mr. D. T., Harlow, Essex
Wilkinson, J., Cadley, Preston
Wilkinson, Mr. S. J., Totton, Southampton
Wilkinson, Vivienne, Hutton, Preston
Willacy, Catherine, (née Syder), Rawtenstall, Rossendale, Lancashire
Willey, Mrs. D., Ashton, Preston
Williams, Mr. D., Fulwood, Preston
Williams, Mr. D. E., Horwich, Bolton, Greater Manchester
Williams, Edith, Deepdale, Preston
Williams, H. P., Lostock Hall, Preston
Williams, Mr. & Mrs. J. R., Fulwood, Preston
Williams, Peter, Lammack, Blackburn, Lancashire
Williamson, Mr. J. K., Hutton, Preston
Wilmott, Shirley, SEN, Preston
Wilson, Mrs. A., Fulwood, Preston
Wilson, E. J., Fulwood, Preston
Wilson, Mrs. Edith M., Goosnargh, Preston
Wilson, Mrs. Valerie, Longridge, Preston
Withers, Callan and Singh, Drs., Preston
Wixon, Edith, Blackpool, Lancashire
Wojnowski, Mrs. R. F., (née Briscoe), Ingol, Preston
Wolstenholme, J., Whitefield, Manchester
Wood, Mrs. Eileen, Bamber Bridge, Preston
Woodhouse, Kathleen, L., Ashton, Preston
Woods, C. J., Penwortham, Preston
Woods, Derek, Goosnargh, Preston
Woods, Mrs. T., Brindle, Chorley, Lancashire
Worden, Mrs. Nessie, Barton, Preston
Worrall, County Councillor, P. H., Fulwood, Preston
Worsick, R. A., Penwortham, Preston
Worsley, Mrs. M., Penwortham, Preston
Wrenhall, Mrs. C. P., (née Richmond), Brewood, Stafford
Wright, A., New Longton, Preston
Wright, Miss H., Southport, Merseyside
Wright, J. B., Chorley, Lancashire
Wright, J. D., FRCOG, S.G.H., Fulwood, Preston
Yates, Miss, Angela, Ormskirk, Lancashire
Young, Mr. & Mrs. J., Lea, Preston

Acknowledgements

IT had been my intention to write a short article on the benevolence of Sir Charles Brown toward his beloved Infirmary for inclusion in the Health District's newspaper, the *Echo,* in 1973 at the request of the newly appointed Public Relations Officer and first editor of the *Echo,* Miss Wilkinson. This, however, was never accomplished for, whilst researching the subject, I was presented with a treasury of information in the form of the original minute books of the Preston Dispensary, just as they had been written, in beautiful script handwriting with a quill pen over 160 years before, and my series of articles on the history of health care in Preston from 1809 until 1948 began, extending over a 13 month period.

My benefactor was Mr. Harry Hill RHA, formerly Deputy Secretary of the Chorley and District Hospital until his appointment as Deputy Secretary to the Preston Hospital Management Committee in 1948 and his appointment to succeed Mr. John Gibson in 1952. Mr. Hill, with the advantage of full knowledge of events from 1948 until his own retirement in 1982, should no doubt have written this account but I am eternally grateful for the help he has given me in so many ways.

My grateful thanks are due also to Mrs. Jean Haworth, personal secretary to the Director of the Public Health Laboratory in Preston for the many hours she spent laboriously deciphering my not always legible script in order to produce the finished typed manuscript.

To the present administrators and officers of the Preston Health Authority my thanks are due for allowing me access to the more recent proceedings of the Authority as published in the *Echo* and other sources. To the editor of the *Echo,* Mrs. Edna Fazackerly, the president and editor of the P.R.I. League of Nurses and to all my friends and colleagues for their encouragement and inspiration over the years, my sincere thanks.

Finally to my wife Carol for her patience, tolerance and guidance over what must have been a traumatic decade and a half, my sincere gratitude and thanks are due for without her assistance and encouragement this volume would never have been finished.

Foreword By Tom Finney

THE CHAIRMAN OF PRESTON HEALTH AUTHORITY

THE story of Preston Royal Infirmary is a story of people. Preston and its people — achievements, generosity, disappointments and at times conflict.

As Chairman of the Preston Health Authority I was very pleased to be asked to write some introductory words for John Wilkinson's book.

It makes fascinating reading. At times, however, the story of health care in the last century is depressing, with scant resources, inadequate facilities and archaic practices making it inevitable that a fair proportion of the news recorded was bad news.

Preston folk have been proud of their Infirmary and this book provides for us a lasting record. The outstanding generosity and unselfish service which it records is quite remarkable. The good side of human nature is represented here in plenty. Many Preston names are fondly remembered. I am sure that as the Infirmary doors finally closed for patients in the Spring of 1987 we shall treasure this book as a record of achievement and care. Preston Health Authority employs 6,000 staff in 1987 and this book records the thousnds also of past decades.

As Prestonians I know that we are proud to be associated with them all.

Introduction

IT has been said that each one of us has a story trying to escape. This story has been struggling to emerge for many years, no doubt from the first day my association with Preston Royal Infirmary began some forty five years ago.

Its telling is now more important perhaps with the imminent closure of the Infirmary after so many years devoted service to the public of Preston. All too often these days, establishments which have been landmarks in the town disappear, quite insidiously in some instances, without the general public being aware of the fact. In recent years, for example, several churches have been either demolished or put to other uses and there are still those who advocate the removal of the Public Hall and the extension of the centrally placed 'glass house' in the town centre.

The first council school ever to be erected in the whole of the British Isles solely for working-class children was recently demolished in Preston. It was erected in 1815 but there is now little trace of its existence. It is for this reason, therefore, that this story must be told now, before the disappearance of what has been an ever present comfort to the sick for over 175 years.

There is need also to place on record the dedication and devotion of countless members of staff of all categories, generation to generation, without whom the Royal Infirmary could not have earned its unique place in Preston's history.

Today it still operates quietly and efficiently, fulfilling a valuable function in the affairs of the Health Authority and without which the divisions of obstetrics and gynaecology, of orthopaedics and pathology would be unable to carry on.

To cover every aspect of the Infirmary's role over such a long period of time would be an impossibility. Therefore, no claim is made that this story is complete; it is a journey moving along the main stream, passing, on the way, many tributaries, any one of which would perhaps disclose other avenues of the Infirmary's past. Everyone associated closely with Preston Royal Infirmary for any length of time has their own reminiscences of their time there and will remember episodes not mentioned here. Suffice it that perhaps in some small way this book will record for posterity the progress of health care in Preston and district and will serve as a lasting memorial to all those who in their own way helped to build a medical service second to none.

The author, in writing this history, is grateful to have had the pleasure and experience of working there for the period 1946-1985 and in so doing has contributed in some small way toward that history.

Chapter 1

'an ornament to the Town . . .' 1809-1869

IT is perhaps necessary for the reader to consider a few relevant facts to put this story in perspective. The earth, we are told, has been around a long time, some thousands of millions of years, and man has lived upon it for about 500,000 years. Recorded history extends back some 7,000-8,000 years but the recorded history of Britain is little more than 2,000 years old. Taking these facts into consideration, the advent of organised health care in Preston, a mere 175 years ago, appears ludicrous but it was not until the year 1809, during the reign of George III, that first mention was made of a 'health service' for Preston. Several towns in Lancashire at the beginning of the 19th century were contemplating the care of their 'sick poor' and it was a prototype set up in Wigan upon which Preston based their scheme for a Dispensary.

In the twelfth century there had been a leper colony in Preston operated by priests in the name of St. Mary Magdalene which, it is believed, was situated in the region of the present day St. Walburge's church and the area to this day bears the name Maudland, a derivation of St. Mary Magdalene.

Preston at the start of the 19th century had a population of around 15,000, the majority of whom were classed as 'poor' and their health care generally must have been a very hit and miss affair, with much reliance on 'wise' men and women, bogus doctors and medicine men probably all intermingled with witchcraft, religion and faith healing; they certainly could not have afforded the charges made by the physicians of the day.

A meeting was held in the Town Hall on October 31st 1809, following a public announcement issued by the Mayor, Daniel Lyon Esq.:

> 'In pursuance of the requisition of several respectable inhabitants of this Borough to take into consideration the propriety of erecting by subscription a Dispensary for supplying the poor with medicine to their relief in case of sickness.'

It was resolved at this meeting that the establishment of such a Dispensary within the town was 'highly desirable and expedient'.

At a meeting of the subscribers to the Preston Dispensary held in the Town Hall on December 5th 1809 pursuant to the public advertisement in the Preston Journal.

Mr. Aspden in the Chair.

The following gentlemen were appointed as a committee for the ensuing year.

William Cross Esq. President.

Dr. St. Clare	Brown Assheton Esq.
Dr. Lowe	Mr. Blanchard
Dr. Robinson	Mr. Jacson Jun.
Dr. Wm. St. Clare	Mr. Winstanley
Daniel Lyon Esq. (Mayor)	Mr. John Baron
Mr. Alderman Grimshaw	Mr. Ralph Aldisson
Mr. Alderman Billock	Mr. James Pedder
Mr. Miller	Mr. Wilson Parker
Mr. John Swainson	Mr. Roger Crane
Mr. George Jacson	Mr. James Crane
Mr. Leighton	Mr. Catterall
J. Addison Esq.	James Aspden Esq.

The Committee are requested to meet on Tuesday next at 11 o'clock - and to hold future meetings from time to time as they shall judge expediate for the purpose of carrying the Institution into effect, and five of the Committee to be empowered to act. Resolved at this meeting that in order to enable the Committee to contract for the intended Building and to proceed in the proposed Establishment the Subscribers be requested to pay their donations and annual subscriptions as early as convenient into one of the Banks in Preston, to the account of Mr. Tomlinson the Treasurer.

One week later on December 12th 1809 another meeting of the committee was held in the Town Hall when it was resolved that:

(1) The four Resident Physicians in this Town and Mr. Tomlinson the Treasurer, to consider and report to the Committee at a future Meeting, the plans of the Building now produced for the Dispensary and any alteration or enlargement of them also the mode of fitting it up and likewise the temporary fitting up of the house taken in Everton Gardens and that such house be made ready as soon as possible for the purpose of the Dispensary till the new Building can be opened and that it also be referred to those Gentlemen to consider and report to the Committee the form of Recommendation to patients to be printed for the use of the Subscribers.

(2) Resolved that the Annual Subscription be always paid one year in advance on the 25th day of October, the anniversary of His Majesty's accession and accordingly that the Annual Subscriptions now paid be taken as payment up to 25th October next when the next years payment will become due.

(3) Resolved that in as much as part of Sir John Shelley's property in Fishergate appears to this Meeting an eligible situation for the Dispensary Mr. Shuttleworth be requested to make an application for the purchase of it upon a ground rent and at the same time to transmit the printed copy of the Resolution of the General Meeting respecting this Establishment and a list of subscribers.

(4) Resolved that this Meeting entertains strong hopes that the funds of the Charity may become adequate to the purpose of a Lying-In Charity as well as a Dispensary. According to the intentions of a former General Meeting and in order to effect so desirable a purpose it is ordered that this Resolution be printed and circulated

immediately and the Ladies are particularly and earnestly invited to take the subject into their Charitable consideration and to honour it with their patronage.

The house at the south end of Everton Gardens was fitted up as a temporary Dispensary and an apothecary was appointed with an 'annual stipend of £100 for house, fire and candles and also bed and bedding except linen'. A Mr. Thomas Collinson was duly appointed to be the first apothecary of the charity.

Everton Gardens was bordered on the west by Tythe Barn Street and on the east by North Road, with Church Street to the south. Spring Gardens was situated on the opposite side of North Road, bordered on the east by Pole Street; the new bus station now occupies this area of the town.

The Mayor, Daniel Lyon Esq., was requested to call a meeting of the taxpayers of the town to enable the overseers of the poor 'to contract with the Dispensary for the medical relief of the poor of the Township'. The amount to be paid was finally fixed at £60 per annum for the Dispensary's facilities. There were about 250 subscribers listed originally, who gave sums annually ranging from 2/6d (12½p) to £10/10/0d (£10.50). The total sum subscribed for the year 1811 was £339/18/0d. The subscriber's donation each year gave them the privilege of submitting patients for treatment at the Dispensary, the number of patients being governed by the sum donated, i.e. £1/1/0d allowed 2 patients etc. The Mayor of Preston had the privilege of recommending five patients at a time and the clergy of every denomination could have two patients at a time over and above any they were entitled to by any subscription they made. It was also stated that the real objects of the charity 'are such sick and lame poor (including poor apprentices who do not live with their masters and mistresses) residing within the Borough as cannot provide medicines and attendance for themselves' and 'that Gentlemen's servants and soldiers are not entitled to any relief from the Charity'.

It became evident early in the affairs of the Dispensary that many of the subscribers were rather loathe to part with their money when the time came to pay and a special sub-committee was formed whose purpose was to visit the non-payers and collect. The special directions laid down for these visits give an interesting insight into Preston's thoroughfares in the early 19th century:

District One. Both sides of Fishergate starting at the Town Hall, Mainsprit Weind (both sides), Pleasant Street, Avenham Street, Winckley Square, Winckley Street, Chapel Street, Theatre Street, Butler Street, Charles Street, Pitt Street, Fox Street, Lune Street, Canal Basin except the north side and to Knox's Plantation.

District Two. Both sides of Friargate commencing at the 'White Horse' and Mr. Arkwright's shop, inclusive to Tulketh Hall and all the streets adjoining on the north side of the Canal and intermediate streets, Back Lane to Derby Arms inclusive and High Street.

District Three. Market place to 'White Horse', Cheapside, Old Shambles, Anchor Weind, New Street, Lord Street Vicarage, Tythe Barn Street, Everton and Spring Gardens, North Road, St. John's Street and the Shambles.

A general meeting of the committee was held in the Town Hall on 4th January 1810, where it was resolved 'that the Dispensary would be built upon ground agreed to be purchased from Mr. Grimshaw by Dr. St. Clare and in the centre lot between Lune Street and the next intended street to the west' (? Fox Street). A further meeting on 10th January 1810 discussed two plans and estimates for the site, one by Mr. Smith and the other by Mr. Roper but nothing was agreed, a further meeting being called for the following Wednesday, 25th January 1810. At this meeting it was resolved 'that a 25 yard square or such quantity of land as may be sufficient to carry with execution the plan produced by Mr. Smith be purchased from Mr. Grimshaw on the understanding that possession of the land could be completed by May 1810, Mr. Grimshaw would also provide a commodious cart road of 3 yards wide at least to the back part of the proposed Building' (this is perhaps still in existence running between Lune Street and Fox Street at the rear of the buildings in Fishergate and is still called Surgeon's Court to this day).

At the next meeting of the committee, called for 7th February 1810, there were insufficient members present to discuss the plans for the proposed new building so this item was left to be discussed at the next general meeting on the 7th March. The rules regarding the recommendation of patients were approved at the February meeting and the secretary was 'requested to give Public notice regarding the delay in opening the Dispensary and to publish the scale of recommendation they had just adopted and approved'. They also agreed that the salary of Mr. Collinson the apothecary for the Dispensary should be paid from the first day of February 1810. A public notice was presented by T. Croft at the *Preston Journal* newspaper office on 27th February 1810:

> The Committee beg leave to inform the Subscribers to the *Preston Dispensary* that owing to the indisposition of Mr. Thos. Collinson the Apothecary, this Institution will not be opened for the reception of patients before Monday 5th March 1810.
>
> Printed forms of Recommendation may be had on application of Mr. Samuel Crane and this Committee take this opportunity of reminding the subscribers who have not paid their subscriptions that their recommendation cannot be attended to so long as their subscription continue in arrear. The objects of this Charity are such sick poor, within the Borough as cannot provide medicine and attendance for themselves, and they must attend at the Dispensary with a Subscribers recommendation at the hour of 10 o'clock in the morning on Monday, Tuesday or Friday. Signed John Taylor, Secretary.

On 7th March 1810, a meeting of the subscribers was held in the Town Hall with Mr. Cross in the Chair. Mr. Tomlinson resigned the office of treasurer and Mr. Samuel Crane was unanimously elected to replace him; Mr. Tomlinson, however, was appointed a committee member for the current year. The main purpose of this meeting, the plans of the new Dispensary building, were not discussed and the meeting adjourned until Wednesday 21st March 1810. It was at this meeting that Mr. Crane the treasurer was authorised 'to agree with Mr. Samuel Blackhurst for the house in Everton Gardens in which the Dispensary business is now carried on and to engage the same to the 12th day of May next'. The secretary was directed to advertise for an apprentice to the Dispensary and, also for a matron, although this post bore nor relationship to the modern idea of a top nursing officer; it would be a housekeeper/cook that the Dispensary Committee would have in mind or, as they described her at the time, a 'female assistant'.

Dr. Robinson and Dr. St. Clare were aked to discuss with the surgeons and man-midwives regarding their assistance in the lying-in charity and they were to discuss with the committee of ladies on the same subject and report back.

Finally the plan and elevation of the new building prepared by Mr. Wren, a local architect, for the sub-committee appointed to look into the project was approved and Mr. Wren was directed to prepare an accurate specification and estimate for submission to the next meeting on Wednesday 11th April 1810.

At this stage therefore progress was being made, albeit slowly, but the temporary Dispensary was finally opened to the public on 5th March 1810 and in the first six months 749 patients were seen. Dr. Robinson and Dr. St. Clare reported to the next meeting on 11th April 1810 their deliberations with the surgeons and man-midwives and it was agreed 'that Mr. Alexander, Mr. Moore, Mr. Farrer, Mr. Fearnside, Mr. Bretherton and Mr. Armistead be appointed to attend as accoucheurs when all such poor women as shall be entitled to relief under the Lying-In Charity'. They would be paid 7/ – d (35p) in each case out of the charity's funds and Mr. Alexander, Mr. Moore and Mr. Farrer would act for the first six months and the other three gentlemen for the succeeding six months.

Four months later, on 15th August 1810, the Committee met 'having examined into the case of Ellen Hall attended in childbirth by Mr. Alexander as a patient of the Ladies Charity, and having heard Mr. Alexander's statement, and also Dr. Robinson in confirmation of it, find there is no cause of complaint against Mr. Alexander in this respect'. The committee also proceeded to enquire into the case of Mary Moon, a woman attended by Mr. Alexander in childbirth who died on the 15th day after delivery, having in the meantime been under the care of Mr. Alexander. It appeared to the committee that Mr. Alexander was not acquainted with the rules of the ladies charity that such patients after childbirth should become patients of the Dispensary and the secretary was directed to send a copy of such rules to the accoucheurs. Further consideration of this subject was postponed until the committee had seen the husband of Mary Moon and heard his statement; the outcome of this whole episode is in doubt.

Mr. Wren, the architect, produced his specification for the new building at the meeting on 11th April and the sub-committee were instructed to 'contract either Mr. Wren or any other architect they may think proper for executing such specification on the most reasonable and proper terms'. It was at this meeting that two names were submitted for the post of matron or female attendant in the Dispensary and a sub-committee was formed to make the appointment and 'to fix finally the terms on which the Matron is to give her services to the Charity'. On the 15th August 1810 an order was signed for £5/5/0d (£5.25), the matron's salary for the quarter ending August 1st. It was also resolved at this meeting that an advertisement be printed and distributed through the town:

> 'Inoculation'. The poor may have their children inoculated without expense by bringing them to the Dispensary on Mondays and Fridays at 10 o'clock.

The first annual general meeting was held at the Dispensary on 21st October 1810, the first item on the agenda being an account submitted by the committee of the ladies charity for payment to the accoucheurs for 40 labourers, at 7/ – d (35p) each, amounting to £14. The treasurer was ordered to pay the amount and it was agreed to continue until the next annual meeting on 25th October 1811 at the agreed sum of 7/ – d. The officers appointed for the year 1810 included a patron - the Rt. Hon. the Earl of Derby; J. S. Aspden - president;

Mr. J. Crane - treasurer; Mr. J. Taylor - secretary. It was ordered that the annual report be printed and distributed among the subscribers and should consist of the following subjects:

(1) A General Introduction.
(2) The Abstract of the Rules.
(3) The form of bequest by Will.
(4) The Officers for the ensuing year.
(5) The Medical Report.
(6) The Treasurer's Report.
(7) An alphabetical list of donations and subscriptions.

This became the form of report which was strictly adhered to each year.

The new building for the Dispensary was ready for occupancy by April 1811 and the committee held its next meeting there on 18th April. It was agreed that payment of the bills would be made and the treasurer was 'requested to provide fire grates and other necessary fixtures and Mr. Miller was requested to see that the back road be completed as soon as possible'. Although it had been agreed at the annual general meeting in October that payments to the ladies charity would remain the same until the following annual meeting, the committee at its meeting on the 3rd May 1811 decided to rescind its decision on being presented with a bill for £25/10/ – d as payment to the surgeons. Dr. St. Clare was to report 'this resolution to the Ladies Committee and report to the next Meeting such allowance as he may agree upon'.

It was also resolved that the Dispensary sub-committee, consisting of Mr. Crane (treasurer), Mr. Smith and Mr. Miller, be requested to order such furniture and fixtures as they shall think necessary in addition to the present stock. The treasurer informed the committee that the bills had been settled and it was agreed that the Dispensary furniture and drugs should be insured in the Royal Exchange Insurance Office, on the building £400, the furniture £100 and drugs £100.

On 16th May 1811 only the president attended for the proposed meeting, so it was adjourned until Thursday 23rd May 1811. Once again the secretary, Mr. John Taylor reported that many subscriptions were in arrears and unpaid and it was ordered that collections should be made. Dr. St. Clare informed the meeting that 'the Ladies Charity expected the allowance agreed upon to continue until the Annual Meeting in October but as they had been unable to extend their charity to a greater number than was first intended they will not require any allowance for the additional number for the current half year'. Dr. St. Clare also informed the committee that John Grimshaw, the owner of the land on which the Dispensary was built, declined to sell the ground rent of £13/15/0d (£13.75) so it was decided to invest £275 in Navy 5% Annuals in the names of the treasurer and Mr. Aspden the president to cover the payment of the annual ground rent. The committee also agreed the indenture of apprenticeship for Mr. Ralph Brackenbury, son of Mr. Francis Brackenbury. He was 'to be articled during the term of 5 years from the 25th day of April last and that he be allowed £10 per annum during the whole term and such further sum during the last three years of it as the committee shall appoint if they shall think him deserving of any increase'. This was one of the recognised beginnings of a medical career at the time but in the case of Ralph Brackenbury it did not last the full five years. In less than two years he had been dismissed for repeated misdemeanours and the committee, in appointing another apprentice, took the decision to insist on a fee of 20 guineas for a 4 year apprenticeship or if no fee was paid then the apprenticeship would be for 5 years.

At the next two meetings of the committee in June and July 1811 so few members attended that no business was conducted. The committee did not meet again until 23rd October 1811 when the annual report was prepared to be submitted to the annual general meeting on the following Friday, 25th October 1811. The balance sheet showed a balance of £564/0/10d after settling all the bills for the ensuing year. The annual meeting was told 'that the poor of all the adjoining Townships receive great relief from this Dispensary without any contribution being made towards its support'. The secretary was requested 'to represent this by letter to the Overseers of the Poor of the neighbouring Townships and to require from each of them a fair and proper contribution and to report their proposals and answers to an adjourned Meeting which will be held for that purpose on Tuesday 26th day of November 1811'. 'It appears to this Meeting that the annual sum of £60 contributed by the Overseers of the Poor of Preston is an inadequate sum, the Secretary is desired to propose to the Overseers of Preston that the annual sum of £120 shall in future be paid by them'. When the overseers objected very strongly to this the committee reconsidered the matter and accepted the sum of £80 instead.

A further complication arose in November 1811 when the committee for the ladies charity, still unhappy about the decision to restrict their finances by not paying them fully for services rendered, instructed the Dispensary committee:

> that as they from the 25th October declined to charging any further debts contracted by the Charity to the Surgery it will not be in their power to continue the salary of 10 guineas per annum to the Matron. Consistent with the economy requisite for the permanent support of the Charity they have made enquiries in some neighbouring Towns as to the salary usually granted in similar cases and find that 5 guineas per annum is considered ample remuneration for the trouble given and services called for by the Charity from the Matron. If the Gentlemen require it they will certainly continue the Matron's present salary until 25th January after which period they resolved at the meeting assembled on the 1st November that no larger sum than £5/5/0d (£5.25) per annum should be given to any Matron.

Throughout these early years such disagreements were not uncommon between the ladies committee and the overseers of the poor with the Dispensary committee. The matron in this instance, Mrs. Hannah Hickson, had no option but to accept a 50% cut in salary. She died three years later, in 1814, and a widow, Mrs. Margaret Haggar, was appointed on 22nd July 1814. In October 1821 because of pressure from the subscribers, who felt that the matron should be a married woman, Mrs. Haggar was dismissed, being given one month's notice, which was later extended until 17th January 1822. An advertisement was issed:

> 'Wanted immediately, a man and his wife as Housekeepers to the Dispensary, without the encumberance of children'.

The newly appointed 'matron' was allowed to employ a Mary Watson as her servant as long as she paid her wages herself out of her own funds but the committee reserved the right to dismiss the servant if there was cause for them to do so.

A list of patients admitted from Preston and adjoining parishes in 1811 consisted of:

Preston	696	Fishwick	1
Samlesbury	15	Brindle	4
Poulton	3	Radburn	2
Woodplumpton	14	Chipping	2
Darwen	4	Horwich	3
Fulwood	9	Longton	2
Elswick	2	Longridge	1
St. Michaels	4	Ormskirk	3
Ashton	6	Blackburn	3
Goosnargh	6	Cuerden	5
Whittle	4	Inglewhite	3
Freckleton	2	Clifton	2
Huddersfield	1	Bowland	3
Hutton	5	Whittingham	1
Broughton	4	Thornton	9
Chorley	3	Garstang	6
Penwortham	6		
		Total	834

The committee received the following letter on the 25th January 1812 from the overseers, Blinkhorn and Lyons:

Gentlemen, The Committee for superintending the affairs of the poor of Preston have ordered us as overseers of the poor to bequest you will have the goodness to investigate a charge of neglect which they hereby prefer against Mr. T. Collinson, Apothecary which they have strong reasons to believe the same to be true. It is respecting the death of the late John Williams, a pauper in the Workhouse. Examination of John Moss, Master of the Preston Workhouse who saith that on Tuesday evening the 7th inst. John Williams, a pauper in the House informed him, this examinant that he was poorly and could not come to his supper and desired the examinant to send him some warm beer. On the Wednesday morning he desired the examinant to fetch the Doctor or else he said he could not live, he added that he had a stoppage in his water and he also desired the examinant to request the Doctor to bring a syringe with him, he said to the examinant that he had had the disorder before and had been cured by being syringed. The examinant accordingly went himself about 9 o'clock in the morning (Wed) to Mr. Collinson and found him at his father's house in the Old Cock Yard, Mr. Collinson was playing on a flute. The examinant informed him of the situation of the man and all that he had requested the examinant to inform the Doctor. The examinant told how extremely poorly the man was and the examinant expected Mr. C. to have followed him immediately to the House and accordingly continued about the House all day himself. Mr. C. did not come until about 5 o'clock in the evening. He saw the man and ordered the examinant to bath him with vinegar and water and to give him a dose of salts in the morning, the Doctor's orders were complied with. The man informed the Doctor of the situation and how he had before been cured of the same disorder he then laboured under by syringing. Mr. C. did not bring any instrument with him, he said he would see the man again.

On the Thursday the man was in great pain and grew hourly much worse. On Friday the man continued still to grow worse and in consequence the examinant went about 3 o'clock in the afternoon to Dr. Wm. St. Clare where he was informed that he was not at home nor had he been for two days. The examinant left word with the Doctor's servant that there was a man in the Workhouse very dangerously ill and requested that she would send the Doctor as soon as he came home. On the Saturday morning about 8 o'clock Dr. W. St. Clare came to the House and saw the man. The Doctor said to the examinant 'it is too late' or 'it is over with him' he is not sure which, 'a mortification has taken place the man is dying', he then desired the man to go to bed immediately. The Doctor wrote a prescription and at the bottom of it 'desired Mr. Collinson to visit the patient every other day'. This prescription was sent to the Dispensary by one of the paupers immediately, the medicine was sent in the forenoon but the direction for Mr. Collinson's attendance was not complied with, the man still continued to grow worse and on the Sunday about 2 o'clock in the afternoon he died. Mr. Collinson never visited him more than once.

The Committee records show that Mr. Collinson's attendances at the Workhouse were:

1811	December 7th	visit to Ellen Bradshaw
	December 11th	visit to Ellen Bradshaw
	December 26th	visit to Ellen Bradshaw
1812	January 8th	visit to John Williams
	January 15th	visit to Samuel Councill
	January 18th	visit to Samuel Councill
	January 21st	visit to Samuel Councill
	January 24th	visit to Samuel Councill

The Committee appointed to superintend the Overseers Office and Workhouse for this Town present their most respectful compliments to the Physicians and Committee of the Dispensary and beg leave to trouble them with the statement and examination of the Master of the Workhouse taken before them this day. It is with extreme regret that they complain of the gross negligence and want of attention which it is too plain have manifested themselves on this occasion in the conduct of Mr Collinson but the dreadful sufferings and agony of which the poor man whose name and case are mentioned seems to have undergone and which in all human probability might have been prevented if due attention had been paid to him, the duty they owe to their situation which they fill as the Committee appointed to attend the Overseers Office and Workhouse and which the Town have a right to expect them faithfully to discharge, as well as the natural claims of Humanity have compelled them to make their complaint and to request that a full examination into all the circumstances attending this unfortunate affair may be entered into by the Physicians and Committee of the Dispensary, as they are the persons who have it in their power to correct the abuse complained of and to prevent a repitition of it. It is most earnestly requested that they will have the goodness to do so.

The Committee for superintending the Overseers Office and Workhouse have ordered the Master of the Workshouse to attend at the Dispensary tomorrow at eleven o'clock. By order of the Committee. Thomas Howard, Chairman.

On Wednesday January 29th 1812 the committee met to investigate the matter. Present at the meeting were the president, Mr. Gorst, the mayor, E. R. Travers, four physicians and seven members. The entry in the minutes stated 'it is the opinion of this committee that the charges preferred against Mr. Collinson by the Poor Affairs Committee for the Town of Preston grounded on the representations made to them and which they have very properly communicated to this Committee has in the fullest investigation failed'. They then passed on to other matters; thus, in one sentence, the charges were dismissed but on February 12th 1813 a letter of resignation was received from Thomas Collinson giving six months notice to the committee who immediately arranged:

for advertisements to be inserted three times in one of the Manchester and Liverpool newspapers also in the Preston and Lancaster newspapers, for candidates to fill the situation, that the day of election be fixed for Wednesday 8th day of July next and that the Subscribers to the Charity be requested not to promise their votes previously to the election, that Dr.'s St. Clare, Lowe and Robinson be requested to draw up a proper advertisement for candidates and to make such private applications among their friends as may tend to secure an able person to fill the situation.

Later, on 20th April, it was decided to advertise even further afield, in Kendal and Leeds, and on the 2nd June 1812 the following letter was received applying for the post from William Hornby.

'Ladies and Gentlemen,

In offering myself as a candidate for the office of Apothecary in this Charity (which office will be vacant in August next) it is equally due to the Subscribers and to myself to state the following particulars: I served my apprenticeship with Mr. Ward, Surgeon at Barton in Lincolnshire. I attended in 1810 St. George's Hospital in London two courses of Anatomy and Surgery with Mr. Brookes (with whom I was a house pupil) and two courses on the practice of Medicine and Chemistry by Dr. Hooper. The following Winter I passed at the University of Edinborough attending the Infirmary there other lectures of Dr. Gregory, Dr. Hamilton, Dr. Duncan, Dr. Rutherford and Dr. Thomson. Since that time I have been assistant to A Surgeon in extensive private practice in Hudderfield.

Tickets to these lectures and recommendations from these Gentlemen I have given to the Secretary to be laid before the Physicians Committee and other Subscribers who chose to examine them. Such are my pretensions; and if I am elected by you I will discharge my duty with fidelity and attention.

I have the honour to be Ladies and Gentlemen,

Your most obedient servant,

William Hornby.

Preston June 2nd 1812.

Another meeting was called on 3rd July 1812 to elect an apothecary but this was not done for some reason until a further meeting on 8th August, where there were two candidates presented. There was no record made of the voting for either candidate but Mr. William Hornby was duly elected in preference to Mr. Sutcliffe, the second candidate, of whom very little was recorded. The election appears to have been cut and dried before it even started.

Two weeks later, on August 26th 1812, the committee had to repeat the whole procedure again, advertising for a replacement apothecary due to the untimely death of Mr. William Hornby. In the meantime the brother of the late Mr. Hornby offered his services until such time as a successor was appointed. On 16th September 1812, Dr. St. Clare put in a nomination for a Mr. John Cooper and Mr. Tomlinson nominated Mr. Thomas Lodge. The voting showed 80 votes for Mr. Lodge and only 2 votes for Mr. Cooper, so Mr. Lodge was appointed apothecary. In February 1813 he made a complaint against the apprentices, Brackenbury and Dickinson, for want of attention to their duty and not keeping proper hours. He also accused Brackenbury 'of taking liberties with the prescriptions by substituting one drug for another and being generally disrespectful'. He made no charge against Dickinson for want of respect; the outcome was the dismissal of Ralph Brackenbury and Dickinson was hauled before the committee and admonished.

In April 1814 Mr. Lodge resigned his position as apothecary due to ill health and he died soon after, early in 1815. The committee had to repeat the process once again and on 22nd June 1814 a Mr. Gilbertson was elected by 43 votes to Mr. E. Thompson's 9 votes.

A House of Recovery was opened on June 18th 1813 as an extension for the Dispensary and the report of the state of the Preston Dispensary for 1813-1814 reported:

> although the patients admitted into the House of Recovery appear small (31 cases) in number yet the Committee are of the opinion that this circumstance by shewing the diminution of contagious fevers in the Town affords the strongest proof in how great a degree the Establishment has answered the intended purpose, for who can say how much the spread of infection may have been prevented by the removal of even a single patient when taken from a crowded unwholesome room to clean and well-aired apartments where only a proper diet and medicines are administered, where the intrusion of unnecessary company is not permitted and where every comfort is bestowed that a person in such a condition can require. The Committee are strongly of the opinion that the discontinuance of this Establishment would soon be followed by such a renewal of infection, as would make its immediate restoration necessary and they hope that no apparent diminution of fever will induce the Overseers to remit so indispensible a precaution.

This was printed for publication by A. Walker at the corner of the Old Shambles in Church Street.

Following the annual meeting in October 1814 the secretary John Taylor received the following letter.

> 'Dear Sir, Having been informed there are two days in the week unattended by any Physician at the Dispensary (viz Wednesday and Thursday) and being conscious of the advantage to be derived from a situation in such an Institution, I therefore embrace this early opportunity of informing you I should be extremely happy in being favoured with the honour and advantage of being appointed to fulfill the situation of Physician to the Dispensary on the aforementioned days. I am Sir, Your obedient and humble servant, Thomas Cunliffe.'

A further letter in similar terms dated 14th November 1814 was received from Dr. Chew. Both these gentlemen were Preston physicians and they each received in reply a copy of the resolutions of the Preston Dispensary committee stating:

> that there does not exist at present any vacancy in the office of Ordinary Physician to the Dispensary in consequence of the present ones being desirous to continue their services to the Charity.

On the 19th November 1814 a long and detailed letter arrived from Dr. Chew renewing his claim for the job of extraordinary physician to the Dispensary, one of his claims being that as he had passed his Doctor of Medicine degree on 12th September 1795 he was senior by medical etiquette to the present holder of the post. The committee at their meeting on 25th November 1814 'found that they have no power under the rules to supply any vacancy now existing in the situation of Physician to the Institution'. They then passed on to instruct the treasurer to see that the word 'Dispensary' was placed on the front of the building.

There followed an unsigned letter dated 23rd November 1814, thus:

> 'Gentlemen, At a public Meeting of Townsmen called for the purpose of taking into consideration the propriety of establishing a Dispensary in the month of October 1809, at the request of those present the four Physicians then practising

in Preston came to an understanding as to the best mode of transacting the business of the Charity. It was agreed that in consideration of the services which the two Senior Physicians had rendered for a great many years to the numerous poor objects of this populous place, that an Honorary appointment which marked a sense of those services and which gave but little interruption to private professional engagements was a compliment to which a fair and legitimate claim had been established. Hence more the distinction into Extraordinary and Ordinary Physicians upon the latter the great weight and burden of business necessarily devolved. The duties of the Dispensary from its first establishment up to the present moment have been discharged by those now in office with perfect harmony among themselves and it is hoped with satisfaction to a majority of the Subscribers. There can be no complaint on their part as to the laborious nature of their situation and they wish to continue to act in the different departments which they at present occupy. If at the same time the Committee and Subscribers are of opinions that a Junior Practitioner in the Town is entitled to promotion over the heads of the Ordinary Physicians who have conducted the business from the origins of the Charity, more especially as such appointment is merely nominal, they will bow with submission to such opinion and they pledge themselves to act with their new associates with the utmost cordiality and to promote to the utmost of their ability the benevolent intentions of the Subscribers of the Charity.'

John Taylor the secretary was inundated with letters on 26th November 1814. First came one from Dr. Chew:

Sir, In your first answer from the Committee to my application to become one of the Ordinary Physicians of the Dispensary, you stated that there is no vacancy. In your second letter last night to my being appointed Extraordinary Physician in place of the late Dr. Lowe, the Committee have now discovered that they have not the power to elect me according to the present rules. I would recommend you withhold the printing of the Rules for the present as I intend to appeal to the Subscribers at large to have them revised and modified.

The second letter came from R. W. Robinson and William St. Clare junior, both of whom had held posts since the Dispensary's inception:

Gentlemen, As the Meeting which you have lately been required to attend must necessarily have been unpleasant it affords us great pleasure to relieve you from all further embarrasment by declaring our acquiescence to the arrangement which shall confer the appointment of Physician Extraordinary upon the Gentleman claiming it, Your very obedient and humble servants, Signed R. W. Robinson and Wm. St. Clare Jun.

The third letter received on the same day was signed by over 30 subscribers and reads like an ultimatum to the committee:

Dr. Chew having laid before us Mr. Taylor's letter as Secretary to the Committee for the Preston Dispensary, in answer to his application to be appointed one of the Physicians Extraordinary to that Institution from which it appears that the Committee have not the power of electing a Physician Extraordinary owing to some deficiency in the Rules. We therefore request that you will call a Meeting of Subscribers at large as soon as convenient to revise and make such alterations in the Rules as may be thought expedient and to appoint a Physician Extraordinary to the Dispensary to fill up the vacancy occasioned by the death of the late Dr. Lowe.

Following this letter signed by so many of the trustees, a meeting of the committee was hurriedly called on November 28th 1814 where it was resolved that a meeting of subscribers to be advertised for Thursday 16th December 1814 and at this meeting Dr. Chew was duly appointed physician extraordinary and the rules were amended to this end.

In January 1815 the committee agreed to allow their apprentice Henry Vernon leave of absence to attend lectures in Edinburgh; in September, however, his father requested his release from his apprenticeship, and so an advertisement was inserted in the *Preston Chronicle* for another apprentice. Henry Vernon, by now a qualified M.D., later applied successfully for the post of apothecary in August 1818, and he served in that capacity until April 1820.

The committee was faced with repeated staffing difficulties during the first few years and a further illustration of this came on 30th April 1816 when Ralph Yates, apprentice to Mr. Lodge the apothecary, 'hath withdrawn and absented himself from his duties and has been guilty of misconduct, negligence and inattention'. He was dismissed and another advertisement placed for an apprentice. So it went on, it seems, almost year by year.

The annual report for 1815-1816 reported:

> 'with regard to the Vaccine Inoculation, the Committee do most earnestly recommend to all parents to make use of this Happy Discovery which is exclusively British for the preservation of the lives of their children. The Committee is sorry to observe that Foreign nations have been more ready to adopt the use of this invaluable preservative than Britain itself and while they have had the happiness to see the Small-pox nearly eradicated the Country which discovered the remedy loses every year a multitude of its inhabitants by neglecting to make use of it.'

This was a period of change and expansion for Preston, of course, with the opening of the Lancaster Canal and the use of gas to light the streets; it was the era of the first railway with Stephenson's *Rocket* and, on a wider field, the victory at Waterloo in the Napoleonic Wars.

The first major crisis for the Preston Dispensary arose in 1823 when the overseers withdrew their annual contribution of £80 and closed the Fever House or House of Recovery. The reason for this was that a Thomas Birchall Esq. had posted a notice of appeal to the quarter sessions against several items in the overseers accounts. They were in turn forced into their action by a meeting of taxpayers although they stated at the time that to provide the kind of service the Dispensary gave the town would have cost the taxpayers far greater sums from other sources. The House of Recovery remained closed for over a year before things returned to normal.

Even in the 1820s the question of rising costs was a problem, one of the largest items of expenditure being that of leeches used to 'bleed' patients, a favoured therapeutic method of the time. The price of leeches had risen in 1823 to 3d each and the treasurer reported that 'as a great proportion of the expenditure was absorbed by the purchase of leeches, greater care needed to be used in their usage'. Rules were drawn up, in consequence that, 'no patient was to be provided with leeches at the Institution's expense for a longer period than four weeks and due to the rapid increase in the population of the Town the use of leeches was to be kept at a minimum'.

In April 1828 Dr. Moore, who practised in Lune Street and whose portrait hangs in the Infirmary's main corridor, was appointed senior physician to the Dispensary and one month later came the first take-over bid by twelve Preston doctors, who offered their services 'to increase the number of Medical Officers and lighten their duties and tend to secure a proper consideration of each individual case, and to render the Institution much more efficient'. This was not very well received by the committee or the medical members already in post and the doctors' offer was politely refused. In January 1829 typhus fever was prevalent in Preston and the townspeople were 'prevailed upon to make sure that all paupers and others infected with contagious disease should go to the House of Recovery in order to contain the infection'.

It was during 1831 that the first re-organisation began, when plans were prepared for a new building to be erected for the institution, the site chosen being the ground on which the present Infirmary stands. At the same time the mayor of Preston, Alderman Mouncey, and other dignitaries were added to the Dispensary committee to form a 'Board of Health' for the town of Preston. Included also were the clergy of all denominations, the church wardens, the overseers of the poor and the medical practitioners of the town. All meetings were to be held in the Town Hall and it is interesting to note that at meetings of this new Board of Health members of the press were excluded.

The town was divided into 10 districts and later into sub-districts and 'visitors' were appointed to each. The visitors were requested to go through the different streets and lanes in their respective districts and report to the Board on the state in which they found them and to put forward suggestions to improve matters. Advertisements were published in the two Preston papers, the *Preston Chronicle* and the *Preston Pilot,* requesting 'the inhabitants of the Town to remove forthwith any nuisance in or near their premises and back yard'. The visitors were also allowed to spend a given amount each year on the purchase of clothing and bedding for the destitute poor of the town. The finances remaining in the Dispensary's funds were used for this purpose and it was recorded 'that any sum not exceeding £30 should be laid out for sheets, any sum not exceeding £10 laid out on bed ticks and less than £20 laid out in chaff' for distribution by the visitors. They were also requested 'to prepare a list of the most deserving cases in their respective Districts who would benefit from such Charity'.

An indenture dated 25th January 1830 made between the mayor, bailiffs and James Dilworth, Adam Blackburn and John Harrison, overseers of the poor in which 'a parcel of Land, being part of the Moor within the Borough of Preston in front of the Workhouse bounded on the North by the Workhouse field measuring 511 feet, on the East by another part of the said Moor measuring 180 feet and on the West by 190 feet and on the South side 461 feet, an area of Land totalling 10,052 square yards' was leased at a yearly rent of 5/ – d (25p) for 1,000 years.

The new House of Recovery was erected on this site and was ready for occupancy early in 1832, just in time to accommodate the victims of a small-pox outbreak which occurred at that time. 3,000 patients were treated during 1832, with 170 deaths.

This, then, was the beginning of todays Infirmary's long and distinguished service to the community of Preston. The committee in its annual report noted:

> that Preston had fared better than many of the surrounding Townships during the visitation of a dreadful pestilence which has been extremely fatal in many of the adjoining Townships. The completion of the new House of Recovery and the

surrounding of it by a spacious enclosure have made that Building at once an ornament to the Town and an admirable presentation against the spread of infectious disease.

Throughout the years, the pattern remained the same; almost an annual change of staff, increases in expenditure, continuous chasing of non-paying subscribers, but all the time a gradual progression in size and stature. As the town of Preston increased in size and importance, so too did the Dispensary, through years of great change in medicine and also the invention of many things which today we take for granted — the opening of the first railway links between Preston and Liverpool in 1838, the first postal service in 1840 and the first successful use of the telephone in 1877.

In 1835 a grievance arose between the medical staff and the committee and to a man the doctors all resigned although they assured the committee they would still carry out their duties; an early example, no doubt, of a work to rule. Ten years later, in 1845, Robert Brown, an honorary physician to the Dispensary for many years and father of Sir Charles Brown, one of Preston's most notable citizens, chaired a meeting in the Town Hall to promote the establishment of an Infirmary or Hospital for the town and while there was some enthusiasm this aim was not achieved until 1869, fifteen years after the death of Robert Brown.

Chapter Two

A Royal Patron

SIXTY years after its inception, the Dispensary and House of Recovery was completely inadequate to serve the greatly increased population of Preston, which had grown from around 15,000 in 1809 to 85,000 by 1870.

A second trust deed was signed on 12th March 1866 for the House of Recovery 'to be solely used for the purpose of an Infirmary for the Borough of Preston and the surrounding neighbourhood or as grounds for the use of patients receiving benefit from the said Infirmary'. The term was for run for 1,000 years at an annual rental of £50. A magnificent bequest of £20,500 by John Bairstow Esq. in 1869 made the necessary improvements possible, allowing the newly appointed board of management to upgrade the building and equipment. H.M. Queen Victoria became patron of the new Infirmary, which was thereafter called the Preston and County of Lancaster Royal Infirmary.

The rules of recommendation still applied as in the original administration; in fact, they were more strictly adhered to than at any time previously. Many patients were refused during the first year of the new Infirmary, both as in-patients and out-patients, for lack of recommendation. The income by subscription in the first year exceeded expenditure considerably but this was the first and last time it was to do so for many years.

The bed state of 24 beds was increased to 30 beds before the end of 1870 and the average occupancy of beds by each patient was 35½ days. In-patients totalled 167, out-patients 2,626. 40 were accident cases, mostly railway accidents, with the remainder being considered 'of a minor nature', mostly from the mills; these were generally compound fractures and lacerations of the fingers and hands, some of which were severe enough to require amputation.

The weekly charge for domestic servants and apprentices was fixed at 10/6d a week and it was reported that all the outlying towns and villages, as far afield as Kendal, were sending patients to the Infirmary without any financial donation toward its upkeep. The salary bill for the first year of the Infirmary's staff amounted to £441/6/11d.

In 1870 Miss Brackenbury, formerly resident in Preston, donated £700 to be endowed as a fund for the purpose of assisting young men entering the medical profession, by means of lectures, books and medical appliances etc. Miss Brackenbury's brother had been the first medical pupil in the old Dispensary in 1810 under Dr. St. Clare senior and Dr. Robinson, being dismissed 'for repeated misdemeanours' two years later.

In 1871 the old Dispensary in Fishergate was closed and amalgamated into the new Infirmary; property and funds amounting to £5,140/15/8d being transferred. Philip Park Esq., president of the Dispensary committee, died in 1871, and also Dr. Walling, one of the longest serving honorary medical officers. A Nurse Oakey also died in 1871 after a few days illness contracted in the discharge of her duties.

A new lodge and approach road were well advanced towards completion and the sum of £773/2/6½d was expended on laying out the grounds 'for the benefit and use of convalescent patients'. The pattern of medical staff changes continued as they had throughout the history of the old Dispensary, the senior house surgeon invariably serving one year to gain experience on the wards and then leaving to set up in private practice. The junior surgeon would then be promoted and after a year, or sometimes less, follow the same course. In an endeavour to remedy this, the Board in 1871 increased the salaries of both senior and junior house surgeons. The results were disappointing, although the rate of changeover did tend to slow down a little.

In 1872 accidents formed 26.3% of the cases admitted, the majority being severe mill accidents requiring surgery. A large number of cases came from county districts, indicating that the Infirmary's value was becoming more widely known and appreciated.

During the year 'a superior microscope' was purchased and also 'a highly scientific instrument for registering the pulse with peculiar delicacy called a spymograph'; these were provided with part of the interest which had accrued from the Brackenbury Fund. Costs were still rising in 1873 and subscriptions from the mills, workshops and churches had once more diminished. Preston was suffering from the aftermath of the Amercian Civil War and the cotton famine that resulted from it.

A private nurses scheme was started with a view to making money for the Infirmary by treating people who could afford it in their own homes. A similar plan had been adopted by Gloucester Infirmary, the object being to train nurses for 'private families'. This necessitated the appointment of ward nurses of 'superior description' capable of training probationers and also a large staff of nurses whose time would be utilised in the Infirmary wards when they were not engaged in private nursing. This was never a paying proposition and was in fact for many years a liability on the Infirmary's resources. Four nurses were employed for private work initially and the cost of their subsistence came to £41/17/2d and their earnings on average amounted to only £23/12/6d each. These figures, for the year 1875, highlight the problem.

E. R. Harris, a member of the Board, offered to provide the funds for an enlargement of the Infirmary by the erection of fever wards. His offer was gratefully accepted and land was assigned for erecting the buildings upon, but many difficulties arose regarding their planning as none of the architect's plans submitted satisfied the Board. Mr. Harris renewed his offer and requested that Mr. Hibbert of Preston, one of the architects whose plans had been rejected on the grounds of excessive space and cost, be invited to submit a modified and less expensive plan. Subsequently Mr. Hibbert was requested to arrange for the erection of the wards, to accommodate 32 small-pox, enteric and scarlet fever cases, at the north-west corner of the Infirmary premises at a sufficient distance from the main building to avoid any danger of the spread of infection. These wards are still in use today. Although they were badly needed for the yearly visitation of plagues and epidemics, they never filled the function for which they were erected as people could not afford the charges made to patients admitted, which initially were 3/–d a day or £1/1/0d a week.

Sixty two small-pox cases and 125 cases of measles were admitted during 1874, many of which proved fatal 'owing too often to the thoughtlessness and neglect of parents'. It was at that time common practice for mothers to take their children to other peoples' houses in the morning, bringing them back home at night when they had finished work in the mills. 'This practice was alone sufficient to produce serious complication to the sufferer and lessen the probability of recovery' it was reported. Diarrhoea was also prevalent in many cases 'which was attributable to the insanitary mode of living and bad housing'. In 1875 it became necessary to close the Infirmary for about eight weeks in order to dinsinfect thoroughly and paint the wards in an attempt to prevent the spread of erysipelas, a very acute inflammatory condition caused by a rather virulent micro-organism which proved a scourge in hospitals generally. Despite this, the number of in-patients continued to rise throughout 1875, one of the small-pox victims being Mr Baines, the dispenser, who had served in the old Dispensary; he contracted the disease in the discharge of his duties.

Increases in nursing staff, both private and ward nurses, created a necessity for separate accommodation and the Board approved a plan to extend the administration department to provide sleeping accommodation for 10 additional nurses. They also approved for a covered area to be provided for horses and drivers of conveyances, the estimated cost being £1,042/15/6d.

In July 1875 a scheme matured following two decrees of the Chancery Court for the administration of the surplus funds from of the Cotton Districts Relief Fund and the Fund for Relief of Distress in the Manufacturing District. The aim was the establishment and maintenance of convalescent homes for poor persons of either sex, resident in certain townships, districts and parishes in the Counties of Lancaster, Chester and York. Homes were eventually opened in Buxton, Cheadle and Southport but for many years these proved unsuccessful. The main reason was, of course, that patients had to pay their own travelling expenses which few people eligible to go could afford, another factor being that in those days for the poor to travel so far from home was a deterrent, even Southport being a long way for most people.

The following year, 1876, saw the completion and opening of the Harris Fever Wards and the completion of additional accommodation for nurses. The number of beds available had again been insufficient and in the early part of the year, extra beds had to be placed along the central passages of the wards to accommodate accident cases. Once again the wards had to be closed for painting and disinfecting because of erysipelas. More space was obviously needed, with separate rooms and beds ready to accommodate highly infectious cases at a moment's notice.

The Harris Fever Wards had been opened without the donor being present (due to ill health) and an epidemic of small-pox in the town made it necessary for the Board to place the accommodation at the disposal of the town's medical practitioners. The wards were placed under the personal charge of the junior house surgeon and strict rules were observed to assist communications with the main building. An ABC telegraphic apparatus was ordered to enable messages to be passed. There was no interchange of nurses, who were vaccinated regularly and special arrangements were made with the sanitation authorities for disinfection and the removal of the dead. The Board insisted that a charge had to be made for patients admitted and they pointed out that their charge of 3/ – d a day or £1/1/0d a week was just half the charge made by the London Fever Hospital. This charge was to prove a stumbling block to the success of the fever wards, which for some years remained virtually empty. People either could not or would not pay the fees, probably the former.

The wards were an added burden to the finances of the Infirmary in that the rate charged had to be subsidised from the Infirmary funds and the medical staff and nurses received higher wages and salaries than the staff employed in the main Infirmary. E. R. Harris, who had for so long been a benefactor both to the Infirmary and the town of Preston itself, died on May 27th 1877 leaving in his will a sum of money for the purpose of erecting and maintaining a convalescent home. The governing body of the Cotton District Convalescent Fund had allocated three beds to the Infirmary at their home in Cheadle, Cheshire, and not one person had availed themselves of the offer of three weeks convalesence, free of charge except for travelling expenses, at any of their homes. The late E. R. Harris's bequest for a separate convalescent home was rejected as the Board felt there was little need for it.

The fever wards remained unsatisfactorily used in spite of the small-pox epidemic during the year; only 33 patients were admitted, at a cost, it was reported, of £87/7/0d, or £2/13/0d per patient. Typhoid fever also prevailed in the town but the wards for those cases remained empty.

During the first ten years of its existence the Infirmary was constantly appealing for funds from the people of Preston in order to keep pace with ever increasing costs of administration and the continuous attempts of the Board to make the Infirmary capable of dealing with the ever increasing numbers of cases which presented as the town grew. Due to short time and bad trade in the cotton industry in the 1870s, collections in the mills and other places of work had fallen very badly. It was still apparent that many people from outside Preston were receiving the benefits without contributing anything towards its upkeep and the income from voluntary contributions which had kept the old Dispensary going for so long was no longer a sufficient source of income.

Despite the shortage of money it was quite apparent that the Infirmary would have to be enlarged. Further land was available on the north side of the Longridge branch of the Lancashire and Yorkshire Railway, which ran alongside the Infirmary's premises. An offer was made for the lease of the land, which amounted to 27,900 yards, at an annual rent of 1½d a yard or £174 a year.

The overseers eventually agreed to lease the land in 1878 at a rent of 1¾d a yard for 999 years. Having acquired the land, another wing was added to the Infirmary to provide separate accommodation for children, who were still being admitted into adult wards, increased accommodation for convalescence and to accommodate another increase in nursing staff. Generally the accommodation throughout the Infirmary was extremely limited and cramped.

The years 1879-1882 found the Infirmary badly in debt. In 1880 beds were restricted to 60, the wages and salaries of the staff were reduced and economies were made on provisions and other necessities. One necessary expenditure the Board felt obliged to make was to replace the straw palliasses with woven wire mattresses for sanitary reasons and a further reduction in the number of beds was considered inevitable.

In 1881 an application was made by the Board to the trustees of the late E. R. Harris's estate for a share of the estate, but this proved unsuccessful. By this time the Infirmary debt had reached £1,556/11/8d but the Board aniticipated that the following year would see the end of their financial difficulties.

Guild year, 1882, proved disappointing as far as funds were concerned, only £140 having been raised from the Guild celebrations in donations and collections. Extensive preparations had been made in anticipation of an influx of casualties from the Guild festivities but only seven casualties appeared throughout the week due, it was claimed 'to the sobriety and orderly behaviour of the people and the excellence of the Police arrangements'. During the summer months of Guild year there was an outbreak of small-pox but spread was prevented by the isolation of five cases, one of whom died; the survivors had been vaccinated.

Another significant link in the Infirmary's history was forged during Guild year 1882. This was the instigation of the Workpeople's Committee and the start of weekly collections in the mills and workshops throughout Preston. It had been attempted in a small way the year before by placing a box near the window where wages were paid at one establishment, with a notice requesting a donation of ½d from all who received more than 8/ – (40p) for their weekly wage. The result was so successful that in Guild year the procedure was adopted throughout the town.

In 1882 £488/2/8d was raised but in 1883 this had risen to £1,021/13/10d and the Board was able to record that the Infirmary debt had been cleared and at the end of 1883 there was a balance of £670 due to the unqualified success of the Workpeople's Fund and also donations given by the millowners themselves. The Board altered the rules to allow two representatives of the Workpeople's Committee to be co-opted on to the Board and in 1899 this number was increased to four members; in 1924 five representatives were elected and a year later in 1925 six members were elected, with the addition of two vice-presidents.

Such, then, was the impact of the Workpeople's Fund, which established a precedent which remained throughout the years until 1948 with collections increasing from £1,447 in 1884 to £2,000 in 1900 and £2,500 in 1914. After World War I, John Gibson, the hospital's secretary, instituted a scheme whereby for a contribution of 2d a week free attention and admission to hospital when needed was allowed for the contributor and his dependents. When I came to the Infirmary in 1946 after World War II the subscription was 4d a week but the establishment of the N.H.S. in 1948 saw the end of this form of income which in the 66 years of its existence had played so great a part in the Infirmary's success.

The Infirmary's first matron, Mrs. Russell, died on 17th September 1878 after a long illness. She had been matron for ten years and the Board individually contributed to a headstone of polished granite for her grave in Preston Cemetary as a memorial. Following her death, the Board decided that the nursing division should be upgraded and 25 persons were interviewed for the post of matron. Florence Nightingale had, through her courage and tenacity during the Crimean War in 1855, shown the way for nursing, both civil and military. She suggested and watched over the founding of a home for training nurses at St. Thomas's Hospital in London in 1860 and in 1862 a training school for nurses at the Liverpool Royal Infirmary. She also helped to establish various institutions for nursing from the East London Nursing Society in 1868 to the Queen's Jubilee Nursing Institute in 1890.

Mrs. Russell's successor was a Miss Le Brun, who had excellent experience as a practical nurse, had good professional training and had been a nursing tutor at the Dundee Royal Infirmary and had subsequently held the post of superintendent of the Infections Hospital at Newcastle-upon-Tyne. Miss Le Brun was appointed to establish a high standard of nursing skill which had not been considered necessary heretofore. Unfortunately, Miss Le Brun decided to leave Preston six months later for reasons which were not recorded and a Miss Dannett became superintendent/matron. She had formerly been lady superintendent of nurses at Manchester Royal Infirmary and under Miss Dannett order and regularity prevailed throughout the Infirmary. The housekeeping and nursing were considerably improved and the whole efficiency of the Infirmary was visible to all.

Miss Dannett instituted the appearance of Christmas trees and presents for the patients in the wards at Christmas 1880 for the first time. Unfortunately for the Board and the Infirmary this capable lady was forced to retire in 1881 in order to look after her sole surviving parent and a Miss Augusta Piggott was appointed to succeed her. Miss Piggott proved a worthy successor and until she retired in 1898 after 16 years excellent service she ruled the Infirmary with firmness but also compassion in that she organised annual outings to Lytham for child patients at her own expense.

The medical officer's report for the year 1884 gives an interesting insight into his findings for that year. Speaking of the death rate in the United Kingdom in general he went on to report:

> we may congratulate ourselves that the death rate among our patients is so low. Indeed when we walk through some of the back streets and see the insanitary condition that exists in them, it excites surprise how the people live at all.

He also recommended to the Medical Officer of Health the removal of decomposing materials deposited on the piece of ground on the north side of the Infirmary, 'due to the unusually hot weather during the summer the obnoxious and injurious odours endangered the health of both patients and officials alike'.

The ophthalmic and aural surgeon reported that 245 cases had been treated, the number of operations having almost doubled from 22 to 36 due to the allocation of four beds in the children's ward. He reported the use of a local anaesthetic, 'cocaine , which was used by the London Eye Hospitals and which was said to eliminate the occasional unsatisfactory effects of chloroform in ophthalmic practices. The dental report showed a total of 634 operations, an increase of 113. A large proportion of these patients were children who were being regarded with increasing importance. A Metropolitan District School had decided to appoint a dentist to attend school one morning a week for the purpose of examining children's teeth at school.

The wages and salary bill for 1884 was £1,210/13/2d and the private nursing services raised £93/9/0d. The continuing success of the Workpeople's Fund allowed the Board to improve the condition of the Infirmary's premises, to increase the number of beds and to replenish the bedding, linen and other necessities. They also established a long needed ward of 20 beds solely for children. This new ward was opened by the mayor, John Forshaw Esq., on 5th June 1884 and in the first seven months 124 children were admitted.

Early in October 1885 a mild epidemic of small-pox broke out in the town, introduced, it was claimed, from Montreal. Prompt action was taken to isolate the 13 cases involved; they were admitted to the typhoid ward which was empty of patients at the time. Only one death occurred, in an unvaccinated infant.

This was the 16th year since the Infirmary had begun and the Workpeople's Fund again showed further increases in donations. The year did not pass, however, without some anxiety. During the first nine months the resources of the Infirmary were strained to the utmost, so much so that it became necessary to restrict admissions except for accident and urgent cases during the first three months of the year. Expenditure eventually exceeded receipts by only £272 and if it had not been for the balance carried over at the start of the year there would again have been a deficit.

A society consisting of 30 members which called itself the Aunt Judy's Work Society was established in 1884 for the purpose of providing garments of clothing, chiefly of flannel and calico, for distribution to very poor patients; boots and second-hand clothing were issued to patients of both sexes on their discharge. The society was formed on the model established by a Miss Gatty in association with the London Hospitals and each member promised to make and supply not less than four garments a year.

The building of a private nurses home was once again raised by the matron, Miss Pigott, who had collected or received promises of £230 towards this aim. £50 was added by the Board and an appeal was made to members of the public for a further £150 to complete the fitting up and furnishing of a house in Stephenson Terrace which had been taken for the purpose. Private nurses were up to this time coming from Manchester and Liverpool as there continued to be a lack of suitably trained nurses locally.

The washhouses and laundry of the Infirmary were reported to be totally inadequate to deal with the amount of work necessary for the efficient running of the Infirmary. The sum of £400 was considered necessary to enlarge them sufficiently to cope with the current work undertaken.

There had been an increase of 222 admissions in 1885, bringing the total to 1,212 in-patients. Out-patients treated were 5,783, an increase of 852, and home visits too had increased by 6,618 to a total of 16,318.

Cocaine was exclusively used for eye and ear patients' operations, chloroform rarely being used. The Infirmary in 1885 acquired another microscope, purchased at a cost of £2/12/8d and wages and salaries increased to £1,355/6/2d.

The seventeenth year, 1886, began with the wards once again having to be closed for the whole of the month of March for disinfecting and cleaning, causing both inconvenience and expense. The matron, Miss Piggott, sustained a broken ankle and was incapacitated for six weeks, though she did not relinquish her charge. There were important changes in the nursing department with Nurse Mahoney becoming matron for the private nurses Home in Stephenson Terrace which opened early in May that year. Nurse Mackay, head nurse in the male wards left to become matron of a small hospital and Nurse Leslie returned from prolonged illness to her former position as head nurse of the female wards. Nurse Palmer became head nurse of the male wards.

Two gifts were donated during the year, a hand ambulance on wheels was given by Alderman Benson, a member of the Board, and a horse-drawn ambulance, built by Messrs. Harding and Co. of Preston, was supplied by Dr. Charles Brown, the first of many gifts he was to give. Lectures were given on ambulance (first aid) work for the first time.

Due to the inadequacy of the laundry and washhouses, blankets and counterpanes were contracted out with the Commissioners of H.M. Prisons. It is interesting to note that as recently as 1973 and again in 1983 the practice of giving hospital laundry to the Prison Authorities was considered as a permanent arrangement throughout the N.H.S.

During the first three months of 1886 there was a continuation of small-pox cases carried over from 1885. A severe outbreak of typhoid in July which lasted until the end of the year meant that the fever wards were busier than they had ever been since they were built; forty eight cases were admitted during the year and there were four deaths, a vast improvement over previous years when the death rate in the fever wards had been almost double that figure.

The number of in-patients again increased, by 27 to a total of 1,239, with out-patients being 5,349, a decrease of 334, and home visits at 15,738 showed also a decrease of 580; the reason given for this decrease was the marked increase in trade which apparently affected the Infirmary's figures; also, the clemency of the weather during the summer and autumn months. The department of ophthalmic and aural surgery noted an increase, especially among children, of cases attributable to malnutrition.

An electro-magnet was added to the Infirmary's equipment which 'proved useful in diagnosing and removing metallic foreign bodies from the deeper structures of the eyeball'; in the dental department, cocaine was used for the first time in the extraction of teeth.

The Infirmary in 1887 was damaged by a fire on the premises which, although covered by insurance, involved the Board in unexpected expenditure. Repainting and cleaning was necessary, beds and bedding had to be renewed and most of the fever wards needed refurbishing. Another expenditure was the need to replace the hot water apparatus.

A course of lectures by Dr. Collinson in connection with the St. John Ambulance Association was enlarged to include the requirements for a hospital

The original notice which advertised the opening of Preston Dispensary in 1810. From humble beginnings, the health care services for Preston expanded and developed.

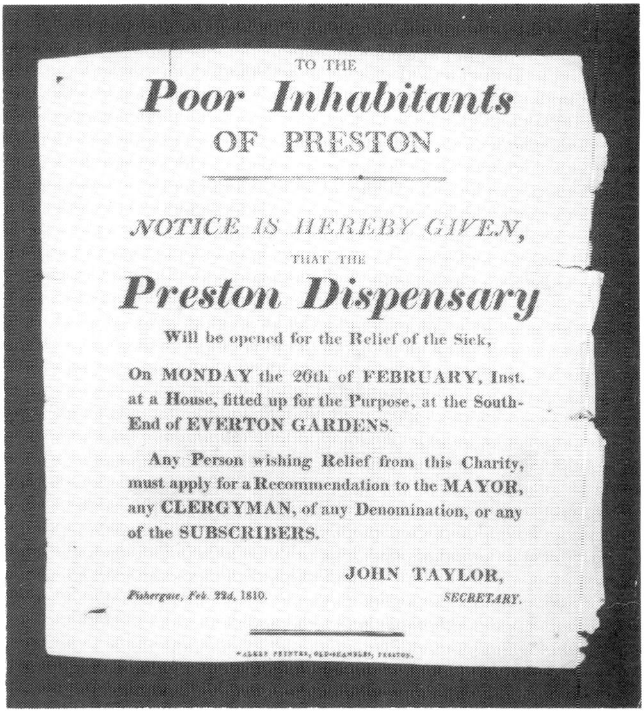

TO THE

Poor Inhabitants

OF PRESTON.

NOTICE IS HEREBY GIVEN,

THAT THE

Preston Dispensary

Will be opened for the Relief of the Sick,

On **MONDAY** the 26th of **FEBRUARY**, Inst. at a **House**, fitted up for the Purpose, at the South-End of **EVERTON GARDENS**.

Any Person wishing Relief from this Charity, must apply for a Recommendation to the **MAYOR**, any **CLERGYMAN**, of any Denomination, or any of the **SUBSCRIBERS**.

JOHN TAYLOR,

Fishergate, Feb. 22d, 1810. *SECRETARY.*

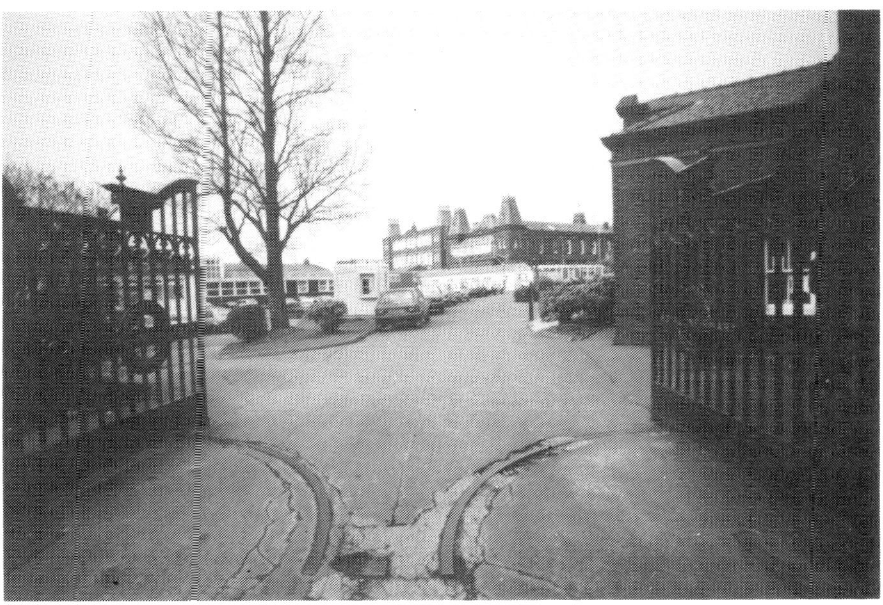

177 years later, Preston Infirmary as it appeared shortly after its closure in 1986.

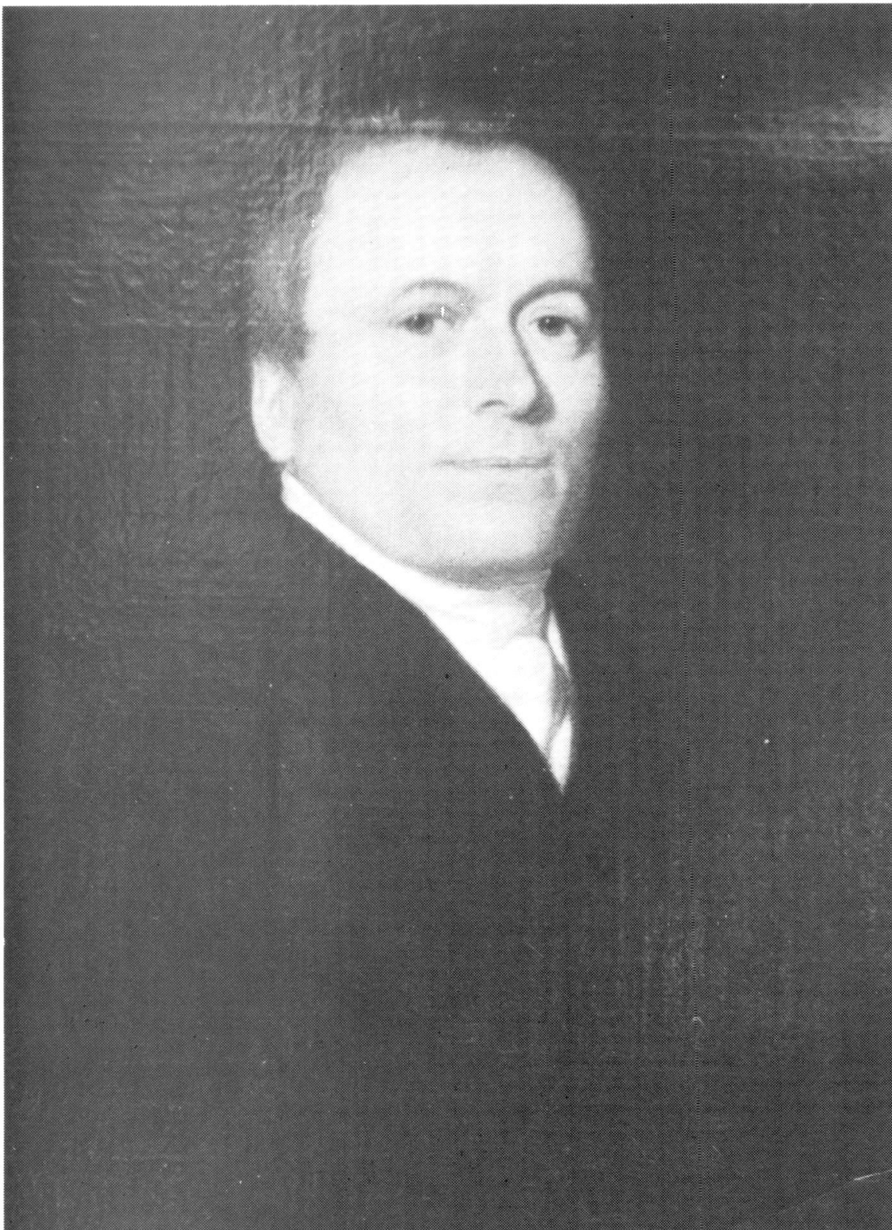

The oil painting of Dr. Thomas Moore, the famous Infirmary surgeon, who died in April 1848 after many years service. The painting later hung in the Post Graduate Medical Centre.

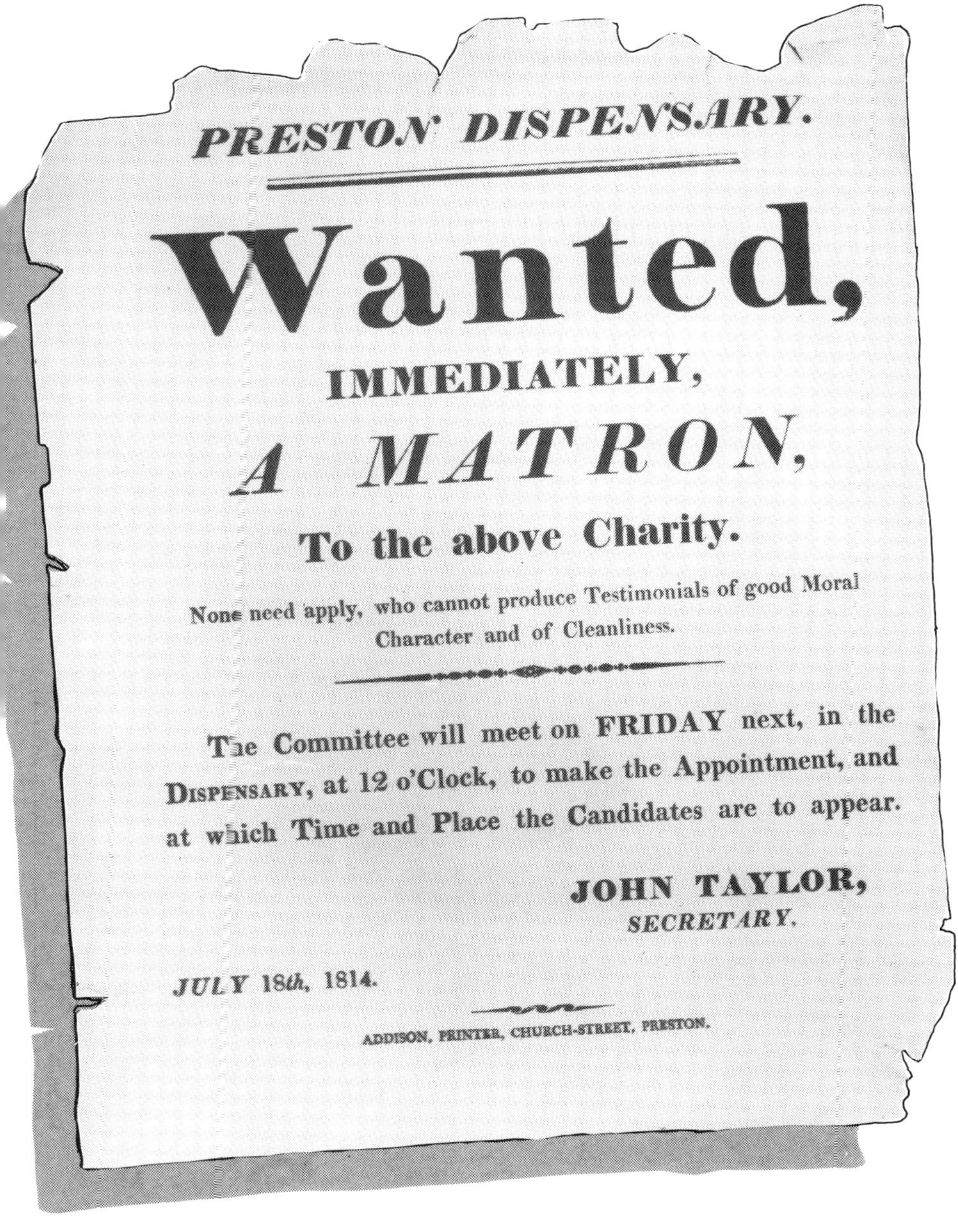

An early advertisement for a Matron for the Dispensary charity. The list of qualifications makes interesting reading.

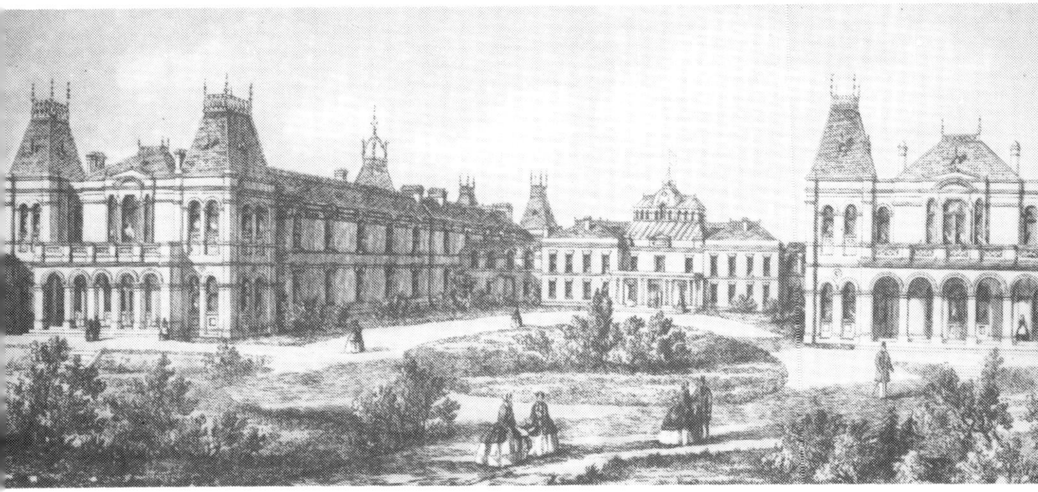

An artist's impression of how the Infirmary was to be developed at the turn of the century. In fact, the actual building, when constructed, was slightly different. Compare the 1925 photograph on the following page.

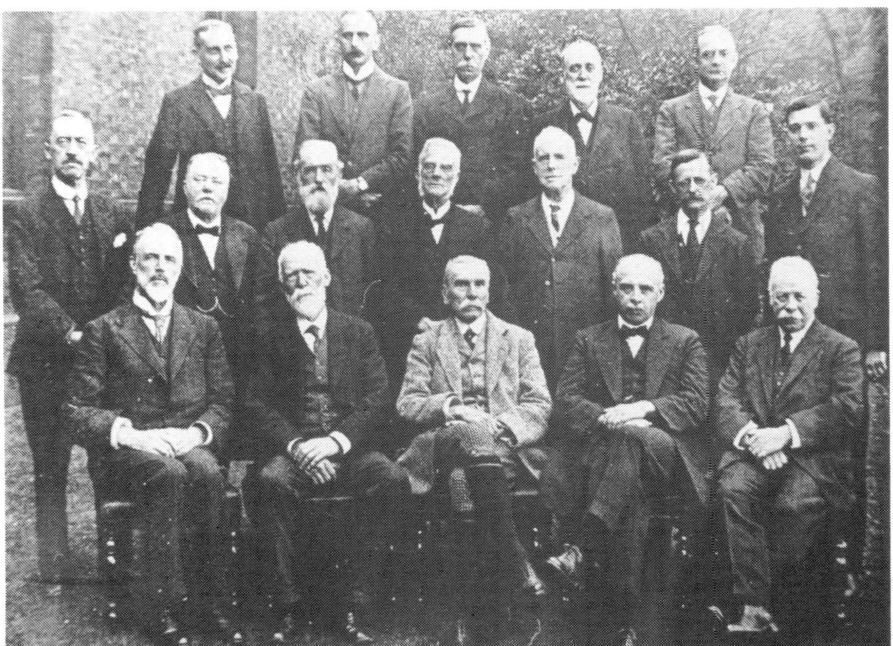

The Board of Management in 1919.

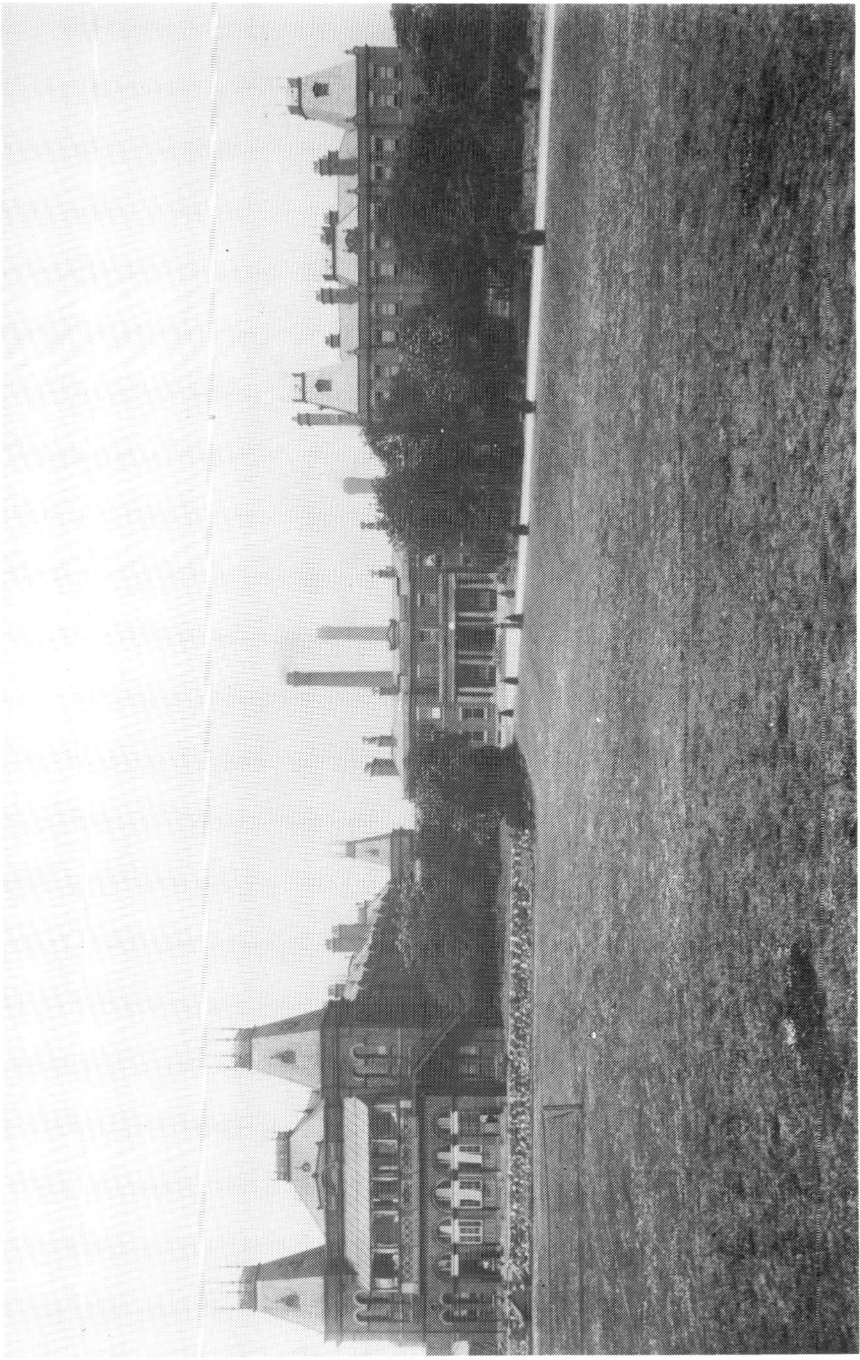

The Infirmary in 1925.

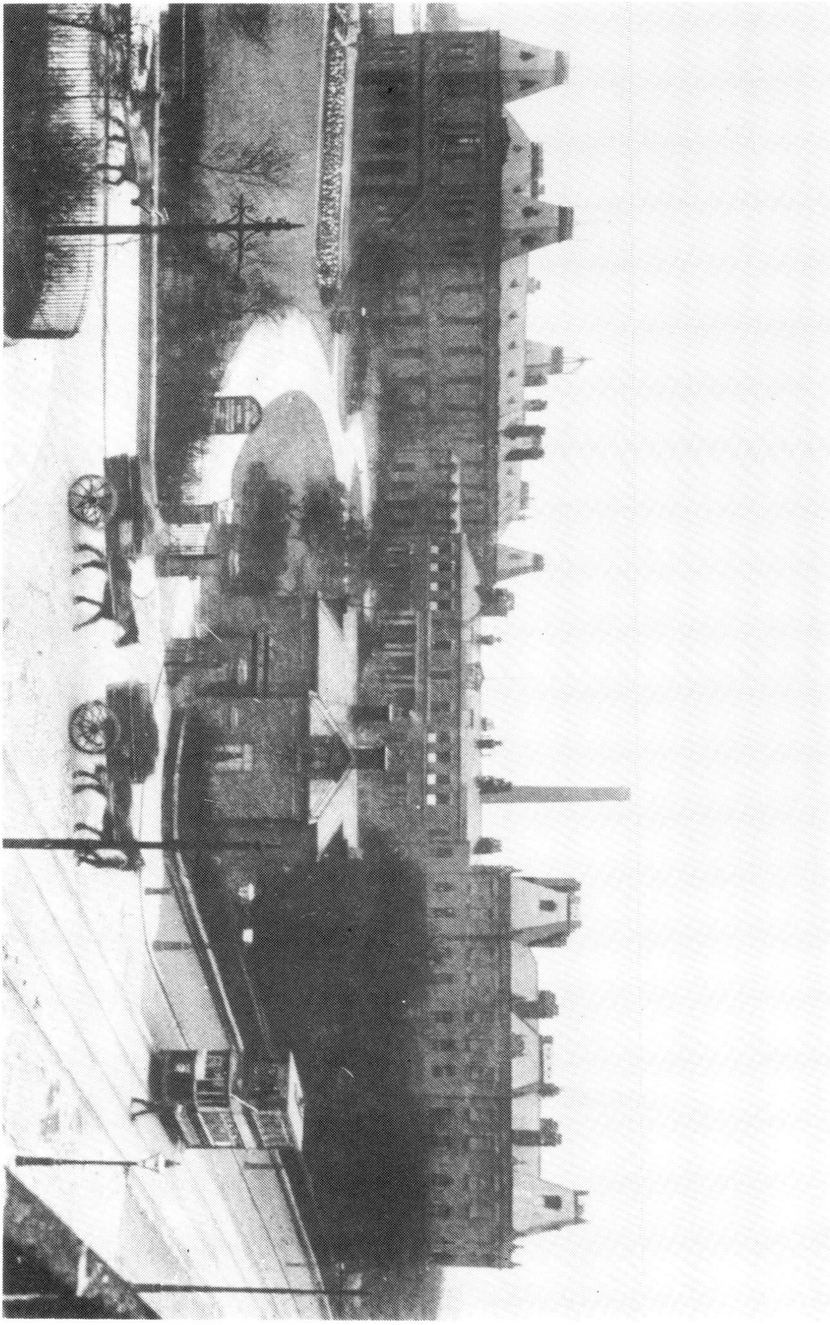

A rare early photograph of the Infirmary, dating from 1910. Note the lodge and the entrance gates, as well as the horse carts and trams on Deepdale Road.

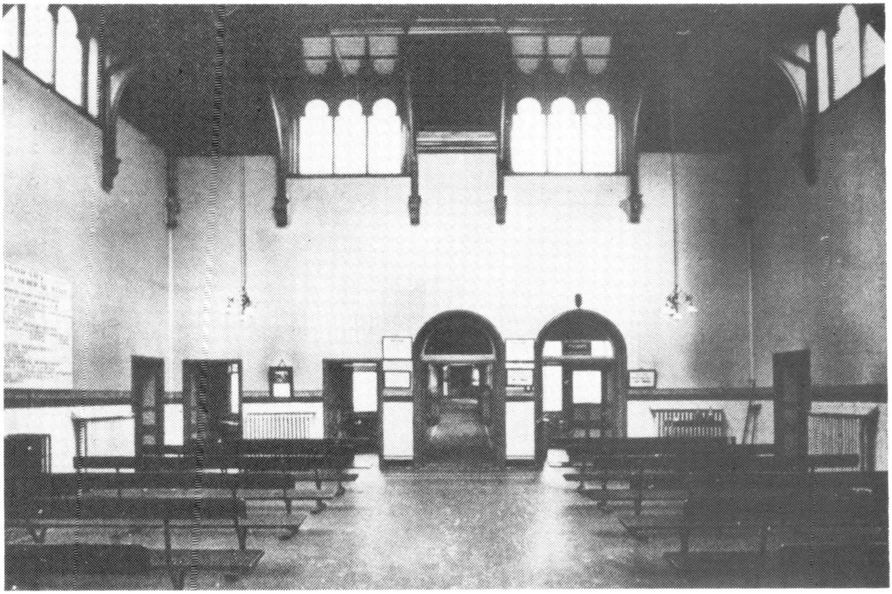

The 'new' Out-Patient Department in about 1901. This hall is remembered by thousands and saw over 80 years' service until Out-Patient services were eventually transferred to the new Royal Preston Hospital recently.

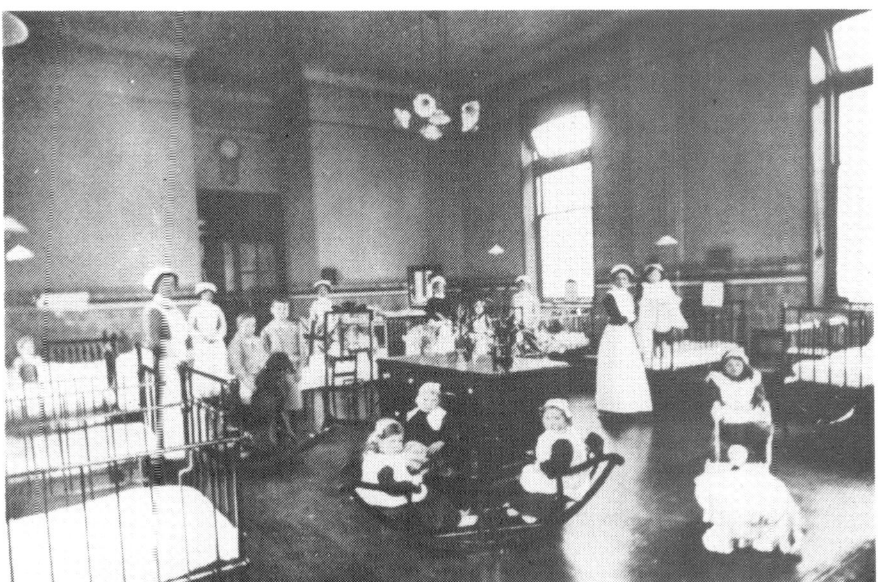

Children's Ward in around 1907.

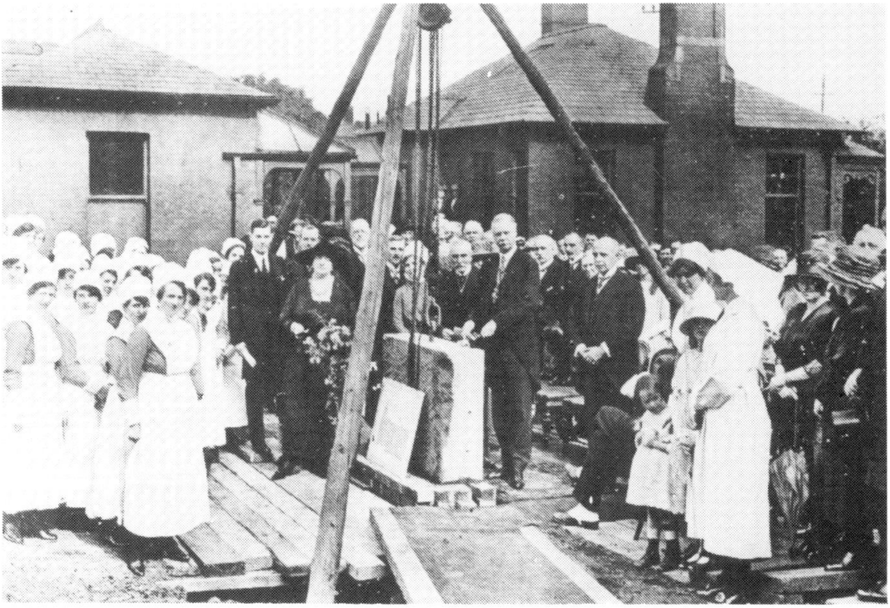

Guild Year 1922. The Guild Mayor, Henry Astley Bell JP lays the foundation stone of the Nurses Home Extension.

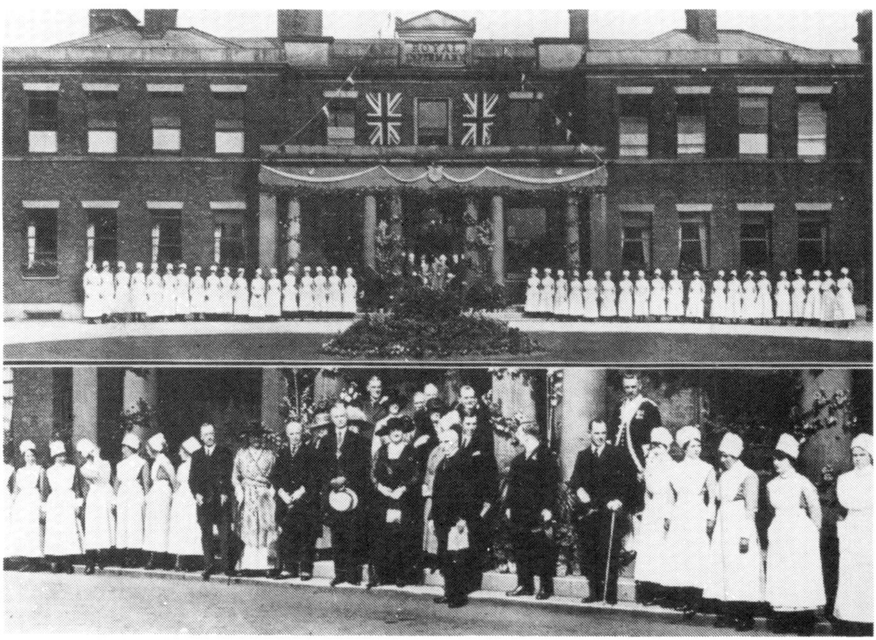

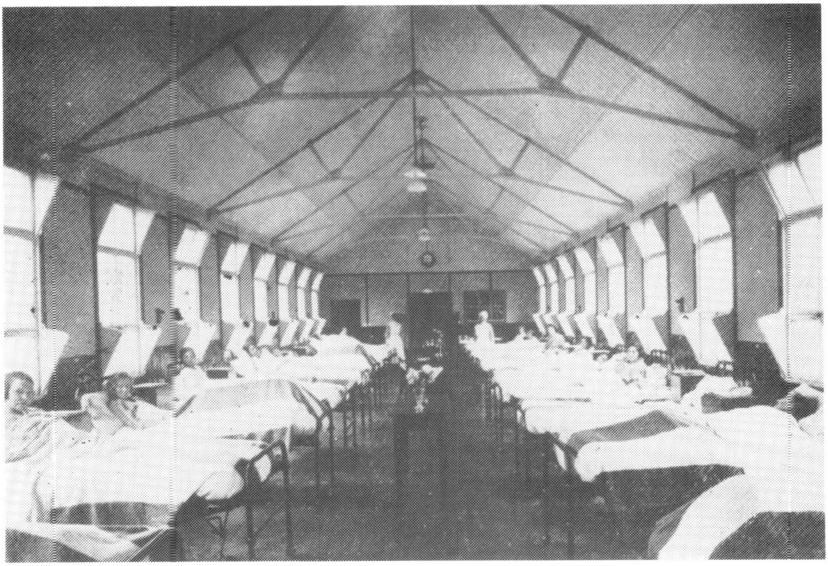

Opened to relieve Women's Surgical, West Ward, seen here in 1926, was built as a temporary ward, but saw continuous use until the hospital closed.

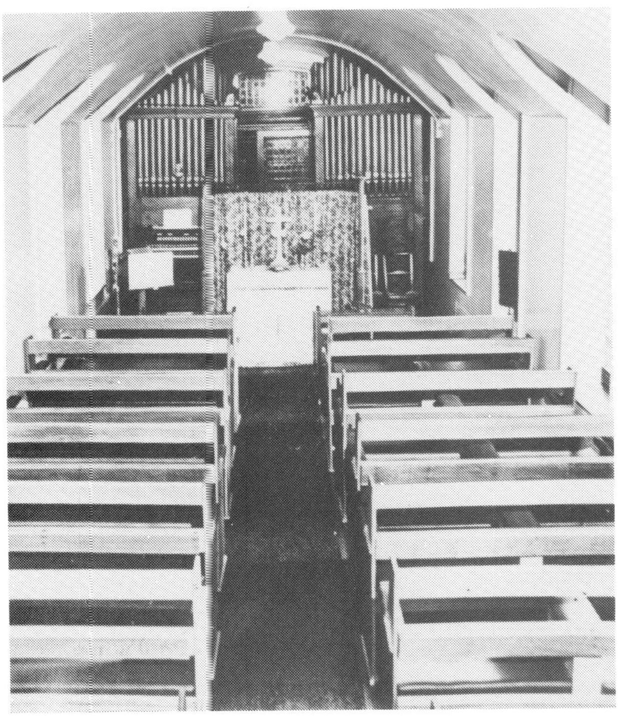

The Infirmary's Chapel.

Photograph courtesy of Lancashire Evening Post.

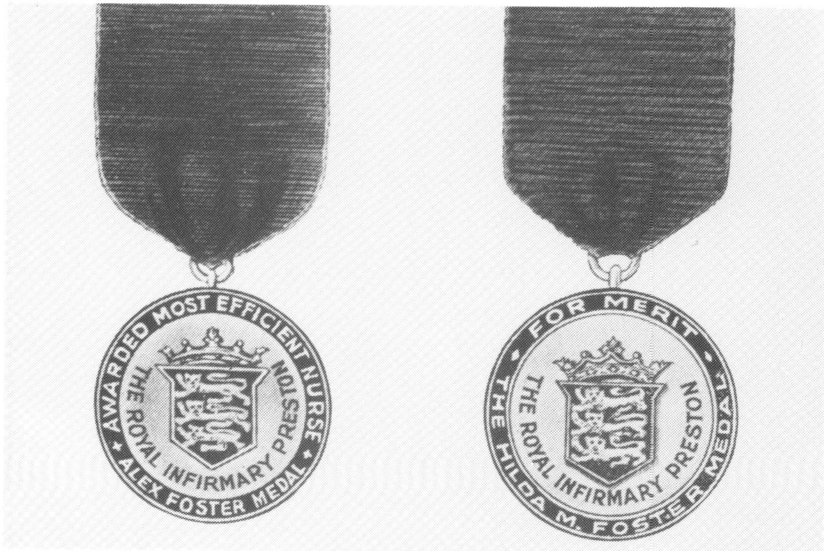

The Alex Foster Gold Medal and the Hilda M. Foster Silver Medal, awarded each year to the most outstanding nurses.

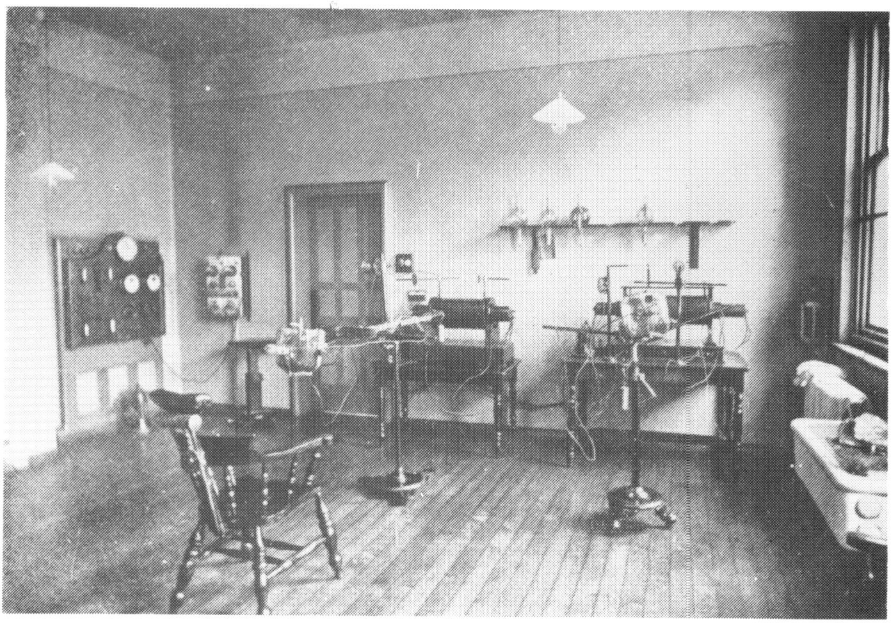

The Radio-Therapy Department, opened in 1908. We can only guess how patients felt being treated with this new-fangled equipment.

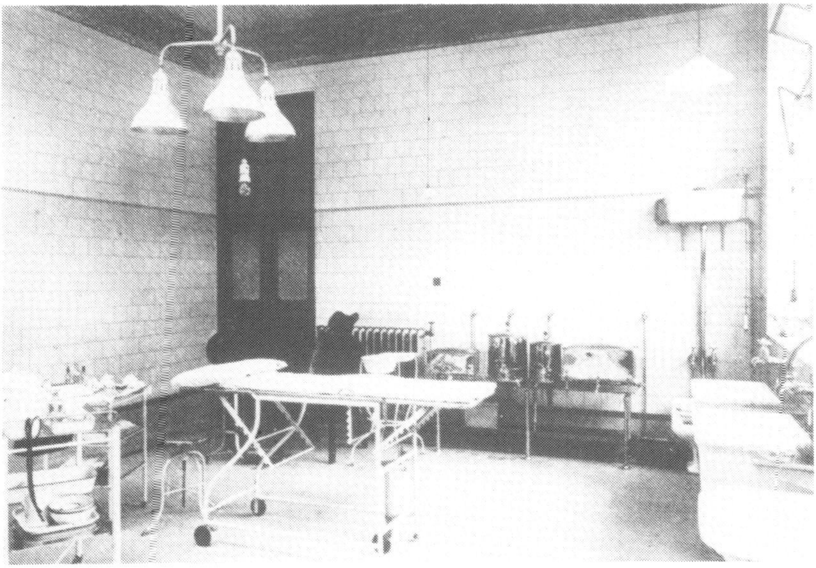

The treatment room in the Out-Patients Department, built in 1901 and in continuous use until the hospital closed.

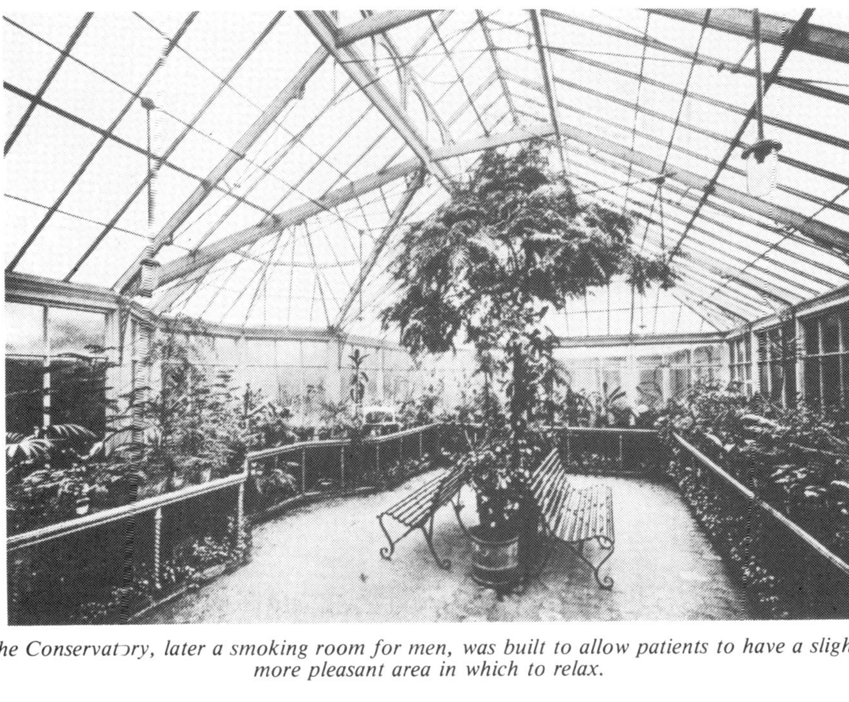

The Conservatɔry, later a smoking room for men, was built to allow patients to have a slightly more pleasant area in which to relax.

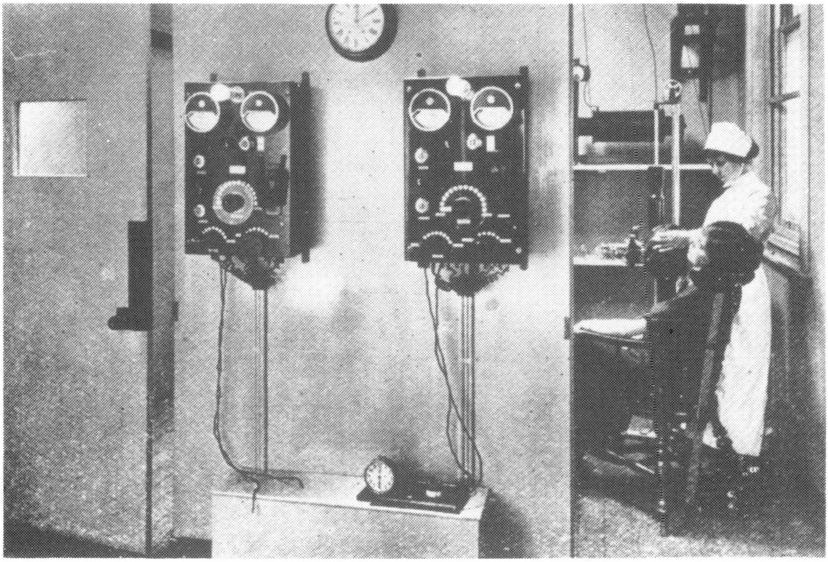

Both pictures on this page illustrate the rather primitive x-ray equipment of the 1920s. Used in the treatment of skin cancers and the like, the single machine which the Infirmary possessed was kept busy at all times.

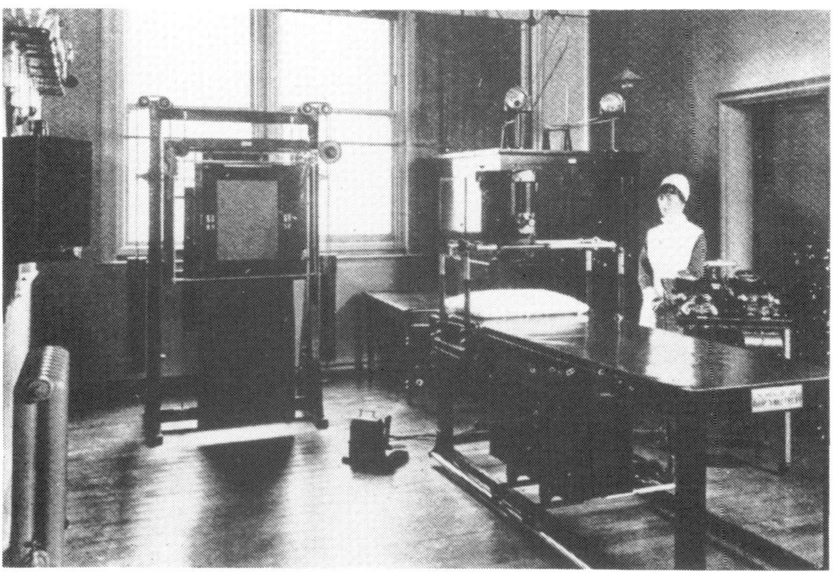

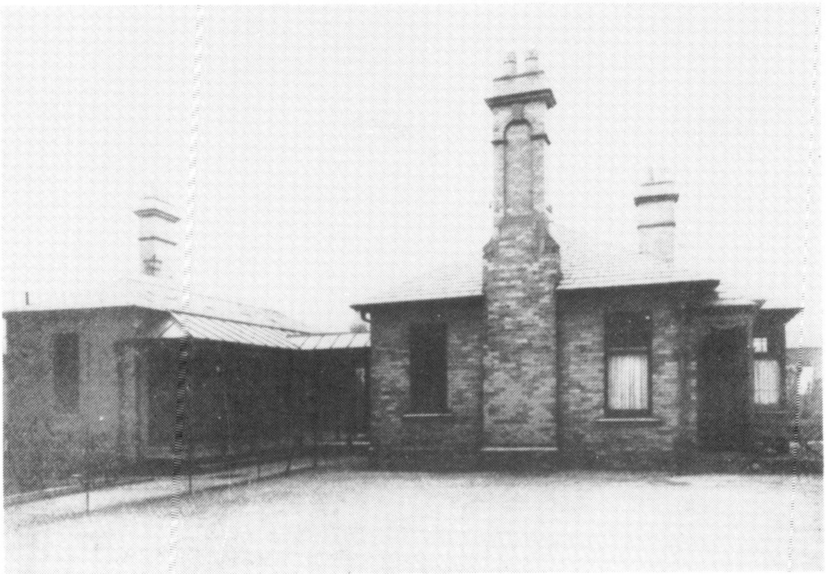

The Fever Wards began to be used, not for the isolation of patients, but for more general purposes and this led to the building of the Isolation Ward above.

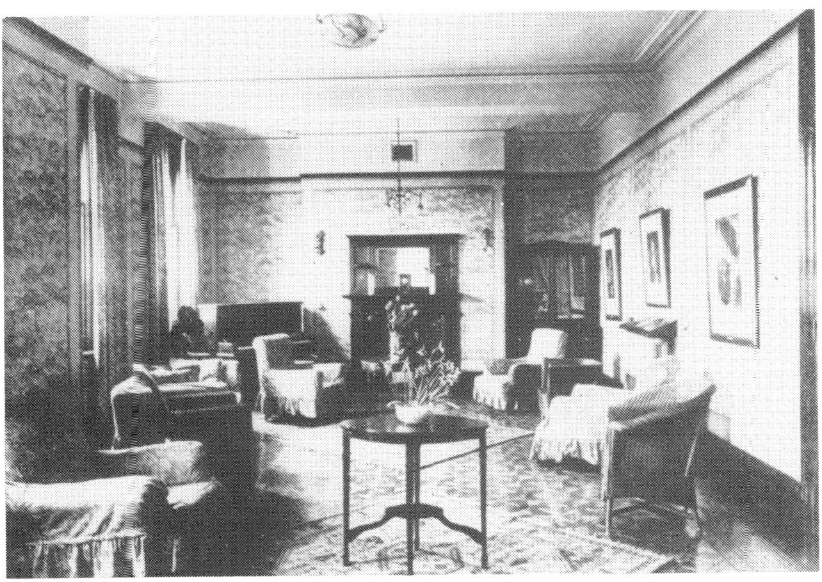

Before the enlargement of the Nurses Home in 1940, this small but plush room was the nurses' sitting room.

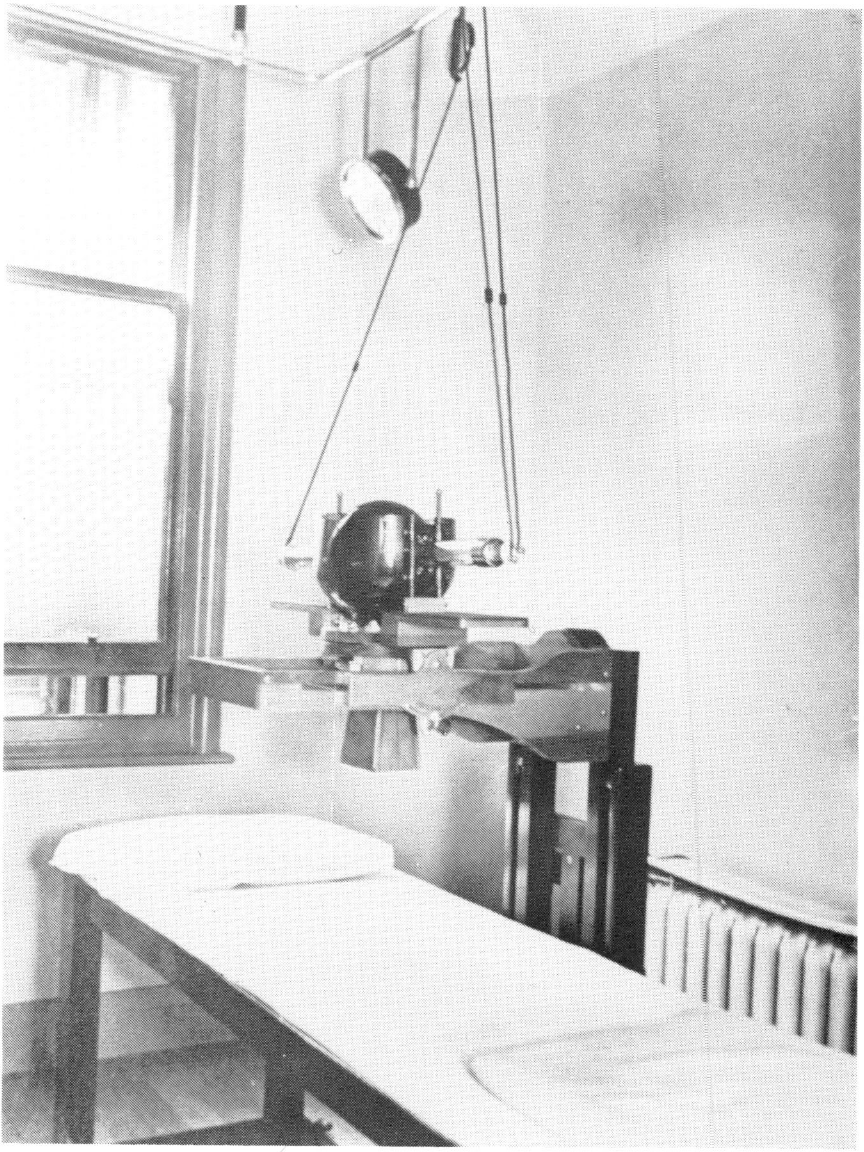

Just how far technology has advanced is evidenced by this early picture of x-ray equipment.
Photograph courtesy of Lancashire Evening Post.

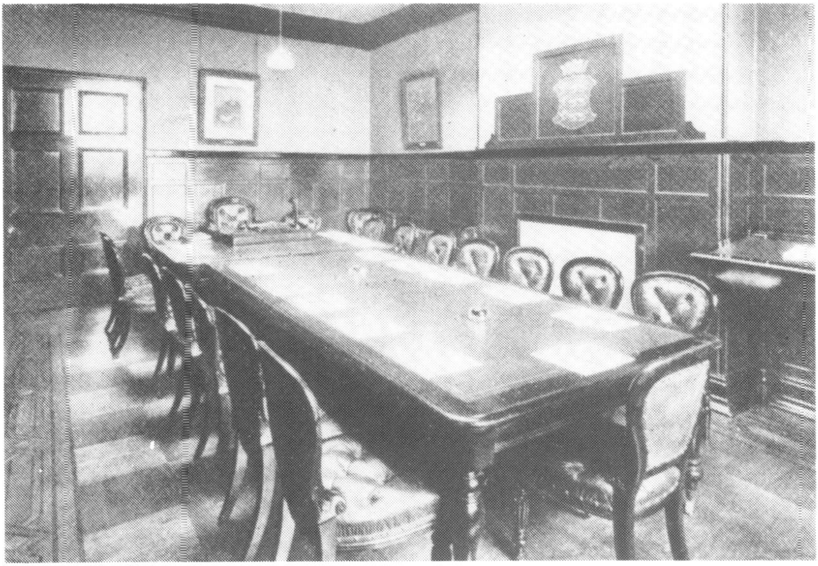

Where all the decisions were made . . . the Board Room in around 1935, before an extension was built for it. The FRI coat of arms can be seen mounted proudly above the fireplace.

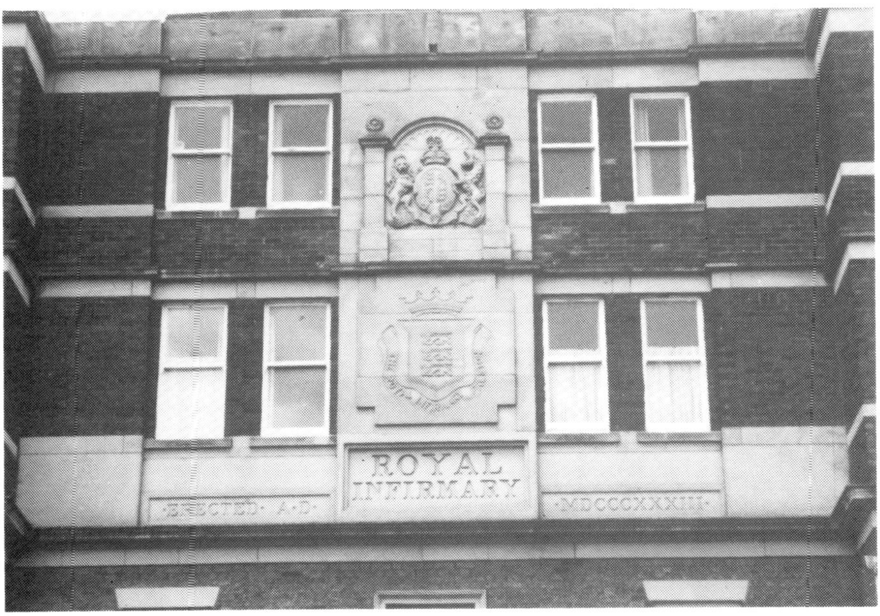

The Infirmary's front aspect showing the stone feature of the coat of arms and the date in Roman numerals, 1833.

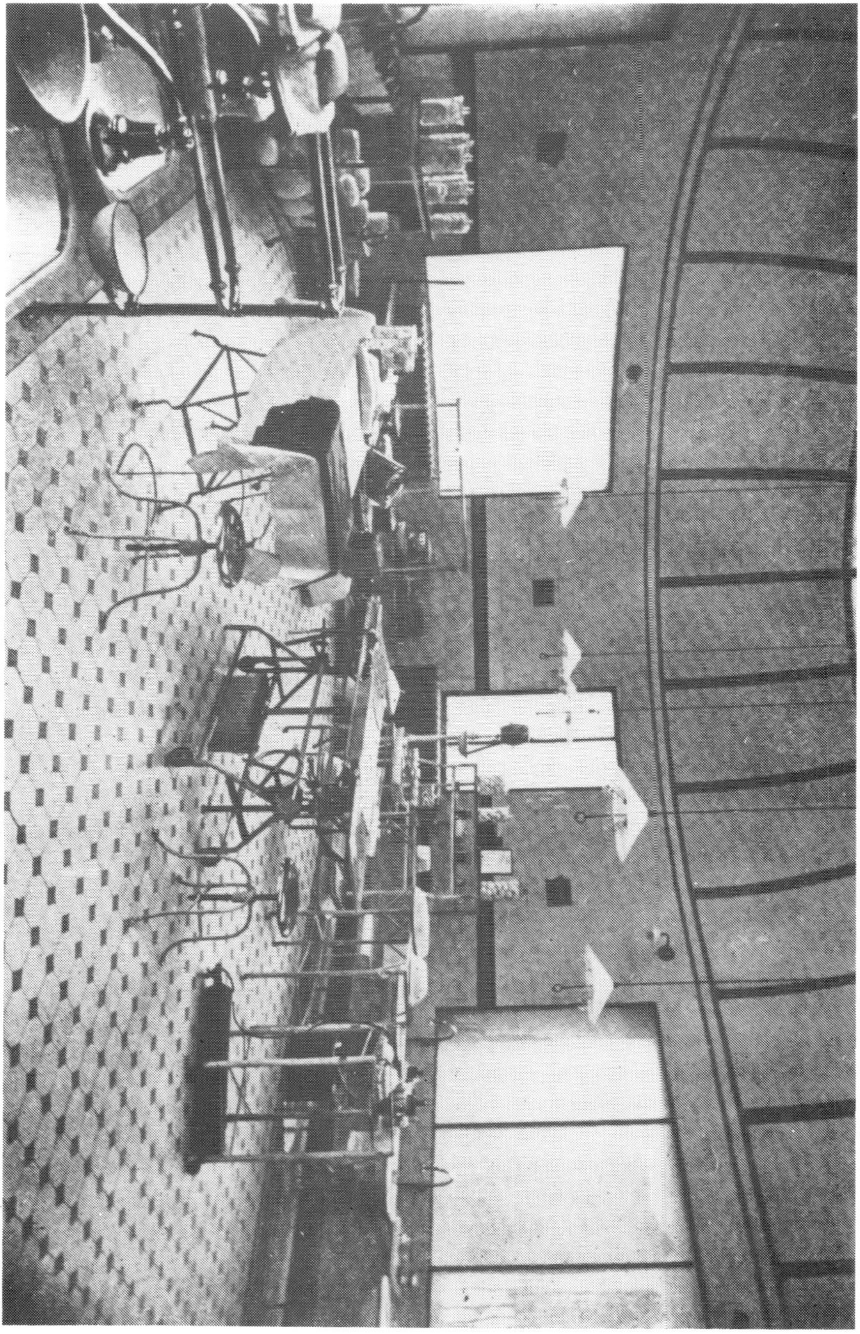

The operating theatre in 1901. The theatre was in use until 1985.

nursing staff. Eleven nurses presented themselves for examination, all of whom were successful, and they each received certificates of proficiency. Other examinations were held for mill operatives etc., and 30 people passed successfully.

The matron, now fully recovered, organised an outing to Lytham for child patients at her own expense; typhoid and scarlet fever were again prevalent and 64 cases were admitted to the fever wards. A large number of deaths from pneumonia was reported and the senior house surgeon, F. W. Collinson, suggested that district nurses would be an advantage in dealing with these cases. The eye surgeon noted an increase in the number of cases requiring removal of the eyeball, nearly all of which were wounds inflicted in the cotton mills by shuttles. One lady aged 91 years, it was reported, had undergone surgery for a cataract with complete success. The fever wards again increased their admissions, to 64 cases, mostly typhoid and erysipelas.

Once more it was noted that outlying districts were using the Infirmary without any financial help toward its upkeep. Of 1,270 patients treated, 985 were from Preston and 285 from outside districts. Fleetwood had begun a Hospital Aid Society in an attempt to remedy this, but patients from Kirkham, Lytham St. Annes, Blackpool, Fleetwood, Poulton, Cockerham, Grange, Dalton-in-Furness, Kendal, Lancaster, Garstang, Longridge, Leyland, Chorley, Hesketh Bank and many other places had been received without financial assistance from any of them.

The year 1888 saw the work of the Infirmary disrupted for five months by a particularly virulent outbreak of small-pox. The children's ward was closed from April 28th until October 3rd; all visiting was suspended and for most of the year the work of the ophthalmic and aural department and the dental department was suspended. The epidemic first appeared on 29th March 1888 and for the first time since they were opened the Harris Fever Wards were used to full capacity. One death from small-pox occurred in the general wards and it became apparent that the proximity of the fever wards to the main Infirmary buildings and the adjoining houses in St. Barabas Place was a hazard in such an outbreak, with so many cases being accommodated at one time for so long a period. The small-pox was confined and no other cases appeared in the general wards and it remained a mystery how the lady who died had contracted the disease. One consequence of the outbreak was a reduction in the numbers of patients arriving from surrounding districts due to the exaggerated reports of the plight of Preston and, also because of this, the convalescent homes refused to accept any case from Preston and district until the outbreak had disappeared.

During 1888 there was an increase in subscriptions received from the mills and workshops and this, combined with the closing of wards and departments for half of the year, resulted in an increase of income over expenditure. This financial situation carried over into 1889, the Infirmary's twentieth year, although due to a remission in trade generally which closed many of the larger mills in the town for several weeks, donations had been £137 less than the previous year. Receipts for the year, however, exceeded expenditure overall by £15/0/9d.

The Brackenbury Library, under the librarianship of Dr. Gilbertson, continued to increase, with the purchase of new works and the latest editions of books on medical and surgical subjects. Another appeal was raised for funds toward improving the laundry and it was reported that the fever wards were still a drain on the Infirmary's resources, as the 3/– a day charge did not even cover the daily expense of operating them.

The ophthalmic and aural department once again requested more beds for their cases and it was claimed there was a need for more wards suitable for the classification of diseases for which no provision existed at that time. Delays were again evident throughout the year in the admission of patients due to lack of accommodation, causing waiting lists of cases awaiting admission. Three nurses contracted typhoid fever but all eventually recovered and convalescent homes were again being used, with Southport proving the most popular.

The death was recorded in 1890 of Dr. E. L. Dixon, one of the original honorary medical officers of the Board. His son, H. L. Dixon, M.A., M.B.B.C. (Cantab), became junior house surgeon. As in previous years, there was a constant turnover of medical staff; Dr. Platt resigned in August, Dr. McNab resigned in May and then Dr. Murdo Rose, the assistant house surgeon, resigned after only a few months to take another position. Most years there was no continuity of service at all.

The matron, Miss Piggott, had now been at the Infirmary for eight years and in that time had stamped a rule of firmness on the place. She gave courses of lectures on nursing in three elementary schools in Preston in an endeavour to encourage a succession of nurses for the Infirmary in later years; the fees she received for this function were given by her to the private nurses home. Changes in the nursing division in 1890 included the resignation of Nurse Hamilton, head nurse in the male wards, being replaced by Nurse Noble who was transferred from the children's ward, Nurse Waddington being promoted to head nurse in the children's ward and Nurse Pitchford appointed head nurse in the female wards replacing Nurse Leslie who had been promoted as matron of the private nurses home. A former matron, Miss Mahoney, who had resigned because of ill health some years before, emigrated to New Zealand.

Throughout 1890 the fever wards admitted only 40 cases and it was recorded that five of these patients died from typhoid. The wards were closed for the early part of the year due to an outbreak of influenza, no fewer than 15 members of the staff being affected. Christmas celebrations were postponed until the New Year for some reason which was not recorded.

The early part of 1891 was extremely cold, with very severe weather, and this gave the Infirmary an adverse balance of £343/19/5d in the end of year accounts due in part, it was stated, 'to the increase of expenditure on fire materials'. Telephonic communication was established for the first time between the main building, the porter's lodge, the Harris Fever Wards and the nurses home.

The private nurses home was proving a vast success, with a constant enquiry for nurses, so much so that it was proposed to increase the number of trained nurses available and the oft proposed district nurse scheme was established. Further changes in the nursing division took place when Nurse Noble, who the year before had become head nurse in the male wards, resigned to take up a post at Netley Hospital. Head Nurse Pitchford transferred from the female to the male wards and Assistant Nurse Whittaker became head nurse of the female wards.

The question of the laundry was raised once more, its enlargement being regarded as absolutely essential; plans and estimates were prepared and tenders requested to remove the mortuary, erect a new mortuary further from the main building and putting a new drying stove and boiler into the now enlarged laundry. The cost of this was approximately £1,000, for which fresh appeals were made.

There had been since its inception as an Infirmary a deficiency of water pressure in the building. A delegate from the Board met the Preston Corporation Water Committee, with the end result that a new water main was laid through the grounds to a cistern on the Infirmary's roof. Despite the considerable cost of this operation, it proved of little advantage as the water pressure remained far from satisfactory for the infirmary's needs. It was suggested that if the Water Board could not find other means to increase the pressure, additional cistern capacity within the building would have to be provided.

An influenza epidemic in the early summer months, not as virulent as the previous years outbreak, resulted in many patients being refused admission as they could not be accommodated; three members of staff were also affected. An outbreak of chicken-pox in the children's ward during April 1891 caused the ward to be closed for three weeks. Thirteen cases of scarlet fever were admitted to the Harris Fever Wards, with two deaths. A record was kept for the first time of anaesthetics given to patients. Chloroform was administered in 203 cases with the times of administration varying from 5 minutes to 150 minutes without mishap in any case. Cocaine had been used in 16 cases with excellent results.

An impartial trial, in conjunction with other similar institutions in the United Kingdom and on the continent, was made of Professor Koch's remedy for tuberculosis. Several cases of lupus were treated it was reported 'with decided temporary benefit. In three cases the new remedy was combined with other methods resulting in the discharge of two cases as cured and one case relieved with the hope that in each case the benefit was permanent'.

The 23rd year of the Infirmary's history, 1892, once again saw continuous staff changes, all three members of the house staff leaving during the year, one member being the junior house officer, Dr. W. H. Pimblett. The deaths were recorded of Mr. J. B. Hallmark, a member of the Board, and also Mr. John F. Clarkson, another of the original trustees of whom there had originally been 25. Henry Silver, gardener of the Infirmary for 20 years, died and also Nurse Hook, who died on 18th August from scarlet fever which she contracted in the Harris Fever Wards. During the summer months steps were taken to meet an expected visitation of cholera but Preston fortunately escaped.

In November the Board was placed in some difficulty by the admission of a case of small-pox from Oakenclough. It was later discovered that the patient had been living in a hut with 60 other men for 8 days. It would have been an embarrassment to have to isolate 59 others and in doing so swamp the facilities of the fever wards. It was resolved that in future more care would need to be taken when admitting patients to these wards from districts outside the Infirmary's area of Preston.

Seven years after its inception the private nurses home was just paying its way but it was openly admitted that improvements would not be made unless the frequent practice of nurses, once trained, setting up on their own was stopped. It became an article of contract that nurses would not be allowed to set up in practice on their own account after completion of their engagement for a stated time or within a certain distance from Preston. More nurses were needed and probationers were sent to other institutions for training.

Water again proved a problem but the Borough Surveyor remedied this and the Infirmary's water supply was much improved. Dr. Brown instigated an annual trip out for nurses to Fleetwood and Blackpool.

The convalescent homes had a bad year in 1892 for the governing body had made it obligatory for patients to pay a fee of 5/– (25p) on admission; consequently very few people accepted convalescence on these terms.

The new mortuary building was completed and declared open. The old mortuary closed on 13th October, allowing for the extensions to the laundry to proceed. The estimated £1,000 for these alterations proved insufficient by over £300 so an appeal was made for further subscriptions to reach the required sum. £826 had been raised by the end of the year but it was then realised that the washing machinery and engine had been in continuous use for 23 years and would not be of much use to an enlarged and updated laundry; they too would have to be replaced. Although the Infirmary's income since 1872 had almost doubled, its expenditure had more than doubled also and the number of patients had trebled:

	1872	1882	1892
Income	£2,836	£4,430	£5,446
Expenditure	£2,604	£4,508	£5,414
In-patients	461	800	1,238
Out-patients	2,353	4,093	5,240
Total	2,814	4,893	6,478

Europe at this time was ravaged by the spread of cholera so once again precautions were taken in anticipation of cases reaching Preston. An epidemic of small-pox occurred in several parts of Lancashire during the autumn of 1892. Preston seemed likely to escape but unfortunately a labourer carried the infection from Warrington to Garstang. The Infirmary was called upon to accept him and he was admitted to the Harris Fever Wards, after strict precautions had been taken to eliminate the spread of the infection; the patient eventually recovered without mishap to anyone. For the first time in 10 years, however, one of the nurses in the fever wards died from scarlet fever; she was taken ill on the ward and died three days later.

The ophthalmic and aural surgeon of the Infirmary gave a fascinating case report of a child aged 7 years who presented as suffering a trivial injury to the eye. Operation revealed the presence of a foreign body in the socket which proved to be the pointed end of a slate pencil which had apparently been embedded in this position for several weeks without attracting much attention. Chloroform was given in 206 cases, varying in times from 5 minutes to 150 minutes; cocaine was used 13 times and ethyl chloride 6 times.

The death was recorded in 1893 of C. R. Jacson Esq., who had been chairman of the Board since the Infirmary's inception in 1869. Mr. Jacson bequeathed

£1,000 to the Endowment Fund. Two of the honorary consultant medical officers also died that year — Doctors Marshall and Gilbertson, both of whom had served the Infirmary since 1869.

Another nurse, Senior Assistant Nurse Mary Johnson, died from tyhpoid fever contracted on the ward. In the nursing division, Nurse Waddington, the head nurse in the children's ward, resigned in January 1893, to be replaced by Nurse Barton, who had been head night nurse, and a Nurse Butler was promoted to become head night nurse.

Although donations and bequests came in thick and fast during 1893, still expenditure outstripped income and it was patently obvious that the Infirmary's income was insufficient to run its affairs properly. The laundry extensions were completed during the year and the cost, including the new mortuary was £1,251/6/10d, of which £827/8/0d had been raised by public subscription; the remaining deficit of £423/18/10d meant a further appeal to the public. There had been a considerable increase in the number of patients, 115 beds at one time being occupied for lengthy periods. There had been increases in maintenance costs such as painting the outside (£100), coal (£50) due to the increase in the cost of coal as a result of the coal strike, and also the £150 it had cost to send laundry to public laundries while the Infirmary's laundry could not cope during alterations and enlargement.

The private nurses home suffered from a scarcity of nurses, it was reported. Four probationers had been trained at other institutions at a cost of £81/2/0d and it was hoped to increase the number of private nurses trained to 20. The largest number of patients since the small-pox outbreak of 1888 was admitted to the fever wards in 1893. Throughout the year there were outbreaks of scarlet fever and typhoid fever and 66 patients were admitted. Another nurse died from scarlet fever with the result that the children's ward was closed for a month. Large numbers of burns cases had been admitted, principally children, many of which proved fatal (out of 32 cases there were 7 deaths). A decrease in out-patient and home-patient numbers was due, it was considered, to the phenomenal summer weather of 1893.

Two cases of serious accidents resulting from explosions were reported by the ophthalmic and aural surgeon. A labourer on Thirlmere pipe tracks had both eyes blown out by dynamite and a well sinker at the Fleetwood Salt Works lost his eye by the premature explosion of a charge of gunpowder used in sinking a shaft. The first death reported by the ophthalmic surgeon was of a young man who presented with faulty vision which he supposed to be due to want of spectacles, but who on examination was found to have a brain tumour. A fund was needed to supply spectacles for poor patients, as it was reported that after long and tedious examination it was found that for financial reasons these patients were unable to avail themselves of the necessary prescribed help.

Income from donations, the mills and workshops increased and expenditure decreased during 1894. The private nurses home had achieved 18 fully trained nurses and there had been a considerable increase in the amount of work carried out by them. The home had become more self-supporting and less of a drain on the Infirmary's resources. The Aunt Judy Society celebrated its 10th birthday and reported 37 members supplying 250 garments a year.

Another death occurred in the nursing division, this time from tuberculosis

(Nurse Brown). Mr. J. A. Forrest, the collector of subscriptions since 1869, resigned and Dr. Riley who had been the Infirmary's Chaplain for 9 years left when he was elevated to the See of Perth in Western Australia.

A large oil painting, *Jacob's Dream,* after Guernico of Bologna, dated 1666, formerly the property of C. R. Jacson Esq, of Barton Hall, was given by his widow to the Preston National Schools' Improvement Fund. The painting was purchased by a few of Mr. Jacson's friends and presented in his memory to the Royal Infirmary, over which he had presided as chairman for 23 years.

On 22nd December 1894 a great storm hit Preston, a stack of chimneys was blown down, crashing through the roof into the female surgical ward. There were some narrow escapes but no one was injured, some of the patients being sent home and others transferred temporarily to the fever wards. The chimney had to be taken down and rebuilt. A covered way from the main Infirmary building to the Harris Fever Wards was deemed essential and a new wing was also envisaged but as it had been said so many times before, 'a benevolent donor or donors was awaited in order to carry out all these ambitious but much needed improvements'. The female surgical ward closed for some time as a consequence of the damage incurred during the storms and gales of the previous December.

With the death in 1894 of the chairman, Charles Roger Jacson, the vice chairman Edmund Birley was unanimously appointed as chairman. He was the sole remaining survivor of the original trustees, 25 in number, who had been nominated on the 12th March 1866. He died soon after, during 1895, as did Mr. J. W. E. Rigby who had been the Infirmary's dispenser for 16 years. He was succeeded by his assistant, Miss Louise C. Holden, who had performed the duties well during the long illness of Mr. Rigby. Surely a unique appointment for those days!

The timetable for nurses and probationers duties was revised 'so as to give some relief in their arduous duties and allow a monthly holiday'. Dr. Brown again gave an outing to the nurses and they were invited in groups to the homes of Miss Salisbury of Myerscough Hall and Miss Pakes of Copp vicarage. Dr. Brown also acted as intermediary between Mrs. R. Holgate-Brown and Miss Horrocks and the Infirmary Board. These ladies had offered the sum of £500 to provide a covered way between the Infirmary and children's ward.

During 1895 there was a great outcry at the lack of operating facilities at Preston Royal Infirmary especially if an emergency operation needed to be carried out at night. Dr. Charles Brown purchased an operating table, made completely of metal to enable constant cleaning and asepsis. However, this acquisition proved an embarrassment for there was no place to accommodate it. Dr. Brown donated the money (£2,700) for the erection of an operating theatre, which was opened for use on 12th February 1901 and proved to be one of the greatest assets the Infirmary had ever acquired and was surely a bargain at such a price, being still in use more than 85 years later.

It must be realised that the progress of surgical technique over the centuries had been terribly slow and there had been no great leaps forward, but just methodical plodding on the part of many dedicated men who would certainly be amazed at the facilities afforded their modern counterparts today. There was little understanding of the problems that retarded the progress of surgery for there was of course no anaesthesia until the 1840s and the need for absolute cleanliness of the hands, the instruments and the site of operation, although recognised by some pioneers, was not practised generally in England. Pyaemia, septicaemia and gangrene were commonplace everywhere in the surgical wards. A compound fracture of the leg in most cases meant amputation and the death rate from septic disease following amputation was between 30% and 50%.

Dr. Ignaz Semmelweiss in 1847 had found that the puerperal fever which was responsible for the deaths of many women in the Lying-In Hospital in Vienna was due to a 'poison' carried from the mortuary by the medical students on their hands etc. He insisted that every student and doctor should wash their hands thoroughly in a basin of chlorine water before entering the maternity wards. The number of deaths dropped dramatically but Dr. Semmelweiss was ridiculed by his colleagues for the nature of the 'poison' was not then understood.

In the same year that Dr. Semmelweiss died at the early age of 47, Joseph Lister began using his antiseptic principle for treating wounds using carbolic acid, the end result being that the surgical wards of Glasgow Infirmary were free for the most part of patients dying from pyaemia and septicaemia. Also, in 1865, Louis Pasteur, a French biochemist, published his work on fermentation and putrefaction and his proof that living organisms were to be found everywhere in the air. Robert Koch, an obscure country doctor who was destined to go down in history as the father of bacteriology, also played a valuable part in the progress of surgical practice. It was Semmelweiss who first grasped the nature of sepsis and asepsis but it was Koch, Pasteur and Lister who finally wrought the miracle which led surgery to hitherto undreamed of procedures.

In the first annual report of the newly opened Preston Royal Infirmary for the year 1870, the senior house surgeon, J. Call. Weddell M.D., master in surgery etc. (Edinburgh), reported on the nature and number of operations performed during the Infirmary's first year.

2 Amputations of forearm, both of whom recovered.

2 Amputations of shoulder, one died and one recovered.

1 Excision of elbow joint, relieved.

3 Excisions of tumour of the breast, all relieved.

1 Abdominal tap, relieved.

3 Amputations of Foot, all recovered.

1 Amputation of leg, under treatment.

1 Amputation of Knee, recovered.

1 Amputation of thigh, died.

2 Amputations of thigh, recovered.

The operation lists for the year 1901 at P.R.I. following the opening of its new theatre consisted of many procedures which today would no doubt be considered as minor operations, 310 general and 190 local anaesthetics being administered. By 1905 more adventurous operations were being undertaken in all departments, with 796 general and 274 local anaesthetics being administered during that year. Only one operation was recorded for gastric ulcer, with the patient failing to recover from the operation. In 1910, 916 general and 534 local anaesthetics were administered and two deaths were recorded as a result, the number of operations, however, on the stomach and duodenum had increased to 18, of which eight had died, nine were cured and one was 'relieved'.

Hospital Sunday in the churches was established in Preston on the last Sunday in January but because the inclement weather seriously interfered with the collection on that day, the clergy were asked to arrange a further Sunday a little later in the year.

A complete apparatus for the production of 'Röntgen Rays' and an electrical battery were purchased with funds from the Brackenbury Fund in 1896, allowing the use of x-rays in the Infirmary for the first time. The battery had connections to the various wards and to the surgery, with the electrical supply coming from a number of cells in the Infirmary's basement. The Röntgen apparatus was as complete as it was possible to be at that time. By means of a flourescent screen made of platino-cyanide of barium it was possible to see the skeleton with the naked eye but the process of permanent photographic record was a rather lengthy procedure.

It was reported that the sanitary arrangements in the Infirmary were unchanged since it had opened in 1869 twenty years before and it was noted that vast improvements could be made in that direction if the funds were made available. In fact, many improvements, both structural and in equipment, were possible but the Infirmary was still operating on a shoe-string. Another wing to the building was envisaged to increase the bed state and so increase the benefits of the Infirmary to the community. Queen Victoria was reaching the sixtieth anniversary of her accession the following year, 1897, and the Board expected great things in the way of financial gain from this event.

Dr. Pimblett resigned to go into private practice, having served for five years as assistant, junior and then senior house surgeon. In the nursing division there were no changes among the senior nursing staff.

A 'framed photographic likeness' of the late chairman was presented by the committee of the Jacson Memorial Fund. The Harris Fever Wards were still reported as a drag on the finances; there had been only 17 admissions during 1896 with the wards remaining completely empty for many weeks. The charge for admission was probably still the reason for this but it was noted that 'the sooner they are endowed and thrown open like the other wards, the better for the health of the town'.

More accommodation was urgently needed in the main Infirmary as 'it occurred all too often that patients were being sent home before they were fully recovered in order to make room for urgent or accident cases'. Beds were also urgently needed for the ophthalmic and aural surgeon's cases. A quote by that surgeon, J. Winkley Landon, states:

> 'Would not the year 1897, when so many other larger towns are vieing with each other to celebrate the longest reign in English history, be a splendid opportunity of leaving to our descendants so lasting a memorial of the unique event as a ward entirely set aside for the treatment of the eye, and which could be christened in such a manner to accentuate the fact'.

Accidents to the eyes were noted from fireworks and whip tops (flick the whip) but there were no serious shuttle wounds from the mills due, it was suggested, to the safety guards which had been put into use during the preceeding few years.

Mr. Buckstone-Browne, of 2 Porter Place, donated an annual sum of £2/2/0d towards the formation of a spectacle fund and a further report was given of the ever widening sphere of cases from far flung places treated in the Infirmary i.e. Burnley, Carnforth, Darwen, Fleetwood, Kendal, Lancaster, Shap, Southport, Wigan etc.

In Queen Victoria's jubilee year 1897, the Board reported that:

> their hopes had been more than realised in that the people of Preston and District, in accordance with Her Majesty's wishes, unanimously decided at a Public Meeting held in the Guild Hall on March 24th, that a Diamond Jubilee Fund should be raised for the benefit of the Infirmary.

By the 31st December 1897 this fund amounted to the sum of £7,899/16/9d by public subscription but other subscriptions had fallen during the year due, no doubt, to the depression in trade and industry and the fact that in the early part of the year a large amount had been raised in Preston and District for an Indian famine relief fund.

Mr. R. F. Easterby, secretary of the Infirmary for 28 years, resigned to take up the duties of county auditor of Lancashire and a well known Prestonian, Mr. Walter Davies, took the office of secretary in his stead. Other changes included Dr. Derham, resigned in January and Dr. W. Murray was promoted to junior house surgeon; he resigned, however, in November to take a post as resident surgeon to the Birmingham General Dispensary. Dr. J. Frank Holden was appointed junior house surgeon and Dr. George Macgibbon became assistant house surgeon. A Nurse Langley died although the cause of her death was not given.

The Board decided that all nurses should wear an outdoor uniform, to be provided at the nurses own expense. The existing staff had the option of wearing it or not as they pleased, but all new nurses were compelled to wear it at all times outside the Infirmary.

The covered way to the children's ward was completed and opened during 1897 and proved 'a great boon in inclement weather'. Mrs. Holgate-Browne who had donated some of the money for this also gave an ambulance carriage to the Infirmary.

The number of accidents treated decreased from 1,202 in 1896, the highest on record, to 991 the lowest number since 1892. Two severe epidemics occurred in the summer and autumn months, typhoid fever and measles, which accounted for an increase in admissions to the Harris Wards to 55 cases, there being only 17 cases in the previous year. Thirty four cases of typhoid fever were admitted, with three deaths. Eight cases of measles occurred in the children's ward during July while the epidemic raged in the town and one patient died, resulting in the closure of the ward to visitors, but no other cases occurred. The after effects of measles was seen in the enormous increase in cases of ulcers of the eyes, 25 cases in all.

One case of typhus fever died in the Harris Wards, an Irish labourer who had just arrived in this country. This disease, generally known as 'gaol fever' had been common enough at one time but at this period was almost unknown. 'Improved sanitation', it was claimed, had stamped it out. There had been a marked improvement in the healing of wounds simply due to absolute cleanliness, the boiling of everything coming into contact with the wound and, of course, the use of antiseptics.

The ophthalmic surgeon, while reporting on the increase of eye cases due to the measles outbreak, also quoted the case of 'a young lady cycling from Preston to Accrington along New Hall Lane when she was struck in the eye by a stone thrown by a young hooligan, completely destroying the eye'.

A system of inviting tenders for the supply of drugs, provisions and dressings was adopted for the first time in 1898, which worked splendidly at a considerable saving overall. Alterations in the Board were made when the number of members representing the Workpeople's Fund was increased from two to four and two further members were added to the Honorary Medical Board. There was an unusually large number of staff changes during the year. Miss Piggott resigned on 31st May after 16 years as matron/superintendent and Miss Leslie, matron of the private nurses home, also resigned after 16 years service. Miss Piggott was replaced by Miss Kathleen Disley, formerly matron of the Boston Hospital, Lincolnshire, but Miss Leslie was not replaced as it was decided that in future the matron/superintendent would be responsible for both establishments. Miss Clara Hoadley, formerly matron of the Cottage Hospital, Goole, was appointed as assistant matron. There was also a complete change round in junior and assistant medical staff during the year. Dr. L. E. Hardy, having served for six years, a record no doubt, resigned and there were five changes overall, with some of the medical men resigning to enrol for the South African War.

An invitation was issued, in the form of a competition, among architects to submit schemes to upgrade the Infirmary. Two of the conditions 'being principally the modernisation and perfecting of the sanitary, heating and lighting should be *sine qua non,* and the whole scheme was not to exceed £12,000'. In 1899 three local architects submitted their designs and these were displayed for public examination in the Harris Free Library. They were judged by Mr. Austin of Messrs. Austin & Paley, architects, of Lancaster, and the first prize was awarded to Mr. F. E. Dixon A.Inst. C.E., A.S.I., who was given the task of putting his scheme into effect for the alterations and upgrading of the Infirmary. This was the decision reached by the Board after lengthy deliberation on how best to use the money from the Diamond Jubilee Fund; however, all their plans failed to materialise. All the competitors were of the opinion that the amount of money (£12,000) was nowhere near sufficient to carry out any of the schemes displayed to the public and the Board eventually disclosed that they were not satisfied anyway with Mr. Dixon's scheme; so they decided on a scheme of their own after visiting some of the most modern hospitals in the country. Their scheme took the course of carrying out all the alterations in phases without interfering with the working of the Infirmary: *viz.*

(1)	Structural alteration to children's ward with repairs to sanitary arrangements etc.	£903/19/0d
(2)	Complete overhaul of sanitary arrangements including drainage	£1,350/0/0d
(3)	Complete overhaul of heating, ventilation, new boilers, steam pipes etc.	£710/0/0d
(4)	Electric lighting (keeping gas as a handy alternative)	£420/0/0d
(5)	Tiling throughout and decorating inside and outside	£700/0/0d

(6)	Relaying all floors	£350/0/0d
(7)	Laundry improvements and tramway to main block	£300/0/0d
(8)	New steam disinfector	£160/0/0d
(9)	Refurnishing throughout	£1,400/0/0d
(10)	New nurses wing with sitting room and dining room for head nurse and sitting room and dining room for nurses and probationers, 43 bedrooms with bathrooms and WCs as necessary	£6,500/0/0d
(11)	New out-patient dept. A one storey block situated at west corner of covered way with waiting rooms, surgery, consulting rooms, dispensary, drug store and other offices	£3,500/0/0d
(12)	Library and board room to be converted from existing out-patient and accident dept. with a new board room, library and waiting rooms; also alterations to entrance hall and basement	£1,250/0/0d
(13)	An operating theatre to be built on the north side of the covered way provided with anaesthetics room, consulting rooms, lavatory, a lift for patients, furnishing and alterations to covered way	£2,587/18/0d
(14)	An isolation cottage away from the main block to be built	£350/0/0d
	The total with 10% added for contingences	£22,530/1/0d
	Plus 5% Architects fee	£1,126/10/0d
	Plus Prize money and Assessor's fees for Competition Plus 2½% quantity allowance on £19,038/4/0d — (some projects already underway with some outlay)	£111/0/0d
	Full total	£24,243/10/0d

Items (1) and (10) of this scheme were already in the process of being carried out with monies supplied by the Diamond Jubilee Fund Committee and it had been decided that the new wing when built would be named the 'Jubilee Wing'. This is still in use today, of course, as Albert and Alice Wards. As we have seen, item (13) was taken care of by Dr. Charles Brown who undertook to finance the new operating theatre to accommodate the operating table he had already purchased three years before.

The Workpeople's Fund raised £2,098/8/10d during 1899, thus breaking the £2,000 barrier, something they had striven for since its inception in 1883 and this was achieved in spite of the fact that other collections were being made for 'war funds' throughout the year in Preston. The Infirmary's income had increased by £357/16/4½d over the previous year but expenditure had also increased by £39/18/5½d, due, it was claimed, to the increase in salaries and wages of the staff. The fact was also noted that the nursing staff had been increased and that the fully trained nurses in the private nurses home had received a salary increase, although the fees for their services had also been increased. Mrs. R. Holgate-Browne at considerable cost renovated the horse ambulance and Mrs. W. J. Hayhurst contributed to the cost of a wire mattress, an India rubber bed and a hair pillow for use inside the ambulance.

In the medical officer's report it was claimed that 'the unusually hot summer had accounted for a diminution of numbers of cases as there was a decrease in the tendency to catarrh and other kindred ailments'.

It was reported that with the death of Mr. Buckston-Browne there was no longer a spectacle fund for poor patients and another donor was urgently needed. In the latter part of the nineteenth century the children's ward was closed for renovation and electric lighting was installed for the first time.

Chapter Three

'a fitting Memorial to a Great Queen . . .' 1900-1939

AT the turn of the century, in 1900, the new operating theatre neared completion and the Diamond Jubilee Wing was almost ready for the roof. Alterations and improvements had been completed in the covered way, the children's ward and the typhoid ward and the male and female adult wards were in the process of upgrading. Contracts were let for refurbishing the wards and the administration department and the total overall cost was estimated to be £28,835/6/6d, of which only £15,893/2/7d had so far been realised, including the Diamond Jubilee Fund. Income from most sources had fallen during the year in view of the 'war fund' and Indian Famine Relief Fund, for which collections were still being made in the town. The Workpeople's Fund raised only £1,887/7/11d, which must have disappointed the Workpeople's Committee having surpassed the £2,000 barrier only the year before. Henry Davies Esq., of Preston, donated £2,000 in memory of his son, Dr. H. Davies, who died from dysentery while serving as a civil surgeon at the front in the South African War. A plaque to commemorate this gift was until recently to be seen hanging in the private wards sister's office.

Following the pattern of previous years, there were changes again in the surgical staff when the senior house surgeon, Edward Young M.R.C.S. (Eng), L.R.C.P. (Lond), resigned; his deputy Edwin W. Falconer M.B.ChB. (Victoria) became senior house surgeon, James E. Helm B.A., M.B., B.C. (Cambridge) became junior house surgeon and H. Hayword Bywater M.B., ChB. (Vict) became assistant house surgeon. Such was the rapidity of promotion that the following year the assistant house surgeon became the senior house surgeon.

In the nursing division there were changes too, when Miss Hoadley, the assistant matron, resigned in February 1900 and Miss Grace Goffin, assistant house matron at Monsall Hospital, Manchester, was appointed to the vacancy. Miss Disley, the matron, resigned in May and Miss Goffin was appointed matron in her place, rapid promotion indeed for Miss Goffin after only three months' service in the Infirmary.

The surgeons reported a large increase in the number of operations carried out during the year and they praised the new operating theatre supplied by Dr. Brown which had made so great an improvement in the surgical field, especially when operating at night. The theatre was officially opened on 12th February 1901 and proved to be one of the greatest assets the Infirmary had yet acquired. It was in constant use throughout 1901 and made it possible over the years that followed to attempt surgical procedures that up to then had been impossible.

Queen Victoria died on January 22nd 1901. When her reign had commenced in 1837 the House of Recovery was in its infancy, having moved to the Infirmary site only 5 years earlier, and during the 64 years of her reign, the Infirmary had grown in size and stature in keeping with the vast changes that had evolved nationally. At a public meeting it was suggested and unanimously agreed that the programme of alterations and improvements at that time being carried out should be dedicated as a memorial to Queen Victoria by the people of Preston. King Edward VII signified his approval of a change of name to the Preston and County of Lancaster Queen Victoria Royal Infirmary.

During practically the whole of 1901, the main wards for adult male and female patients were closed, undergoing a thorough renovation and in consequence there was a large decrease in the number of admissions. Only 798 admissions were allowed, the lowest figure since 1883. There were, however, more out-patients treated (4,665) the highest for over five years and the number of visits made to patients' homes rose to 13,556. There was no reduction in staff or other permanent establishment charges so that the cost per bed per week rose to £1/13/6½d in 1900; with such limited accommodation available, only the more serious cases were admitted and, since many of these died shortly after admission, the death rate figures were very adversely affected. The out-patients' department was described as 'draughty, badly lit and wanting in accommodation and out of keeping with the rest of the building'. It was also suggested that patients needed protection from the weather when being removed from the ambulance.

By the end of 1901 all the alterations and improvements in the wards had been completed at a cost of £32,500 and in Guild Year 1902 Lord Derby laid the foundation stone of a new out-patient department. The nurses home had been opened and the private nurses establishment in Stephenson Terrace was transferred into the new quarters. It was during this period that Dr. Brown commenced his many benefactions to the Infirmary; he donated a clock for his new operating theatre, a piano and pianola for the benefit of the patients, a billiard room for the medical staff and a bagatelle board and other games for the nurses recreation room. In 1903 he erected a conservatory for use as a smoke room and sitting room for male convalescent patients and he also supplied a magic lantern for entertaining the patients and for use occasionally for medical lectures to the staff. The following year he donated a second conservatory as a memorial to his sister. This became the smoke room for male patients and the other was used as a day room for female patients. Also in 1904, he donated a complete and up-to-date x-ray department which allowed treatment for previously hopeless cases to be carried out for the first time. These included cases of lupus, rodent ulcer and leukaemia, all of which were successfully treated in the latter part of the year.

Dr. A. Rayner was appointed honorary medical and surgical electrician in charge of the new x-ray department. Dr. J. Winkley who 22 years previously had commenced the ophthalmic and aural department in the Infirmary retired in December 1904 and died 19 months later in July 1906. Another member of the staff long associated with the Infirmary until comparatively recent times was Miss M. E. Withers who became dispenser when her predecessor Miss Holden retired in 1905.

In 1904 a full report of all the improvements and alterations carried out as a memorial to Queen Victoria was issued. The total income from various sources such as the Diamond Jubilee Fund (£7,848/4/6d) and public donations (£20,903/9/6d) amounted to £34,864/7/0d and the Infirmary was 'recognised as one of the best equipped Hospitals in the Country, outside London and a fitting Memorial to a Great Queen from the people of Preston and District'.

In 1907 the Infirmary was assessed for the first time since its inception for local rating purposes, the rateable value being fixed at £306. A deputation from the Board were successful in obtaining a reduction of this figure to £200. The finance committee of Preston Corporation was asked to donate an annual subscription to the Infirmary's funds and when they agreed to donate £52/10/0d this practically covered the amount of rates which were payable.

In his report for 1907 on the work being carried out in the x-ray and light department, Dr. Rayner emphasised the necessity for alterations and enlargements to his new department. 333 patients had been seen in the department as against 267 in 1906; 280 radiographs and screen examinations were carried out in 1907, with 210 the year before, but the number of patients actually receiving radium treatment had dropped from 57 in 1906 to only 46 in 1907. Only one x-ray apparatus was available for all purposes at the same time, which accounted for the fact that although the number of patients attending for examination had increased (287) as against those attending for treatment (46), the latter invariably had to wait for long periods of time while the day's examinations were carried out before they could be treated. It was imperative that at least one separate apparatus was available for treatment cases only as the x-ray therapy was a very slow process. Each patient required from 10-20 minutes exposure at each sitting and the number of sittings could be limitless. In 1904, for example, 22 patients had between them 520 sittings and in only 14 of these cases, was there some evidence of improvement.

The outcome of this report by Dr. Rayner was the installation of a further piece of x-ray apparatus in 1908 which allowed the radio therapeutic work of the department to be increased. The method of measurement of Keinbach, Saboraud and Benuoist was used in every case, making it as possible 'to measure both the quality and quantity of the dose of x-rays used as it is to measure medicine in a minim glass'. This resulted in increasing the exposure time from the old 10 minutes standard up to 40 minutes, so reducing the number of exposures needed. A permanent nurse was appointed to the department to learn the complicated techniques of radiography.

The Workpeople's Fund which had started in 1882 as an experiment raised £2,633/5/3d for the Infirmary in 1907. The total sum raised over the 25 years since its inception was over £50,000, indicating the interest taken by the working people of Preston and their appreciation of the value of their hospital.

Tiling of the administration block, the main entrance, the corridors and the ophthalmic ward was carried out at a cost of £657/7/0d; alterations to the ophthalmic ward (£84/12/0d) and the administration block (£560/0/0d) were also carried out during 1908. The following year a new x-ray department was in course of erection and Dr. Charles Brown continued his benevolence with the installation of three new observation wards. A new electric lift was installed at a cost of £301/5/7d.

The Board in 1909 announced the death of Dr. Moore, the senior consultant medical officer who had served the Infirmary since 1869.

The new x-ray department was opened and one of the Harris Fever Wards was converted into a medical ward with a complement of 16 beds, bringing the total bed state of the Infirmary to 138. Dr. Brown donated new beds and bedding for this 'new' ward and at the same time new cots were purchased for the children's ward with money donated by Mrs. Holgate-Browne and Miss M. M. Horrocks.

There was a complete change of medical staff during 1910 and Miss Marks was appointed assistant matron. Miss Goffin, who had been matron for 13 years, resigned to get married in 1912 and Miss Marks became matron, a position she held until the end of the Second World War. Edward Pyke, a member of the Board since 1869, died in 1911 and also William Hilton, who was a founder member of the Workpeople's Fund.

Due to the continuing increase in the Infirmary's workload, the rules of the Infirmary were revised to allow for an increase in the medical staff and subsequently a year later to the rearrangement of the medical and surgical divisions into two separate bodies for greater efficiency. On July 12th 1912 the National Insurance Act came into operation, adversely affecting the income by subscriptions, the Workpeople's Fund and private nursing. Alterations were made in the rules of admission from January 15th 1913, in that no insured patient could be treated at the hospital for any ailment that could be treated at home by a general practitioner. The old form of recommendation was scrapped and a new form issued. This change of rule did not decrease the number of cases admitted, but the nature of the cases were more serious and, in consequence, the surgical division continued to increase. In 1913 great difficulty arose in obtaining medical staff and it became apparent that higher salaries were needed to attract them. The following year, after the outbreak of World War I, the situation was critical and for two months the Infirmary had no resident doctor. So many staff, including nurses, left for war service that it became necessary to appoint two senior students to act as residents under the supervision of the honorary medical staff; two assistant anaesthetists were also appointed. This shortage of staff persisted throughout the four years of the Great War. On the outbreak of war in August 1914, a medical ward of 20 beds was placed at the disposal of the military authorities and by the end of the year 60 cases had been admitted.

In the x-ray department, both Dr. Rayner and Dr. R. Williams left for military service in 1917 and Sister France ran the department in their absence, for which she was later awarded the Royal Red Cross. Major Rayner received the O.B.E. for his war service and Miss Charlesworth, the assistant matron, was mentioned in despatches on her return to duty in 1919 after 5 years' service army nursing overseas. The x-ray department, it was reported, proved invaluable in the location of bullets, shrapnel etc.

A pathology department was opened for the first time in 1914 and Dr. J. B. Tindall was appointed pathologist; unfortunately, Dr. Tindall died in 1917 and the pathology department remained without a pathologist until Guild year 1922, when Dr. K. M. Duncan M.B., F.R.C.S (Eng) became honorary pathologist.

In September 1913 the Infirmary had been inspected by Sir Henry C. Burdett K.C.B., K.C.V.O., an eminent hospital authority and subsequently he published an excellent, glowing report in the publication *The Hospital* dated October 3rd 1914 which is well worth reading as it gives an excellent description of the Infirmary of seventy five years ago, reflecting credit on the staff of that time.

In 1918 a massage department was commenced and two V.D. clinics were opened, so many patients attending the latter that two medical officers were needed for each clinic instead of one. Lostock Hall, with its 6½ acres of grounds, was given to the Infirmary by Messrs. Geo. & R. Dewhurst Ltd., for use as a convalescent hospital. Mr. Walter Davies, secretary for 21 years, resigned and Mr. John Gibson became secretary with an office at the Infirmary, instituting the office of secretary as a full time post for the first time. Lord Ashton of Rylands, Lancaster, donated a gift of £2,000 to help balance a deficiency in the Infirmary's accounts. The income for the year 1918 topped £10,000 but escalating costs due to the war meant that the expenditure also exceeded £10,000 for the first time.

The following year, 1919, was the Infirmary's jubilee year, fifty years of service to the community of Preston and district, during which time 58,800 in-patients had been treated and 246,100 out-patients seen. It had grown from a cottage with 24 beds into a general hospital of 144 beds with specialists in ear, nose and throat, x-ray, massage, electrical and skin, pathology etc. Its equipment and administration were renowned and yet even further enlargement was envisaged.

Dr. W. H. Pimblett was promoted from assistant to full physician with charge of medical out-patients. Dr. T. H. C . Derham was appointed medical officer in charge of the massage department and Dr. A. Toulmin became assistant surgeon with charge of surgical out-patients in collaboration with Dr. R. Williams and Dr. Cedric Pimblett became assistant anaesthetist and home visitor.

King George V conferred a knighthood on Dr. Charles Brown in 1919, an honour thoroughly deserved by one who had contributed so much to the success of the health care of Preston since 1869.

Income during the Infirmary's jubilee year soared to nearly £15,000 but expenditure kept pace. Lord Ashton made a further donation of £5,000 towards the cost of building an additional male ward of 20 beds and it was proposed to erect a new massage department, a unit for genito-urinary diseases and also to re-equip the laundry with new washing machines and hydro-extractors.

The hours of duty for probationer nurses were reduced from 70 to 60 hours per week which entailed additional nursing staff and in consequence extensions to the nurses home; at the same time the salaries of nurses were increased, which must have left them feeling that 'they had never had it so good'.

By 1920 waiting lists for admission had appeared for the first time and the building of a new ward of a 'semi-permanent character only' was commenced for the admission and treatment of ex-servicemen being discharged from a V.A.D. hospital in Moor Park. This ward was still in use until quite recent times as East Ward. A further reduction in nurses duty hours was envisaged from 60 to 56 hours, but this was postponed until further extensions could be made to the nurses home. The Infirmary's income in 1920 reached over £20,000, the Workpeople's Fund donating almost £4,000 and the Alexander Rose Day collections, inaugurated in the summer of 1919, raising £944/13/10d. The cost per week for each in-patient had risen to £6/14/4d.

All the proposed extensions and alterations were progressing, but a new extension to the nurses home to include lecture facilities was needed urgently. Alterations to the boiler house, the installation of fuel economisers and the provision of more beds for male patients were also proposed when finances allowed. East Ward was officially opened in July 1921 with 17 beds and during the year all the Infirmary's departments increased their workloads so that waiting lists for admissions continued to increase. Lostock Hall was formally opened in June by Lt. Commander H. Dewhurst M.P., with 43 beds for women and children and this had some effect in relieving the pressure on the Infirmary and reducing the waiting lists but the situation regarding male surgical wards was far from satisfactory; another ward for these cases was an urgent necessity but a financial non-starter.

The Workpeople's Fund in 1921 increased its donation to over £6,000 and the Infirmary's total income realised £28,000 but, as in previous years, expenditure outpaced income and in 1921 topped £30,000. A verandah was built on the south side of the women's surgical ward and a new telephone system installed and the large front lawn was drained. The new electro-massage department was almost completed and Sir Charles Brown donated £500 towards the cost of alterations and furnishings at Lostock Hall and he also gave £2,000 for the erection of a treatment centre for V.D. cases.

A decision was made to convert the female medical ward into a maternity department with 12 beds and this was accomplished the following year, 1922, Preston's Guild year. Its object was to provide accommodation for expectant mothers who were either homeless or had only unsuitable surroundings or for abnormal cases. There were 10 maternity beds, a delivery room and an ante-natal clinic attached to the out-patient department. 51 cases were admitted during its first year, 1922, and 50 babies were born.

The nurses training school issued examination results for the first time and six nurses successfully passing were awarded certificates and badges.

During Guild year, 1922, more patients were treated and more operations performed than ever before in the Infirmary's history. This was due mainly to the vast increase in the number of accident and emergency cases admitted. Most of the accident cases were caused, it was claimed, by the increase in motor traffic appearing on the roads of Preston. At this time up to 150 cases a week were being admitted which the wards could not properly accommodate and the need for further accommodation became acute. Waiting lists had doubled in number although women and children were transferred to Lostock Hall as soon as they were considered fit to do so and without this facility the situation would have been hopeless. All the Infirmary's departments were increasing by over 10% a year and it became imperative to increase the accommodation available so that in 1923 plans were prepared for a new block of 72 beds in three wards with the addition of smaller wards of two beds for patients who desired private ward treatment at actual cost.

This plan was formulated by 1925 when Princess Mary opened the new nurses home and laid the foundation stone of the new patients block. In September 1922, the Guild Mayor, Henry Astley Bell J.P., laid the foundation stone for an extension to the nurses home which was to provide a further 30 bed or sitting rooms, a dining room, lecture, reading and recreation rooms.

The following year, extensions were completed to the ear, nose and throat department adding 10 more beds and the operating theatre was enlarged and improved by the addition of the latest equipment available. The x-ray department was also entirely re-equipped and the number of staff increased but in spite of all this it was reported that there was a need for another operating theatre, an increase of 30-40 staff, a new pathology department and extensions to the kitchens.

The Infirmary was approved by the General Nursing Council as a training school for nurses in Guild year, 1922, and the training curriculum had to be revised to meet the requirements of the Council's syllabus. Eleven nurses succcessfully passed their final examination and gained their certificates and badges. During 1923 the Central Midwives Board was approached to seek approval for the Infirmary as a training school for midwives and this also was granted one year later in 1924. The maternity department was increased to 17 beds and during 1923 admitted 258 cases; 215 babies were delivered, but 43 were still or prematurely born.

Dr. F. W. Collinson resigned from the honorary surgical staff on 30th April 1923, but he became a vice-president of the Infirmary and remained a member of the honorary consultant staff.

The Workpeople's Fund, supplemented by a free maintenance scheme of weekly contributions, raised £16,755/10/1d during 1924. This scheme, which had been inaugurated during 1921, guaranteed free treatment when hospital treatment was necessary to any weekly wage earner and his dependents who contributed to the scheme. Any worker over 19 years of age regularly contributed 2d a week, those under 19 years 1d a week but any patient not covered by the scheme was asked for a contribution to the Infirmary's funds according to their means. The scheme covered either out-patient or in-patient treatment or admission to the wards for the contributing members and his family and proved very successful as far as employees in mills, workshops and business establishments were concerned but people working in shops, offices, business houses and smaller workshops were not as willing to join the scheme and it was many years before the aim of the scheme to include all workpeople in Preston and district was realised. An indication of the success of the scheme can be seen in the donations actually raised during this period:

1920	£3,810/2/8d
1921	£6,260/19/10d
1923	£11,227/17/6d
1924	£16,755/10/1d
1926	£20,000 +

In 1924, an agreement was reached with the Ministry of Health and Preston Corporation for the treatment of V.D. New buildings were added to the out-patients department for the treatment of gonorrhoea and when these opened attendances increased fourfold. The resident medical and surgical staff were increased from 3 to 4, *viz.* resident surgical officer, house physician, senior house surgeon and junior house surgeon.

In the Infirmary training school for nurses all the nurses who sat their final examinations passed the oral, written and practical tests, reaching a very high standard with an average mark of 82½%. Four nurses successfully entered the first state examination of the G.N.C. in 1924. In England and Wales 107 nurses sat their preliminary examinations; 10 nurses from the Preston school passed this exam and later the same year successfully passed their final examinations, a very good record indeed for the Infirmary's school. The chairman of the Board, Mr. Alex Foster J.P., and his daughter Miss Hilda M. Foster respectively donated funds for the provision of gold and silver medals to be awarded to the most efficient nurses completing 3 years training.

Miss Rossiter was appointed assistant matron and tutor. The nursing staff of 1924 consisted of matron, assistant matron (who acted as sister tutor), a housekeeping sister, 5 ward sisters, 1 theatre sister, 2 x-ray sisters, 2 masseurs, 6 staff nurses (4th year training), 40 probationer nurses and 10 fully trained nurses for private nursing.

Tenders were invited for a new patients wing, a new pathology laboratory, additional consulting rooms and the lengthening of the children's corridor to link up the four wards on the north side of the Infirmary, namely medical, orthopaedic, ophthalmic and East Ward, the first three mentioned being, of course, the original Harris Fever Wards opened in 1875. The nurses home annexe, the V.D. department, a hard tennis court and a verandah for the children's ward were all completed in 1924 and extensions to the kitchens with a stairway to connect the maids home were also in hand. A semi-permanent ward was opened to relieve the pressure of surgical waiting lists until the new patients wing was completed. This was West Ward which contained 22 beds for female surgical patients and which today 60 years later is still fulfilling its semi-permanent function, although no longer for patients.

The pressure of work continued to grow throughout the 1920s, with a never ending call on the Infirmary's facilities and the administration was constantly trying to keep pace with the annual increase in numbers of patients. In view of the trade situation in Preston and the country generally, culminating in the General Strike of 1926, it was a credit to the Infirmary's Board that they attempted the ambitious schemes that were in hand at that time. The finances for the proposed extensions which included, of course, increases in staff and other expenditure, had to be found by public subscription as in the past but in Preston at that time there was wide unemployment. Despite this, however, the Workpeople's Fund in 1926 raised over £20,000 and a whist drive organised by the Workpeople's Fund committee in the Majestic Rooms, attended by over 1,200 people, raised £61/6/5d. This money was used for the provision of headphones and other comforts for patients and this event became a permanent means of raising money for this purpose, with increasing success. This surely must have been the forerunner of today's Hospital Welfare Society which continues to this day to supply amenities for the Preston hospitals.

Sir Charles Brown died in November 1926; he had been associated with the Infirmary since its inception in 1869, being the honorary medical officer until 1886 when he became an honorary consultant. During his years at Preston Royal Infirmary he had given gifts and benefits to the Infirmary at a cost of more than £40,000 and on his death the executors of his will donated the residue of his estate to be endowed for Lostock Hall Continuation Hospital, amounting to the sum of £26,000. In the same month, November 1926, the new light department was opened by Professor Leonard Hill, the operating theatre was very near completion and the new patients wing, increased to 80 beds, had its roof on and neared completion.

Two houses, numbers 88 and 90 Stephenson Terrace, were purchased for the use of night nursing staff to alleviate overcrowding in the nurses home. The pathology laboratory with their microscopes and incubators had been kept busy during 1926 having made almost 4,000 examinations throughout the year. This statement will, no doubt raise a chuckle among my erstwhile colleagues but I hasten to add that the laboratory staff at that time consisted of two technicians and they did not have the sophisticated apparatus of today at their disposal.

The increase in workload throughout the Infirmary's departments can perhaps be illustrated by the rise in numbers of patients over the years, from 7,010 in 1914 to over 21,000 patients treated in 1926. The following year, 1927, there was no respite with over 4,000 in-patients and 17,867 out-patients, or an average of 555 a day, and 5,051 operations were performed. The laboratory also increased its quota by a further 610 tests over the 1926 figure, the new premises for the laboratory were opened and the work was re-organised to accommodate specimens from the local authorities and general practitioners.

Mr. W. H. Graham was appointed to the resident medical staff in 1927 and W. W. Galloway Esq. J.P. of Bilsborough Hall presented the 'Willows' in Ashton as a convalescent hospital for male patients, with a donation of £2,000 toward the cost of conversion.

In spite of the continued depression in the staple cotton and engineering industries of the town, the Workpeople's Fund continued to grow and in 1927 £22,000 was raised, with £23,108 the following year. The Fund covered 920 firms in Preston and district and their whist drive at the Majestic Rooms raised £61/15/11d, with over 1,400 people attending. Sixty pairs of headphones were purchased for the Infirmary and a wireless set for the Willows Continuation Hospital, which was opened on 11th October 1928 with 25 male beds. Electric wiring throughout the Infirmary was replaced into steel conduit from the wooden casing they were originally placed into and a new boiler was installed in a temporary position awaiting the erection of the new boiler house. It was in 1927 that a new private automatic telephone system linking all the wards, departments and services was installed. The new patients wing was now almost completed and by the end of 1928 the childrens ward was in use. The male and female wards (Green and Brown) were expected to be ready early in 1929 and then it was presumed the days of waiting lists would have disappeared for ever. When the new wing was offically opened by H.R.H. Princess Mary in August of 1929 it did alleviate the strain on accommodation and for a time the waiting lists were reduced, but so many people were attending out-patient clinics that long waits to be attended to were inevitable.

In 1929 the trustees of the estate of the late Alderman Thomas Parkinson gave the Infirmary £10,000. This was the cost of the new childrens ward, which was dedicated to his memory. The Workpeople's Fund continued to grow with employees of 939 establishments participating in the scheme but a further appeal was issued in 1929 to all 'black coated' workers and farm labourers to join the ranks. By 1931 the number of work places involved had risen to 1,125 and there were also 1,044 individual contributors.

Dr. F. B. Smith was appointed pathologist in 1930. He remained in charge of the laboratoryuntil his retirement in 1948.

In 1931 a propaganda film on the Infirmary was produced and shown in the Preston cinemas. This gave the public an insight into the Infirmary and its departments with a view to generating interest, both financial and ethnic. This film still exists today and was recently transferred to safety film from the highly flammable cellulose film originally used; it is immensely interesting to compare the Infirmary of fifty years ago with todays counterpart.

The need for a new maternity department was raised in 1931, the existing facilities being totally inadequate and it was claimed that a new department would release beds for a male medical ward. Extensions were also needed to the nurses home and in consequence of the extra workload generated from local authorities and G.P.s, the new laboratory needed to be enlarged. New equipment was needed by the x-ray department so an appeal was made by the Workpeople's Committee to the social clubs of Preston and within a very short period of time £800 of the £1,600 needed had been raised. By 1932 the pathology laboratory had been extended and further extensions had been made both to the x-ray and out-patients departments.

In the early 1930s trade continued to decline and unemployment to rise, with cotton mills and other factories in Preston closing down, the consequence of which was a decline in the source of income from the Workpeople's Fund. Thirty cotton mills which had donated some £3,250 per annum five years before had closed completely in 1933; nevertheless a radium department was commenced in that year, followed in 1934 by the laying of a foundation stone for a new maternity hospital. The nurses home was extended further and building commenced for a new orthopaedic department.

Despite the general depression in trade, all records were broken in 1935 by the Workpeople's Fund, when £26,009/8/11d was raised, allowing a mobile x-ray machine to be purchased for use on the wards, a boon to staff and patients alike and emergency lighting was installed in the operating theatres.

A lady house surgeon was appointed for the resident care of maternity and ophthalmic cases, a rather odd combination of specialities, the significance being that she was the first lady doctor to be appointed to Preston Royal Infirmary.

King George V, the Infirmary's patron, died in 1935. He held Preston Royal in some esteem as he had sent a yearly gift of grapes and sometimes venison for members of the staff. H.M. King George VI conferred the Royal patronage upon the Infirmary, which meant that every sovereign since its foundation in 1869, sixty seven years before, had so honoured the Infirmary and its staff. Miss Marks, the matron, reached her jubilee year in 1935, having been appointed assistant matron in 1910 and matron in 1912.

The new maternity hospital was opened on 4th September 1936 by the Countess of Derby, accompanied by her husband, the R.H. Earl of Derby K.G., the Infirmary's president. A large gathering of subscribers and donors attended the opening ceremony and a very enjoyable and memorable afternoon was held. The new hospital contained an antenatal department, wards containing 43 beds, labour rooms, nurseries, an operating theatre and staff accommodation. It was visited before the official opening by many thousands of people who expressed satisfaction generally with the beauty of the building and the excellence of the equipment and facilities. It was one of the most up to date maternity hospitals in the United Kingdom when the first patients were admitted on 1st October 1936, the only flaw in such an accomplishment being the fact that £5,000 was still needed to meet the cost of the new building. Negotiations with Preston Corporation and Lancashire County Council resulted in those two authorities agreeing to give financial assistance towards the appointment of a consultant obstetrician whose duties would include the setting up of antenatal clinics for all expectant mothers in the two authorities.

Mr. Alex Foster J.P., first elected a member of the Board of Management in 1907, vice-chairman in 1918 and chairman in 1923, was obliged through ill health to relinquish his office and he was succeeded as chairman by Mr. W. F. Ascroft M.A., D.L., J.P., in May 1936.

The aggregate number of patients treated throughout 1936 was 38,286, the daily average being 970; 322 in-patients and 648 out-patients; the average stay of each patient in the Infirmary was 16.4 days while the average stay at Lostock Hall Continuation Hospital was 18 days and at the Willows, 15.8 days.

The Nurses Training School continued to flourish and from 100 applicants for training 27 candidates were selected. Nineteen nurses entered the final state examinations of the G.N.C., with fifteen of them passing. In the preliminary state examinations, 34 nurses entered with 28 passes and fourteen pupil midwives obtained the diploma of the Central Midwives Board. The annual distribution of the medals and prizes for nurses was included in the opening ceremony of the new maternity hospital with the Countess of Derby presenting the awards.

Mr. W. W. Galloway J.P., who joined the Board in 1900, and who had given many generous gifts to the Infirmary, including the Willows Continuation Hospital, died in 1936.

The old maternity ward was renovated and enlarged at a cost of £5,000 and became the female medical ward with 42 beds. The male medical ward, which occupied East Ward at that time moved into the old female medical ward with 24 beds. Another move was the segregation of fracture and orthopaedic cases from purely surgical cases to meet the requirements of the orthopaedic surgeons appointed two years previously (B. J. McFarland M.D. and E. Bell Jones F.R.C.S.; thus the old East Ward became the orthopaedic ward.

A portable electric cardiograph was purchased for use in the wards and the out-patients department; also purchased were a shortwave diathermy, new electric tables for the electro-massage department, new Hanovia lamps for the light department and a new piece of apparatus for the administration of anaesthetics in the operating theatres. Further microscopes and milk testing equipment for the laboratory were supplied in response to the large increase of work generated by public health authorities. Over 18,000 examinations were carried out in the pathology department during 1936.

The annual ball and whist drive held in the Public Hall in Preston on 24th October 1936 raised £50 for the Benevolent Fund for patients amenities. A second ball arranged later in the year coincided with an influenza epidemic and raised only £2/4/2d.

In 1937 there were the first signs of enhanced income from the Workpeople's Fund due in part to the increase of contributions from 2d to 3d a week and also an improvement in trade throughout Preston and surrounding districts. Many firms, including some of the larger ones, such as Leyland Motors, increased their subscriptions as soon as the committee recommended they should do so but there were still, however, pockets of resistance to change. The Fund's contribution rose dramatically, from £30,077/7/10d in 1937, £35,988/18/0d in 1938, £42,902/1/5d in 1939 and £43,245/12/10d in 1940. During 1938 the scheme was expanded with many other similar schemes throughout the country whereby any member could receive treatment for himself or his dependents even outside the Infirmary's area. An 'iron lung' was added to the Infirmary's equipment in 1938 through the generosity of Lord Nuffield and two new departments became established, a heart clinic and dermatological (skin) department.

Largely due to the allocation by the Trustees of the late W. W. Galloway of £30,000, the Board established a Special Extensions Fund for the erection of orthopaedic and ophthalmic wards and extensions to the nurses home, the kitchen and the administration offices. Other additions during the same year included a new garage and ambulance, a new corridor to medical wards and new deep x-ray therapy apparatus.

This was a period of great anxiety, with the possibility of war in the air and precautions already being taken to meet as far as possible any emergencies that might arise through enemy action. It was the time now called the 'September crisis', which culminated in Prime Minister Chamberlain's meeting with Adolph Hitler, which event managed to defer the advent of war for twelve months. The Infirmary was designated by the Ministry of Health an A1 Hospital for the treatment of civilian casualties arising from aeriel bombardment and arrangements were made for the evacuation of patients, supplying extra beds, the stockpiling of stores and the formation of mobile units ready for despatch to any district where they may be needed. Air raid shelters for the use of patients and staff were set aside and remnants of these were still to be seen until recent times in the basement corridor connecting the Infirmary buildings to the maternity hospital.

A voluntary hospital scheme was recommended by Lord Sankey, in which all voluntary hospitals would group themselves into regional areas, so co-ordinating their services on an area basis. The Infirmary, being the largest hospital in the north and east Lancashire/Westmoreland group, was expected to play a leading part in the administration of the region.

The chairman of the Board of Management became Sir William Ascroft M.A., D.L., J.P. in the New Year's Honours List.

Chapter Four

Growing regional importance 1939-1948

MANY of the ambitious schemes laid down by the Board in 1938/39 had to be abandoned with the outbreak of World War II in September 1939. These included a private patients wing, a neurological clinic, a neurosurgical centre and a new x-ray department. The nurses home did get extended before the war began but the proposals for orthopaedic and ophthalmic wards were shelved until the end of the war; and as events turned out, they were never realised.

The Workpeople's Fund became a member of the British Hospitals Contributory Schemes Association in 1939 and the committee released all members of H.M. Forces from further payment of contribution if their war pay and allowances amounted to less than their civilian pay while their dependents remained within the benefits of the scheme. My own pay as a soldier in September 1939 was 2/ – (10p) a day, which was considerably less than my civil pay; therefore, the release from contributions would have applied to most members of the scheme who joined the Armed Forces. The annual ball was not held in 1939 due to a ban by the government of the day on all night functions.

Blast walls were erected around the wards and operating theatres and all windows were protected with tape to minimise the effect of shattering glass during air raids and several practices were arranged and carried out with the first aid and ambulance services during 1940. Although the air raid sirens were sounded constantly during the autumn and winter nights in Preston there were no casualties from air raids. Nevertheless, each night and all day on Sundays teams of volunteer workers, both men and women, were standing by in the Infirmary ready to assist the staff if the need arose. This was the period known as the 'phoney war' when nothing of a warlike nature seemed to be happening anywhere.

In July 1939, the pathology laboratory commenced building up a roll of blood donors for emergency blood supplies. 1,100 donors were enrolled by the end of 1939 and this had increased to 3,000 donors by the end of 1940, most of the blood taken being processed as plasma. Quantities of this were issued to areas such as Liverpool and Manchester where casualties from air raids had increased the demand for plasma above the locally available supply. In October 1940 the Emergency Medical Services of the Ministry of Health organised a transfusion service on a regional basis and in the north-west the existing local efforts of Preston Royal Infirmary became an outstanding factor in the success of the scheme in the region with the Preston Laboratory acting as the blood transfusion centre for central Lancashire.

The staff shortages which had been experienced during the First World War was again evident early in the Second World War. Dr. F. B. Smith, the consultant pathologist, returned to the laboratory after 'inactive service' overseas in October 1940 but many of the permanent members of staff were still absent; Mr. H. S. D'Arcy, a nursing orderly, was killed in action with the Royal Navy and other members on active service included:

Major Wm. Simpson R.A.M.C. consultant obstetrical surgeon
Major R. B. Guyer R.A.M.C. assistant radiologist
Miss W. Hall Q.A.I.M.N.S.
Miss E. Hall, Princess Mary R.A.F. nursing service
Miss F. Radcliffe Q.A.I.M.N.S.
Miss M. Hind, territorial nursing service
Miss R. Welsby, territorial nursing service
Miss N. Houghton, overseas nursing service
Mr. S. Grimshaw, R.C. Signals, administration department
Mr. T. Flevill R.A.M.C., nursing orderly
Mr. W. Walsh R.A.F., nursing orderly
Mr. J. Birkett, South Wales Borderers, barber & porter
Mr. J. Roebuck R.A.M.C., porter
Mr. A. Southworth East Lancs Regt., painter
Mr. B. Moore, Pioneer Corps, painter

Lord Nuffield gave £1,250,000 to set up a trust, the object being to assist the voluntary hospitals in their efforts to implement the recommendations for an improved hospital service made by Lord Sankey's Commission. With the formation of the Regional Hospital Services in co-operation with local authorities, the seeds of the National Health Service were planted, finally to come to fruition in 1948.

In spite of the war, the general work of the Infirmary progressed unabated, 6,879 in-patients being admitted in 1940, while the out-patient department received 35,554 patients requiring treatment. The total number of out-patient attendances in all the Infirmary's departments during 1940 was 216,976 and this figure rose to 237,013 during 1941 and 255,326 in 1942.

In 1941 Mr. W. Allison Davies C.B.E., J.P. was appointed vice-chairman of the Board and Mr. R. T. Easterby J.P. became joint honorary treasurer. Mr. R. Cunliffe Shaw M.Sc. F.R.C.S. was appointed full surgeon and Mr. G. M. Arnott F.R.C.S.E., assistant surgeon, both appointments being temporary for the duration of the war and one year afterwards. The matron, Miss M. A. Marks, founder of the Preston Royal Infirmary League of Nurses in 1929, was recognised in the Birthday Honours List with the M.B.E., Mr. K. M. Duncan

F.R.C.S. who had served the Infirmary as a member of the visiting surgical staff for 30 years and as senior surgeon for 20 years, died early in 1942. He was held in great esteem by the people of Preston not only for his surgical skill but also for the kindness and understanding which endeared him to his patients.

Dr. R. P. A. Rigg joined the Royal Army Medical Corps serving as a medical consultant and Dr. W. M. Simpson R.A.M.C., the Infirmary's consultant obstetrical surgeon was promoted to assistant director of medical services (A.D.M.S.) for the Caribbean area which carried the rank of Lieutenant Colonel. Mr. J. Eastwood Sykes F.R.C.S. was appointed medical officer to the V.D. treatment centre and Mr. J. E. Delory M.Sc. (London) left the Post Graduate Medical School in London to become the Infirmary's first biochemist in 1942. Mr. Arthur Toulmin F.R.C.S.E., the senior surgeon, resigned at the end of 1943, having served the Infirmary for 29 years as surgeon, assistant surgeon, anaesthetist and resident medical officer; he became a vice-president of the Board in his retirement and also an honorary consultant surgeon. Mr. J. M. Arnott F.R.C.S.E., the assistant surgeon, was promoted to surgeon and with the resignation of the visiting orthopaedic surgeon, Mr. B. L. McFarland M.D., M.Orth. (Liverpool) F.R.C.S.E., Mr. Arnott agreed to perform this appointment also on a temporary basis.

The aggregate number of out-patients in 1943 again reached over 250,000 and a new orthoptic department for the treatment of squint in children was opened on 1st January 1944. The fourth year of the war produced a record of progress when the Board took the decision to establish a rehabilitation centre to facilitate the recovery and return to employment of injured patients. A building licence was obtained, which was no mean feat in wartime when all projects requiring materials needed for the war effort were strictly vetted, and the erection of the new building was commenced.

In February 1944 the then Minister of Health issued a White Paper containing suggestions for a proposed National Health Service. This proposal to establish a free hospital service by means of payment from the proceeds of proposed security insurance and from local rates, was not welcomed by the Infirmary's Board of Management or by the representatives of the Workpeople's Fund. They foresaw a lowering of the standard of treatment and attention which patients would receive in state-run hospitals and their only consolation was the fact that discussions were to take place between the Minister and representatives of the British Hospitals Association and the British Hospitals Contributory Schemes Association in the early stages and they hoped to modify the government's plans to include their own continuance. The Board of Management were not anxious regarding the future of the Infirmary which they felt would be an essential part of any improved health and hospital service.

In consequence of these proposals looming, a Hospital Service Planning Committee was formed for Lancashire consisting of representatives of local authorities, universities and the voluntary hospitals and one of their first objects was to request that the Ministry of Health make a factual survey of the hospital services of the County. The Ministry agreed to this but insisted that the area be extended to include north Wales, Cheshire, Westmorland and Cumberland. Two surveying officers were appointed by the Ministry and eventually similar surveys were arranged throughout the United Kingdom to obtain a complete survey on all hospital services.

After D-day, in June 1944, war casualties were admitted in large numbers, with 150 beds being requisitioned for this purpose. Albert and Alice Wards were used mainly for military casualties but on occasion they spilled over into other wards. During this period there was a constant intake of wounded who arrived, usually at night at Preston station in Red Cross trains, to be ferried to the Infirmary in converted single deck buses or small ambulances, nursed the whole time in transit by Infirmary nurses. The walking wounded were sent to other hospitals in the area. The number of requisitioned beds was reduced to 100 on January 1st 1945 as the number of casualties from the war in Europe lessened but military casualties, and indeed wounded prisoners-of-war, who were placed in Alice Ward under armed guard, were still evident in the Infirmary until the end of war.

When Germany surrendered on 7th May 1945, followed by Japan on 10th August, the former event was celebrated by a service in the Infirmary chapel, a special tea arranged for the patients and a dance organised for the staff. All the irritating reminders of the war years were quickly discarded, the covered windows and sandbagged walls and, of course, the blackout. Redecoration of the wards was commenced and as there were still 50 beds being held for the military authorities efforts were made to have them released as soon as possible. Throughout the war years the Infirmary had treated some 6,749 members of the forces, including 1,149 wounded from the battlefields overseas.

The rehabilitation centre was completed and opened on 9th March 1946 by the R.H. George Tomlinson M.P., Minister for Works, and was described as 'one of the finest Departments of its kind in the Country'. The orthoptic department opened in the board room in 1944, moved into its new premises in No. 26 Stanleyfield Road and two more houses in Stanleyfield Road were purchased, opposite the out-patient entrance, numbers 25 & 28, with a view to possible further extensions to the Infirmary. Another purchase in 1945 was a large dwelling house known as the Preston Nursing Home which was situated in Garstang Road (numbers 1 & 2 Alfred Terrace); this was converted into a hostel for nursing trainees, so making room for additional nurses in the Infirmary's quarters. Some reorganisation of the administration department was made and a catering officer appointed, Mr. H. Gillet and with the appointment of a supplies officer, the Infirmary Stores and Supplies Department were also reorganised.

Lt. Col. William Simpson R.A.M.C., the obstetric surgeon, died while serving in the Caribbean and Dr. J. H. Taylor who had served the Infirmary as honorary ophthalmic surgeon for 21 years, also died in 1945. Dr. A. E. Rayner O.B.E., who had been a member of the Infirmary staff for 41 years during which time he had organised the expansion of the x-ray department, resigned his position as radiologist and was appointed the first honorary consultant radiologist to the Infirmary, a post he held until his death in 1963. Other members of the staff retiring soon after the war included Dr. W. Sykes (ophthalmic and aural surgeon), Mr. W. A. H. McKerrow, surgeon, and Mr. T. H. C. Derham, the medical officer to the physiotherapy department for 21 years. Dr. R. P. A. Rigg returned from war service to take up his post as visiting physican. My own association with Preston Royal Infirmary began in this period when on 11th April 1946, having just returned from overseas service, I joined the laboratory staff, serving with Dr. F. B. Smith and Dr. R. T. Cooke.

Dr. A. H. Issacson the resident medical officer, was accepted for membership of the Royal College of Physicians. Older members of the Infirmary staff would agree that Dr. Issacson, a fine cricketer who reputedly had played for the Gentlemen of Ireland team, was the mainstay of a fine cricket team that the Infirmary boasted in the years following the end of the war. The team included other stalwarts such as Mr. Richardson from the administration office, a rather young Norman Sutcliffe, Ted Wareing, a fine wicket keeper from the boiler house and a very much younger 'yours truly', with other members of the laboratory staff.

In view of the impending retirement of so many of the specialist staff during 1945 consideration was given by the Board to a scheme for upgrading the specialities by appointing a consultant physician, an obstetrician/gynaecologist, an assistant obstetrician/gynaecologist, an orthopaedic surgeon, a urologist and a paediatrician and they also separated the specialities of ophthalmic and aural into distinct departments. With the co-operation of Preston Corporation, the Board arranged to share the services of an ear, nose and throat surgeon.

Miss M. A. Marks M.B.E., the Infirmary's matron for 34 years and founder of the Preston Royal Infirmary League of Nurses in 1929, retired on 31st December 1944 and at the same time Miss S. F. Rossiter, the assistant matron also decided to retire, having served in the Infirmary for 20 years. Miss N. Livesey became the new matron and Miss M. Cheese, assistant matron. Miss Livesey was formerly matron of the Royal Victoria and West Hants Hospital, Bournemouth, and with her appointment it was decided that all three hospitals (Preston Royal Infirmary, Lostock Hall and the Willows) would be amalgamated under her direct administration. Miss Ogleby was appointed senior sister tutor and later became principal tutor, the post she held until her retirement in July 1969. Toward the end of 1945, both Miss A. M. Ronson, matron of Lostock Hall and Miss E. B. Rice, matron of the Willows became seriously ill. Miss Ronson resigned and was succeeded by Miss Marian Eyre who was appointed assistant matron under Miss Livesey; Miss Rice unfortunately died and was succeeded by Miss Rudd.

The Workpeople's Fund continued to flourish and in 1945 raised almost £58,000 but with the National Health Bill becoming more imminent the future of the Fund was in doubt. There was considerable feeling among the contributory scheme workers that the organisation which had carried out such excellent work and engendered so much interest for so many years should be retained to represent and act as the mouthpiece of the workers in all matters affecting the future administration of the health and hospital service. The Minister of Health, during his discussions with the representatives of the hospital contributory schemes, had expressed the view that 'ways may be found to continue the Scheme in order to cover additional benefits and assistance to the Voluntary Hospitals which may not receive the full cost of treatment rendered by them under the Government Scheme'.

The report of the surveyors appointed by the Ministry of Health to consider the hospital requirements of the north-west region was published during 1945. One of the recommendations of the report was that Preston should be developed as a 'sub-metropolitan consultative centre' and that the Infirmary should occupy a central part in such a development. The National Health Bill at this time was before parliament and it provided that the Ministry of Health would take over all hospitals in the country, both voluntary and local authority (i.e. Sharoe Green Hospital) as well as the invested funds of the voluntary hospitals, excluding the teaching hospitals, and administer them as part of a National Health Service through regional boards and local management committees. This new National Health Service began to operate in its new format from July 5th 1948.

It was a matter for regret that the war had prevented the Infirmary's administration from proceeding with much needed extensions and improvements for which financial provision had been accumulated over the years. These included the provision of another medical ward, an ear, nose and throat ward, a new orthopaedic department and the nurses home. The provision of a private patients wing was also considered at that time an absolute necessity. There was sufficient money available for a brand new purpose-built general hospital prior to the handing over of resources at the commencement of the N.H.S. and the land for such a venture was available adjacent to the Infirmary, extending from Stanleyfield Road to North Road.

At a meeting of the Hospital Management Committee early in 1947 the chairman, Sir Wm. Ascroft emphasised the necessity to secure, if possible, the much needed extensions which the war had prevented the Board from proceeding with. It was hoped that the government would allow these extensions even in the short time available before the implementation of the National Health Bill which was at that time before Parliament. The Board consulted an eminent firm of hospital architects, Adams, Holden and Pearson of the University of London, who were asked to survey the Infirmary's buildings in conjunction with Mr. Alfred Lillie, the Infirmary's architect, the object being to prepare a report and master plan for the future development of the Infirmary which the Board would then submit to the Manchester Regional Hospital Board.

The final report, issued in January 1948, following several visits to Preston by the architects throughout 1947, makes very interesting reading; it emphasised the restricted nature of the Infirmary's site and stated:

> the aim must be to build at least one new Hospital on a suitable site. The Royal Infirmary site, though larger and better than those of most of the Voluntary Hospitals would not, even if cleared, be nearly large enough for a Hospital such as this District is likely to require. The Municipal Hospital at Sharoe Green being quite unsuitable as the nucleus for a first class Hospital.

The report went on to express the need for the expansion of the present out-patient department at the Infirmary stating:

> the present site is well situated for the convenience of patients and staff and such a central position has so many advantages that it would not be advisable (even if it were possible) to entirely remove the Hospital from its present site.

The survey suggested some rebuilding of the existing Royal Infirmary building by adding a further storey to and remodelling the existing Albert Ward block and adding a complete new surgical block to the north of Albert Ward. Among other recommendations of the report were enlargement of the boiler house, the laundry and the mortuary and the provision of an animal house; the erection of a new out-patient clinic with a complete new entrance following the removal of the medical and ophthalmic wards and East and West Wards; the existing out-patient department would become a casualty department with a department of pathology, a public health laboratory and other departments on the floor above. The old Harris Fever Ward being used as a medical ward was to be adapted to become a new light department and there was also a recommendation to lengthen the existing rehabilitation department, opened in 1946, to include a physiotherapy department. Another recommendation was 'to add another storey to the existing Maternity Home. This building is of recent erection and is in every way up-to-date so that there is every reason for retaining it on the Infirmary site'.

The most interesting recommendation was a suggested upgrading of the Infirmary's convalescent home at the Willows in Ashton by the erection of 4 ward blocks of two storey height, each block containing 50 beds (units of 25 beds on each floor) giving a total of 200 beds. The formal gardens on the 6 acre site, stated to be the finest in the county, would remain untouched and the 'Willows' House itself would become a staff house and this, it was suggested, would be capable of being extended. Under the heading of accommodation for staff the survey stated:

> the alterations to the Royal Infirmary outlined do not show any additional provision for Nurses and staff. There is a prevailing feeling nowadays that except for probationers in their first year or two, the rest of the Nurses and staff are better out of the Hospital precinct, this gives them more freedom and is better for their health, both mental and physical. We therefore recommend that accommodation for the above should be obtained outside the grounds of the Royal Infirmary. If this is done it would be in line with the policy of many other Hospital Boards who are looking to the future.

The report was submitted to the Minister for Health and the Manchester Regional Hospitals Board, but was never implemented entirely, although many of the recommendations were carried out during the first ten years of the new administration under the National Health Service. If the full recommendation had been allowed at that time then Preston would have had its new district general hospital rather than have a wait of 34 years. The Board continued to press for the improvements and extensions outlined in the report but in the postwar era very little could be achieved because of the difficulty in obtaining the necessary building licences and materials. They did, however, re-equip the x-ray department with more up to date equipment and added a small extension containing 8 beds to East Ward for E.N.T. patients. A new 'calling' system was installed, a new electric passenger lift provided and all the wards received refrigerators and many other improvements. A nurses hostel for 12 nurses was established with the purchase and conversion of no. 4 Highgate Avenue, Fulwood. Larger projects than these now had to be approved at a higher level and plans were submitted to the Ministry of Health for a new physiotherpay department and pathology laboratory and also the no. 2 operating theatre. Schemes were also submitted for improving the main kitchen at the Infirmary and for the installation of central heating for Lostock Hall Continuation Hospital and the Willows.

The Board of Management was to be dissolved on 5th July 1948, to be succeeded by the already formed Manchester Regional Hospitals Board. The Workpeople's Fund still flourished and expressed their wish that they should continue to maintain their organisation within the new administration; in the last year of its existence, 1947, a record sum of £64,613/10/6d was raised.

The Earl of Derby K.G., who had been president of the Infirmary for 40 years, died in 1947 and other long serving members of the staff were also departing. Dr. F. B. Smith M.D., director of the department of pathology retired after 18 years service his successor being Dr. A. A. Miller M.A., M.D. (Oxon) D.P.H., D.T.M. who retired in 1968 and died ten years later in 1978. Another departure from the laboratory at this time was Dr. G. B. Delory M.Sc., D.Ph., the biochemist, who left to take up a new appointment as assistant professor in biochemistry to the University of Manitoba in Winnipeg, Canada. Mr. G. M. Arnott F.R.C.S.E. returned to Scotland and Mr. D. J. Davies F.R.C.S.E. left to go into private practice.

The Board gave permission to the Nurses League to place a stained glass window in the Infirmary chapel 'in gratitude for the devoted lives of two of its members A. M. Ronson and E. B. Rice' and a memorial plaque was placed in the main corridor of the Infirmary recording the services rendered to the hospital and the Nurses Training School by Miss M. A. Marks and Miss S. F. Rossiter. The Board also placed on record appreciation of the service rendered by the superintendent, Mr. John Gibson M.B.E., whose untiring work for so many years had been the mainspring of the Infirmary's administration.

Thus the Infirmary passed into a new phase after 76 years of voluntary service to the community of Preston with so many changes having evolved since its early beginnings in 1809 as the Dispensary in Fishergate, its upgrading in 1829 to a House of Recovery and in 1869 as an Infirmary, trying at all times to keep pace with the constant changes in modern techniques in medicine for the improvement of the health care of the people of Preston, in an atmosphere of financial restriction.

Chapter Five

A National Health Service 1948-1968

WHEN the National Health Service Act became operative on 5th July 1948 the Hospital Management Committee took over the responsibility of operating 10 hospitals and 3 dispensaries. These were:

VOLUNTARY HOSPITALS

The Preston Royal Infirmary (396 beds) the principal general and maternity hospital.

Lostock Hall Continuation Hospital for Women and Children (45 beds) opened in 1922.

The Willows Hospital, Ashton (26 beds for men) opened in 1928.

Chorley and District Hospital, a general and maternity hospital of 76 beds, opened in 1933 when the old Rawcliffe Hospital in Gillibrand Street was closed. The latter was opened in 1893 to replace a dispensary for the sick poor, founded in 1828.

LOCAL AUTHORITY HOSPITALS

Sharoe Green Hospital, Fulwood, a general and maternity hospital with a mental wing (358 beds) which was administered by the Guardians of the Preston Union up to 31st March 1932 when, under the Local Government Act 1929, it was transferred as a public assistance hospital to the Corporation of Preston, who appropriated it in 1936 under the Public Health Acts.

Preston Infectious Diseases Hospital, Deepdale Road (89 beds, 54 for fevers and 35 for pulmonary tuberculosis). This hospital had been administered by the Corporation of Preston since its erection in 1907.

The Chestnuts Sanatorium, Ribbleton (30 beds for TB patients) was opened in 1920 and administered by the Corporation of Preston.

Fulwood Infectious Diseases Hospital (50 beds) was erected in 1904 and administered by a joint board appointed by local urban and rural councils.

Eaves Lane Hospital, Chorley (184 beds for chronic sick, mental deficiency and maternity patients and also accommodation for 174 non-sick and casual inmates). This was administered by the Guardians of the Preston Union from its opening in 1871 until 31st March 1932, when it was transferred as a public assistance institute to the Lancashire County Council.

Heath Charnock Hospital, near Chorley (111 beds) 72 beds for Infectious Diseases — 23 of which were occupied 'temporarily' by chronic sick patients and 39 beds for TB patients. This hospital was opened in 1898 and had since been administered by a joint board comprised of representatives of Chorley Corporation and surrounding urban and rural councils.

Local Authority Out-Patient Clinics. The Preston clinic at 2, North Road, Preston, administered by the Corporation of Preston.

County Tuberculosis Clinics at Walton's Parade, Preston, and St. Thomas' Road, Chorley, both of which were administered by Lancashire County Council.

This list illustrates the enormity of the task which the Hospital Management Committee had undertaken at the outset of the National Health Service, to administer such varied and widely scattered establishments.

One of the first duties of the committee was to appoint a secretary to act as chief executive to the committee and the man chosen was Mr. John Gibson M.B.E., J.P., F.H.A. who had been superintendent and secretary to the Infirmary for 30 years. Further senior appointments included a deputy secretary, a finance officer and an engineer. The new committeee met fortnightly for the first three months but, owing to the large amount of business which had to be transacted, it was found necessary to divide the workload into sections. Eight sub-committees were formed, holding their first monthly meetings in September 1948, and dealt with catering, establishments, estates and development, finance and general purposes, finance (accounts), nursing, supplies and welfare.

There was a generalised centralisation of services, based on the Infirmary, with all the senior officers engaged being previously employed in, and transferred from, the individual hospitals which now formed the Group and they were not replaced in their former place of work. It should be realised that a great deal of extra work was placed on the staff by reason of the comprehensiveness of the service, involving many functions which until then had not been attempted i.e. the supply of surgical appliances of every kind, spectacles, hearing aids, the making of arrangements for ambulances and the payment of expenses of patients travelling from a distance and many other services.

The committee decided that there was no longer a need for the maintenance of the infectious diseases hospitals in the Preston district and as from 1st January 1949 concentrated such treatment at the Deepdale Hospital. The Fulwood Isolation Hospital (known as Longsands) was declared redundant and after a thorough renovation involving the renewal of all engineering and electrical services and refurbishing it opened in November 1949 as a continuation hospital. Forty orthopaedic patients from the Infirmary were transferred, which greatly relieved the pressure on beds in the Infirmary and reduced the waiting lists which were rather large and growing larger all the time. In order to secure co-ordination of the services and lessen the cost of administration, the work of the TB clinics in North Road and Walton's Parade were amalgamated at the latter clinic, the North Road premises then being used as the centre for the mass miniature radiography unit.

Dr. W. A. Simpson, who had been a member of the senior medical staff at Preston Royal Infirmary for 10 years, tendered his resignation to the Regional Board and the Group lost the services of several medical officers who secured promotion to other areas. The deaths were recorded of Dr. F. K. Bradley, veneriologist for 7 years, Mr. D. C. Wiseman, obstetrician/gynaecologist for 6 years and Mr. A. E. J. Berry, the dental surgeon who had served for many years at the Infirmary.

A Medical Advisory Committee was set up to assist the Management Committee; this was composed mainly of consultants representing all the specialities, but it also had G.P.s, representatives of the public health medical officers and a member of the dental staff among its membership. Its principal function was to advise on all matters pertaining to the practice of medicine, in particular scientific and ethnic matters but medical staffing and special equipment were also matters on which advice was given.

The H.M.C. set up a Group works department using the workmen employed at Preston Royal Infirmary as a nucleus. This staff comprised 44 craftsmen, joiners, plumbers painters, engineers and electricians, together with their apprentices and labourers.

A considerable number of schemes for the development and improvement of the services had been submitted to the Regional Board in Manchester. In the period 1948-1952 a new biochemistry laboratory had been erected in the pathology department, a rontgenoscope room had been completed and also additional x-ray plant had been acquired. A new dental department was completed and also a urological operating suite and, at the request of the Ministry of Health, a new hearing aids diagnostic and distribution centre was opened in September 1948 where deaf patients from the north and north-east Lancashire areas attended for tests and the fitting of hearing aids; by the end of 1952 9,000 hearing aids had been issued by the centre. A chiropody service was instituted in December 1948 for long stay patients, as a result of which patients were given periodic attention which rendered relief to many sick and bed ridden elderly people. During this period also modernisation of the children's ward was in progress, but many schemes still awaited either starting dates or were in a preparatory stage. These included a Group pathology laboratory, a general operating theatre, ENT operating theatre, a physiotherapy department, another extension to the x-ray department, extensions to staff accommodation, ventilation of the kitchens and extensions to the boiler house.

The impact of an unprecedented demand for treatment upon accommodation and staffs which were really inadequate for the task began to take its toll and despite great efforts the waiting lists for treatment and admission became longer.

The policy of the Ministry of Health was to improve the out-patient diagnostic and treatment facilities in order to reduce the number of patients requiring in-patient treatment but the accommodation in the out-patient department was much too small to cope with the greatly increased volume of work. Extensions to the out-patient department were needed but the state of the national finances and the increase in the housing and re-armament programmes had delayed, it was reported, the progress of capital schemes for hospital extensions. The formation of the Group supplies office at the Infirmary had made it possible for the H.M.C. to purchase and enter into contracts on an extended Group basis, as a result of which considerable savings were made.

Attention was given by the welfare sub-committee of the H.M.C. to the need for supplementing the work of the doctors and nurses by helping the patients to occupy the daytime hours in bed with interesting pursuits. The most important of these activities was the inauguration of a library service which proved a great boon to in-patients, organised by the public library committee of Preston who carried out the service throughout all the hospitals in the Group; the H.M.C. contributed to the cost of this service but only nominally.

Funds were made available with grants arising from donations made by grateful patients and members of the general public and also from the interest arising from the Central Endowment Fund formulated from all the endowments and funds of the former voluntary hospitals and distributed by the Ministry of Health to all hospitals and regional boards for the provision of extra amenities for patients and for research. These funds were used, on occasion, to provide a motor coach outing and for the showing of films to patients etc. The Preston and District Hospitals Welfare Society carried on the tradition of the former P.R.I. Workpeople's Fund and continued to raise funds to provide concerts, film shows, easy chairs, games and other materials for patients. The Ladies Linen League carried on its tradition as a voluntary welfare organisation, organising egg collections and raising funds to provide curtains for cubiclising two womens wards at the Infirmary in order to provide privacy for the patients and relief from the chore of screen carrying for the nurses on the wards. The Womens Voluntary Services in Preston also rendered their assistance in the field of welfare for patients by distributing library books and taking 'trolley' shops around the wards. At the time of the changeover to the N.H.S., there was very little in the way of social services carried out in hospitals. The H.M.C. endeavoured to correct this defect by instituting an almoners service to see to the social needs of patients.

Although the National Health Service Act 1946 provided for a comprehensive and 'free' hospital and consultant service, Section 5 of the Act provided for 'the continuation of beds in private wards which could be occupied by patients desirous of choosing, and paying the fees of, a particular specialist, at the same time paying the statutory maintenance charges'. Section 4 of the Act introduced a further kind of patient who 'desiring privacy may occupy a bed (if available) in a single ward in return for the payment of a charge of either 12 shillings or 6 shillings per day according to accommodation but such payment does not entitle to the privileges of a private patient or to priority of admission or visiting, though the services of the specialist or registrar available at the time are received without charge'. It was emphasised, however, that these 'private' and 'amenity' beds were only available provided they were not required for other patients on medical grounds. The Infirmary set up a unit containing 26 private and 12 amenity beds.

After serving for 34 years as chief executive hospital officer, Mr. John Gibson M.B.E., J.P., F.H.A. retired from active professional work on 31st March 1952. For thirty years he had been superintendent and secretary of the Preston Royal Infirmary and its auxillary hospitals and since June 1948 had been secretary and chief executive officer for the Preston and Chorley Group of hospitals set up in the N.H.S. Of the many stories which could be told regarding Mr. Gibson and his endeavours during his long service on behalf of the Infirmary and its patients, perhaps one episode could be recorded here. During the depression of the early 1930s he decided that the Infirmary could save money at Christmas by raising their own turkeys rather than buying them. The staff at Lostock Hall Continuation Hospital were given the responsibility of raising these young turkeys to maturity in time for Christmas. The birds were allowed to range freely through the hospital's grounds and Mr. Gibson, being one of the few in those days with a motor car, made weekly visits to observe their progress. All seemed well until one evening just before Christmas when a turkey sat in the centre of the drive, forced him to stop his car and repeated bleeping of the car horn failed to shift it. The bird could not move of its own volition, apparently, as all the turkeys had contracted some disorder which meant the whole flock had to be destroyed. Undeterred however by this catastrophe Mr. Gibson repeated the same exercise the following year, substituting geese for turkeys, but this failed too for similar reasons just before the festive season began. The experiment was not repeated again.

Mr. H. Hill R.H.A., formerly secretary to the Chorley and District Hospital until becoming deputy secretary to the H.M.C. in 1948, was appointed to succeed Mr. Gibson and Mr. A. W. Cunliffe A.H.A. became deputy secretary with Mr. J. R. Hindle A.C.A., A.H.A. as finance officer to the Group. The senior medical, surgical and dental staffs for the Group in post at the end of 1952 were as follows:

Physicians	
Dr. D. M. Anderson M.D., F.R.C.P.E.	Consultant
Dr. B. F. Brearley M.D., F.R.C.P.	Consultant
Dr. R. P. A. Rigg M.D., Ch.B. (Edin)	Senior Hospital Medical Officer
Dr. O. K. Guyer M.R.C.P.E.	Senior Hospital Medical Officer
Paediatricians	
Dr. A. Gordon Hesling M.R.C.P., M.R.C.S., D.C.H.	Consultant
Dr. W. Griffel M.D.	Chest Physician
Dr. H. Villiers L.R.C.P. (S.I.)	Chest Physician
Dr. S. J. Sutton M.D., D.P.H.	Chest Physician (M.M.R.)
Venereologists	
Dr. J. F. Mackay M.B., Ch.B.	Consultant
Dr. S. Ball M.R.C.S., L.R.C.P., M.B.Ch.B., D.P.H.	Senior Hospital Medical Officer
Pathologists	
Dr. A. A. Miller M.A., M.D., D.P.H.	Consultant
Dr. A. F. Ollerenshaw M.R.C.S., L.R.C.P.	Senior Hospital Medical Officer
Surgeons	
Mr. R. Cunliffe Shaw M.Sc. (Man) F.R.C.S. (Eng)	Consultant
Mr. Ian M. Orr F.R.C.S. (E)	Consultant
Mr. S. Newsom F.R.C.S. (E)	Consultant
Obstetricians and Gynaecologists	
Mr. R. M. Corbet F.R.C.P. (I) F.R.C.S. (I) F.R.C.O.G.	Consultant
Mr. W. H. Tod M.R.C.O.G.	Consultant
Mr. W. A. Robson M.R.C.O.G.	Assistant Consultant
Urological Surgeons	
Mr. W. H. Graham F.R.C.S.	Consultant

Orthopaedic Surgeons	
Mr. R. S. Garden M.Ch.(Orth) F.R.C.S.E.	Consultant
Mr. N. A. G. Covell M.Ch. (Orth) F.R.C.S.	Assistant Consultant
Ophthalmic Surgeons	
Mr. S. S. Sumner F.R.C.S. (E) D.O.M.S.	Consultant
Dr. D. Plum M.R.C.S., L.R.C.P., D.O.M.S.	Clinical Assistant
Ear, Nose and Throat Surgeon	
Mr. J. A. Kersley F.R.C.S.E., D.L.O.	Consultant
Thoracic Surgeon	
Mr. F. Graham Bryce M.D., F.R.C.E., D.P.H.	Consultant
Dermatologist	
Dr. Paul Meiring M.R.C.P.E.	Consultant
Anaethetists	
Dr. J. A. Gray M.D., D.A.	Consultant
Dr. D. J. Lyall M.B., ChB., D.A.	Senior Hospital Medical Officer
Radiotherapist	
Dr. R. Gibb M.B., Ch.B., D.M.R.T.	Senior Hospital Medical Officer
Radiologists	
Dr. T. Harrison M.B., Ch.B. (Edin) D.M.R.E. (L'pool)	Consultant)
Dr. R. B. Guyer M.B., Ch.B. (Edin) D.M.R.E. (L'pool)	Consultant
Dental Surgeon	
Mr. E. H. Cooper F.D.S	Consultant
Psychiatrists	
Dr. A. R. Grant O.B.E., M.D., J.P.	Consultant
Dr. C. S. Parker M.D., D.P.H.	Consultant

The chairman of the Hospital Management Committee, Mr. W. Allison Davies C.B.E., J.P., M.A., died while a patient in the Infirmary on May 30th 1956; he had been the chairman of the committee since it was first appointed in 1948 and it was recorded at the time 'that his wise councils and long experience of hospital management will be missed'. He was succeeded by Mr. J. H. Maltby J.P. as chairman with Mr. G. H. Warburton-Steel becoming vice-chairman. Mr. Maltby unfortunately died shortly afterwards on 5th January 1958 to be replaced as chairman by Mr. W. Holden J.P. who had been a member of the hospital management committee since July 1954.

There followed a period of change among the H.M.C. membership, due not only to the deaths of several long serving members of the committee but also to the number of members who were required to retire under an 'age rule' directive of the regional hospital board. Early in 1958 the vice-chairman Mr. G. H. Warburton-Steel had to retire from office under this 'age ruling' but he was later awarded the O.B.E. in the 1959 Birthday Honours List in recognition of his public service to the Preston and Chorley Hospitals. Mr. J. Tomlinson succeeded Mr. Warburton-Steel as vice-chairman.

The neurosurgical department at P.R.I., set up on 1st September 1955 with the appointment of Mr. G. K. Tutton Ch.M. (Vict) F.R.C.S. (Eng) as consultant neurosurgeon, was playing an important part in the provision of hospital services in the area, with the head injury service for the northern part of the Manchester region being centred in the Infirmary. The building of a neurosurgical and nueroradiological department to accommodate these services was completed and, towards the end of 1955, Dr. D. T. Irwin was appointed part-time consultant radiologist and Dr. G. N. Mulliner, part-time anaesthetist with their main duties to be in association with the neurosurgeon. The development of this service was so rapid that the regional hospital board found it necessary to give additional assistance. In mid 1958, Dr. N. S. Gordon was appointed consultant neurologist, spending one whole day every week in Preston and later, toward the end of 1958, Mr. R. A. Daws F.R.C.S., F.R.C.S. (Edin) was appointed as an additional consultant neurosurgeon.

It was during the period 1955-1957 that other capital schemes were completed at the Infirmary with the provision of twin operating theatres, a new ventilation system to the main kitchen and extensions to the x-ray department. A new pathology department was in course of erection which would also include a public health laboratory, and a connecting corridor was built from the main hospital extending to the physiotherapy department and through to the new Group laboratory which, on completion, opened in November 1958.

The cost of these schemes and the expansion of neurosurgery together with the completion of the twin operating theatres placed the committee in a predicament when it was realised that they had insufficient funds to meet the needs of staff and equipment. At the end of May 1956, the finance officer gave a statement to the H.M.C. showing an overspending of £13,254 covering the first two months of the current financial year, due in no small measure to the increased number of nurses employed in Preston Royal Infirmary where the number of 299 full-time and part-time nurses was the highest there had ever been and represented 42 more nurses than were in the establishment at the same time in 1955. The largest overspending items for the first two months of 1956 were as follows:

Salaries and Wages	£5,682
Drugs	£2,367
Medical and Surgical Instruments and Appliances	£1,005
Provisions	£858
Domestic repairs and renewals	£670
Uniforms	£499

In November 1956 a deputation from the hospital management committee visited the Manchester Regional Hospital Board to discuss the serious financial position which, despite stringent economies, was not improving. The situation was discussed at length between the H.M.C. and the officers of the R.H.B. but it was the publication of the revised estimates for 1957/58 issued in January 1957 that finally persuaded the M.R.H.B. of the seriousness of the situation and they allowed an increased allocation of funds.

One decision taken in view of the financial situation was that no official ceremony could be held to lay the foundation stone of the new pathology/public health laboratory and at the same time no ceremony was held for a similar function for the new casualty department at Sharoe Green Hospital. In September 1956 the Infirmary was visited by Dr. Godber, deputy senior medical officer at the Ministry of Health. He visited the wards and departments and discussed problems with the hospital secretary and the consultants. On his return to London he wrote to the H.M.C. stating that he now appreciated more fully the problems and was well aware of the need for improvement in the service. Later, on 17th January 1957, a further visit was made by two senior officers of the Ministry of Health, together with Dr. Marshall of the M.R.H.B. The outcome of this visit was the extensions to Sharoe Green Hospital, the enclosing of the new corridor from the main building of Preston Royal Infirmary to the pathology department and the eventual purchase of part of Astleyfield Mill in Stanleyfield Road for use as a Group store. This was finally completed in July 1957 and in the same month a quotation was accepted for the provision of 10 internal extension points on the Infirmary's telephone switchboard, at a cost of £189.

In 1956 the Regional Board decided that it was necessary for the consultant paediatrician, Dr. G. Hesling, to concentrate his work in the Preston Group and when a new appointment was made for Blackpool it became possible for Dr. Hesling to hold daily out-patient clinics for children at the Infirmary, so reducing considerably the waiting lists for young patients.

In March 1957 Dr. A. F. Ollerenshaw, who had been senior hospital medical officer in pathology was appointed by the M.R.H.B. as an additional consultant pathologist in anticipation of the new pathology laboratory in course of erection at that time and the expected increase in laboratory investigations.

Miss N. Livesey, matron of Preston Royal Infirmary for 12 years during which time great improvements in the nursing service had been effected, retired in August 1957. Miss E. M. Watt S.R.N., S.C.M., M.T.D. was appointed as Miss Livesey's successor and following a visit by an inspector of the Central Midwives Board to the maternity department, four additional midwives were appointed to the unit and Sister Phillips was designated deputy maternity superintendent.

In the autumn of 1957 the secretary, Mr. H. Hill, reported on the effect of an influenza epidemic affecting both staff and patients in all the hospitals of the Group. It had been necessary to suspend visiting and to limit admissions of patients to emergencies only. In the Infirmary there had been a maximum of 54 nurses suffering from flu and the writing room had to be used as a sick ward and later West Ward also was used. The opportunity was taken to close the twin operating theatres to carry out urgent maintenance, including painting and the same action was taken at Sharoe Green Hospital where 17 nurses were suffering from flu. The medical wards had been extremely busy, with admission of influenzal pneumonia cases and because of the shortage of nursing staff and other staff a great strain had been thrown on the staff on duty. The grateful thanks of the Hospital Management Committee was 'conveyed to all members of the staff who had worked under heavy strain for several weeks past'.

The committee continued to give much attention to the problems of large scale catering and the natural tendency for hospital food to become monotonous. The staffing in the catering department at Preston Royal Infirmary was remarkable for the very low turnover of staff, due, no doubt, to the very successful apprentice cook scheme initiated by the catering officer, Mr. H. Gillet. The scheme continued to train cooks to a high standard but inevitably once qualified they left to take up senior appointments elsewhere in the hospital service. While there had been some difficulty during the 1950s in recruiting staff, the quality of personnel had been very satisfactory. Difficulties had however been found with regard to the employment of qualified dieticians due, in the Committee's opinion, to the fact that these posts did not carry a sufficiently high grade to attract suitable applicants. The responsibility for the preparation of special diets therefore remained with the general kitchen staff until early in 1961 when a Group dietician was finally appointed.

July 1958 saw the coming into effect of a 44 hour working week for all grades of ancillary staff e.g. porters, domestics, ward orderlies, storekeepers etc., employed in hospitals, which inevitably led to the employment of extra staff and the rearrangement of hours of duty of those already in post in the Infirmary. There had been a fall, nationally, in the number of people entering some of the professional and technical branches of the hospital service, particularly in radiography, physiotherapy and dietetics. The situation regarding the shortage of radiographers at Preston Royal Infirmary had been a source of worry for several years but it was hoped that this situation would be relieved by the re-opening in September 1959 of the School of Radiography in Stanleyfield Road, after a break of 5 years. There was an overall increase of 100 members of staff recorded in March 1959 which was accounted for by the reduction in the working week of ancillary and works staffs and nursing staffs, improved staffing standards, new departments being opened and extensions to older departments which necessitated increased establishments of staff. Ancillary and works staff were now working a 42 hour week.

In an attempt to improve the conditions of service for nurses, the Ministry of Health had issued a circular recommending all hospital management committees to introduce an 88 hour fortnight for all nursing staff. This had to be achieved at no additional cost in nursing budgets which the Infirmary's committee found impossible to implement, for, in the year ended 31st March 1959, the committee had overspent on nurses salaries throughout the Group by £9,400. Representations were made to M.R.H.B. for a revised nursing establishment and following a visit to Preston by the Board's representatives, an increase was allowed to the establishment of all the nursing staffs in the Group but the Board granted authority for only one instalment of 21 nurses and added a further £8,400 to the estimates for 1959/1960. The Preston committee hoped that further instalments would be allowed as soon as possible to increase their present establishment of nurses (701) to the new ultimate figure of 830.

The implementation of the 88 hour fortnight for nursing staffs was not achieved until 1962 and even then it did not apply to the night nursing staffs. The main problem facing the H.M.C. was the need to recruit more nurses, qualified or otherwise, as a number of beds had to be closed because of a shortage of nurses, and a further reduction to 42 hours with an award of increased holidays in 1964 did little to ease the difficulty.

During the late 1950s the Hospital Management Committee found it difficult to attract house staffs, in particular pre-registration house surgeons. In some more senior appointments, e.g. pathology and anaesthetics, the field of choice was very narrow. The M.R.H.B. agreed a change in establishment for the Infirmary by the substitution of a registrar instead of a senior house officer in the department of urology. It was hoped that new and upgraded medical residences would go some way towards easing the shortage problem and a review of junior posts was carried out by the Royal College of Surgeons in 1958.

It was a recognised fact that 40% of junior posts were filled with doctors qualified outside Britain and that the National Health Service would not survive without their valuable assistance; efforts, however, were being made locally and nationally to ensure that the language barrier, obviously quite often a disadvantage between doctor and patient, was overcome. The late 50s/early 60s period saw the spread of what became known as the 'brain drain', with many newly qualified doctors taking more rewarding posts overseas.

It was also a period of rising cost of living which raised the cost of healing the sick, so much so that in 1958 the Minister of Health introduced a hospital costing scheme to investigate national, regional and local costing. The Infirmary was selected to provide a comparison of costs, with similar hospitals throughout the country, using finance as a basis of efficiency. It was gratifying to the H.M.C. that the costs of running the Infirmary and other hospitals within the Group compared very favourably with their counterparts in the scheme. It was found that by bulk buying great savings could be made and it was reported that the savings on drugs and dressings alone, over a four year period, was estimated to have been £89,200. Cost consciousness was running nationally throughout the National Health Service as the cost of maintaining patients had become a national problem.

The Infirmary's expenditure from 1955-1959 was as follows:

1955	£292,455 out of a Group Budget of	£753,055
1956	£341,451 out of a Group Budget of	£871,420
1957	£397,772 out of a Group Budget of	£961,065
1958	£425,486 out of a Group Budget of	£1,042,350
1959	£460,470 out of a Group Budget of	£1,119,300

The cost of fuel, light, power, water, laundry all continued to rise, from £89,658 in 1960/61 to £101,302 in 1962/63. Subscriptions and donations to the Endowment Fund fell by £539 in 1962/63 when compared with 1960/61 and legacies to the Infirmary fell to their lowest recorded figure of £278.

The finance sub-committee of the H.M.C. reported in the annual report of 1964/65:

> The Committee are anxious that the constant battle against increased costs and the economies being made should not result in a curtailment of the services provided to our patients. There is a danger of this happening if inadequate accommodation is not replaced with larger and up-to-date buildings but the present economic situation and curtailment of Government spending may dictate a policy of restriction of capital development of the service and it must be faced that this will inevitably result in a lowering of the standard of service provided. Difficulties are being experienced in maintaining existing services because of cuts in expenditure and any further pruning of financial resources could be very serious. There is a limit to which economies can be made and if the principle of a 'free' Health Service is to be defended then the money must be allocated.

In the same report they stated that 'The national drug bill is substantiated at our local Group level where the costs of drugs and dressings during 1964/65 was £191,404, an increase of £21,942 over the figure of £169,462 in 1962/63, representing an increase of 13% in two years'.

Chapter Six

Modernisation and change 1968-1974

IN February 1968 the resuscitation unit in the emergency department was presented with two special electric clocks and a photometer by the Preston Ladies Circle 231 and new beds, curtains and curtain rails for Brown Ward, easy chairs for Albert and South Wards and a television set for the children's ward were donated by the Preston Royal Infirmary Comforts Leagues who had made their contributions for the benefit of the Infirmary's patients for so many years.

The nursing and medical staff in January 1969 jointly produced a most successful revue and pantomime, the script having been written and whole show produced by Mr. Allen, the surgical registrar. Sisters, doctors and nurses formed the cast, ably supported back stage by other colleagues and on three consecutive nights, appreciative audiences of friends and colleagues were amazed and delighted by the high standard of the performances and the enthusiasm and obvious enjoyment of those taking part. Programmes and refreshments were provided at a small cost and a silver collection was made during the intervals at each performance. Just over £100 was raised and one week later, on the occasion of the doctors' and sisters' Christmas dinner, a cheque for this amount was presented to matron, Miss N. M. Dixon, who decided that as Human Rights Year had just drawn to its close the money should be sent to the British Council for Aid to Refugees.

In May 1968 a tender from D. Whittle was accepted for the supply of 12 C.S.S.D. units at a cost of £86/10/0d (£86.50) per unit. This resulted in a vast expansion in the central sterlization supply department (C.S.S.D.) during the early months of 1969, with these units being put to use in most wards and departments throughout the Group. It became a popular innovation especially among the nursing staffs in that it removed the tedium of having to sterilize equipment by boiling on the ward and it certainly cut the risk of cross infection which had heretofore been a chronic problem in hospitals.

Alterations to West Ward with the addition of further storage space for linen at the end of the ward resulted in sister gaining more space in her tiny office with the removal from it of the linen supplies. Progress, in the form of bed curtains and C.S.S.D. units however, resulted in the loss of three beds to the ward, highlighting the critical situation regarding female surgical beds generally in the Infirmary. Albert Ward had all its old fashioned beds replaced by a modern, easily manipulated type of bed which could be adapted to almost any nursing position required and East Ward was closed for general upgrading, modernisation, redecorating and the introduction of C.S.S.D. units. The small theatre too was upgraded and extended using an area which previously provided bath and toilet accommodation for the ground floor private patients wing. A new outer doorway was made which avoided opening immediately opposite the swing doors leading into the theatre itself and which led into an extended anteroom large enough to accommodate a bed which on occasions was essential for neurosurgical cases. A corridor was constructed behind the theatre by which nurses could travel from the autoclave room to the sluice without having to pass through the theatre itself while operations were in progress, which had been the practice before.

The private patients unit moved in August 1968 to the old cubicle wing off the main Infirmary corridor. The six cubicles on each floor were transformed into four rooms, each with its own toilet and bathroom shared between two patients. The furniture was modern and each room had essential equipment such as piped oxygen and a suction apparatus available. The resulting rooms were small but truly luxurious accommodation, at a price; one disadvantage was the fact that the unit was split on two floors adding to the problems of the staff whose office was situated on the ground floor. A new extension to the pathology department, consisting of a waiting room for patients, three offices and two small surgeries was constructed and when operable, filled a much needed gap in the laboratory's accommodation.

In June 1968 it was decided to call for information from other hospital management committees regarding the provision of creche nursery accommodation for children of hospital staffs. This subject arose because of repeated requests that such a facility should be made available to staff in the Preston Hospital Group but no such provision was ever made.

Late in 1968 there was a great deal of discussion on the Green Paper on the 'Administrative Structure of the Medical and Related Services in England and Wales' issued by the D.H.S.S., being the first indication of the Department of Health's views on the re-organisation of the National Health Service. The document was not wholly acceptable to the majority of the Hospital Management Committee, who felt that the present structure of the N.H.S. needed to be fully investigated before any major changes occurred. It was recorded that the 'Green Paper did not quantify the proposals but first impressions would definitely appear to indicate a considerable increased cost'.

The junior medical staff review for 1969/70 was issued in December 1968 and its proposals included a senior house dental officer whose duties would be shared between Preston and Blackpool and also two general practitioner clinical assistants for two sessions each week for the maternity department at Preston Royal Infirmary. The M.R.H.B. was approached early in 1969 with a request for an additional consultant in obstetrics and gynaecology and also for a second paediatrician.

Mr. A. Toulmin F.R.C.S. (Ed) J.P., who for the greater part of his life had been associated with P.R.I., first as house surgeon, later a junior consultant and for many years as a senior consultant, died on 3rd March 1969. For his high ethical standards, his never failing interest in the nursing staffs both as a lecturer and an examiner in surgery, generations of Preston Royal Infirmary nurses would remember him with affection and gratitude. The death was announced in January 1969 of the former chairman of H.M.C., Mr. Warburton-Steel, followed quite soon afterwards by the death of his wife.

Members of the Regional Hospital Board visited the Infirmary in March 1969 to inspect the basement corridor and the storage of medical records and, following on from this visit, in May an urgent request was sent to the R.H.B. for alternative accommodation for medical records; one outcome was the installation of a sprinkler system as an urgent priority.

This was the 'Pay as your Eat' period when, due to pressure from the Department of Health and Social Security and nursing organisations, it became necessary to put into practice the payment for meals by ticket system for resident and midwifery staffs. No further deductions were made from salary in the case of non-resident staff and all resident staff together with non-resident student nurses or non-resident pupil nurses under 21 years of age were issued with a voucher which they presented in the dining room. All other non-resident staffs were required to buy specially printed tickets to produce in exchange for meals taken. There was much antagonism to this change of procedure and a great deal of dissatisfaction was expressed in the local press requiring prompt action on behalf of the Hospital Management Committee in terms of an explanation, by the committee's secretary. The members of the H.M.C. considered junior nurses no doubt had cause for dissatisfaction but regretted they had not been approached on it directly. They informed the Regional Hospital Board that they considered the financial position of junior nursing staff needed improving in view of 'Pay as you Eat'. A further outcome of this situation was that the standard of residential accommodation of ward sisters in the Infirmary had to be improved to include the provision of a kitchen in which they could prepare their own meals, a facility they had not enjoyed until 'Pay as you Eat' came along.

Student nurse, M. S. Turner, of the P.R.I. School of Nursing, won a Duke of Edinburgh gold award which was presented to her at Buckingham Palace on 21st July 1969. Also in July the thanks of the county ambulance authority were conveyed to Dr. Hall and Dr. Salpeker of the accident and emergency department for the work they had carried out in training some 200 ambulancemen.

A request was made in September 1969 for the appointment of a consultant neuro-pathologist and for an additional histopathologist for the laboratory in view of the vast increase of work in these specialities. A new innovation came in December 1969 with the introduction to the Preston and Chorley Group of resident clinical clerkships, whereby four students from medical schools would be accommodated at the beginning of the Lent term, the arrangements being made between the dean of the medical school and post-graduate clinical tutor.

A re-organisation of office accommodation and medical staff quarters in the Infirmary followed yet another visit by R.H.B. representatives and the Regional

Board was asked to consider an allocation of funds for this purpose. Staff shortages throughout the hospitals in the Group at this time due to an influenza outbreak caused great concern with so many staff having succumbed. Many volunteers offered their help in the wards and departments following a campaign in the local press and when things returned more to normality the thanks of the H.M.C. were issued to all volunteers and also the staff for their efforts in maintaining a full hospital service at a most difficult period. Late in February 1970 thanks were also issued by the R.H.B. to all staff and volunteers across the region.

In March 1970, the executive council for the County Borough of Preston requested 'open access to the Physiotherapy Department at Preston Royal Infirmary be made available to all General Medical Practitioners', but the request was not approved; at the same time the H.M.C. had made a request to the M.R.H.B. seeking their approval for the establishment of a unit for nuclear medicine at Preston Royal Infirmary; the outcome of this request is in doubt.

Mr. R. S. Garden, consultant orthopaedic surgeon was granted an honorary fellowship of the Royal College of Surgeons of England for his outstanding and distinguished service to the speciality of orthopaedics, early in 1970.

A full re-organisation of Hospital Management Committee sub-committees was effected in April 1970, namely:

(1) Finance and general purposes
(2) Staffing, medical, allied services and patient care
(3) Buildings, services and equipment

This followed discussions on the second Green Paper on re-organisation of the National Health Service and the consequent need to amend standing orders accordingly.

More financial assistance was sought from the Regional Hospital Board for the introduction of new nurses uniforms proposed by the Department of Health and Social Services who recommended that six uniforms should be issued to each nurse instead of the current two uniforms. An allocation of further monies from the R.H.B. was essential to meet these additional costs. A revised list of schemes costing up to £5,000 was received from the R.H.B. which included £1,000 for improvements to the Group offices and £4,000 for the storage of medical records in P.R.I. Other larger schemes were mentioned, including £15,000 for a radio isotope scanning unit and £7,000 for the dental department extensions, both of which were scheduled for commencement in 1971/72. In October 1970 the R.H.B. agreed on a scheme to provide additional accommodation in the pathology laboratory at an estimated cost of £7,780 and also agreed to the establishment of a senior house officer for the accident and emergency department at P.R.I. instead of a junior hospital medical officer.

A report was received from the Regional Hospital Board early in 1971 on its proposal to adopt, in the construction of appropriate parts of the new Preston Hospital, a form of hospital building construction developed in Oxford, which made extensive use of prefabricated building elements. It was also noted in the report that the R.H.B. proposed the deletion of the laundry from the plan of the new hospital which raised protests from the hospital management committee members, the only outcome of which was a meeting between the Secretary, Mr. H. Hill, the Deputy Secretary of the R.H.B. and a member of the Home Office Staff, to discuss future laundry arrangements for the new hospital.

A staff dispute due to a disagreement concerning conditions of service arose in April 1971 when the works staff, joiners, fitters, electricians and plumbers declined to cover the Good Friday/Easter Monday period. The H.M.C. were obliged to arrange for cover to be obtained from independent contractors and as the dispute continued throughout 1971 and into June 1972 before being resolved, emergency cover from private sources persisted.

In May, further attempts were made to re-establish joint consultative committees whereby management and staff representatives would regularly meet to discuss local problems. These committees had been set up at the start of the National Health Service in 1948, but they never achieved the purpose intended for them, no doubt because of the climate within hospitals at that time where liaison between staff and management had not been encouraged. The management side of the joint consultative committee was constituted for the year ended 31st March 1972 and staff were invited to appoint their representatives. One of the main reasons for the lack of success of J.C.C.s in the early years of the N.H.S. must have been without doubt the failure of staff representatives to communicate with such dignitaries as the chairman of the H.M.C., the matron and other persons of high authority who comprised the management side of the committee.

The climate within the hospital unit was vastly different at that time and many of the practices which are commonplace today were undreamed of then and in many instances were punishable with instant dismissal without hearing or redress; such was the power wielded by the administrators. The aims of staff/management consultative machinery were stated as being:

(1) To promote the closest co-operation and provide a recognised means of consultation between the Health Authority, its Senior Officers and its staff.

(2) To give staffs a wide interest in and greater responsibility for the conditions under which their work was performed; to make suggestions for the improvements of the general arrangements for the comfort of the staff, their recreation, entertainment and dietry.

(3) To prevent friction and misunderstanding.

It was to be many years before these committees achieved any success in terms of full co-operation between management and staff.

A consultative document on the re-organisation of the N.H.S. together with a foreword written by the Secretary of State for Social Services was issued to all members of the Hospital Management Committee in June 1971. The following month the views of the R.H.B. on this document were received. They agreed in principle to co-terminal boundaries for area health authorities and local authorities in the new structure but there was a special case to be put for County 10 (Lancashire), which covered a vast geographic area including five existing County Boroughs with a population of 1.3 million. The M.R.H.B. felt that it would be advantageous if this area could be divided into a number of area health authorities. In January 1973 concern was expressed when the long awaited proposal for the re-organisation had been issued proposing a single area health authority for County 10 (Lancashire) embracing Preston and Chorley, Blackpool, Blackburn, Burnley, Lancaster and Ormskirk. Representations were made to all the M.P.s of these areas stating 'that it would not be to the benefit of the patient, the efficiency of the service or in the interest of the public generally' and called on their support for opposition to a single area health authority.

The Hospital Management Committee were informed that waiting lists were increasing yet again and at a time when they would normally be expected to decrease (June 1971). The same information on waiting lists was tackled at regular intervals, the subject being raised again in November 1971 and December 1972, still posing problems to the present day. Another subject discussed in July 1971 was the provision of a new national nurses uniform which would be introduced over the following three or four years.

The annual church service for hospital staffs was held in Manchester Cathedral on Sunday 31st October 1971. An interdenominational service arranged by the Regional Hospital Board was held, following which a request was sent by the Hospital Management Committee to the R.H.B. 'that as it was Preston's Guild Year in 1972 would they allow the service for that year to be held in Preston?' This was not to be, however, as the R.H.B. had already made arrangements for the service in 1972 to be held in Leigh, a venue they could not change.

A meeting was held in September 1971 between the chief public health inspector, the smoke abatement officer and an assistant engineer from the R.H.B. to discuss smoke emissions from the boiler plant at Preston Royal Infirmary in contravention of No. 13 Smoke Control Order. Their decision was that a complete reorganisation of the boiler house and conversion of the boilers, possibly to oil firing, was the only solution. In July 1973, the chief public health inspector again raised the question of emission of smoke and grit from the Infirmary's chimneys. Attempts were then made to remedy the problem using the existing boiler plant but as this was then more than 40 years old, little success was expected from the exercise. The matter was referred to the Manchester Regional Hospital Board.

Representatives were invited from the Hospital Management Committee to visit the R.H.B. on 18th November 1971 to discuss the present and future aims and objectives of the National Health Service and the impact that these would have on the revenue allocations for 1972/73. The chairman, Mr. J. Tomlinson, secretary Mr. H. Hill, treasurer Mr. J. Hindle, the chief nursing officer and chairman of the medical executive committee were elected to represent the H.M.C. at the meeting. Later it was decided that as it would be impractical for these members to be committed to attend what later turned out to be some 28 meetings in all, the chairmen of the sub-committees should be given the dates and invited to attend those meetings convenient to them.

Arrangements were made for open days to be held in P.R.I. on 6th and 7th October 1971. Details were given in October of an outbreak of salmonella poisoning in some hospitals in the Preston Group, the source having been traced to a milk supplier. The policy of the H.M.C. was that only heat treated milk was purchased for use, but it transpired that resident staff had been purchasing untreated milk privately; the outbreak was quickly brought under control.

The patients' day room with accommodation for relatives was opened on 31st October 1971. An appeal was made by the Preston and district schools and other organisations regarding the raising of funds for the Preston hospitals during

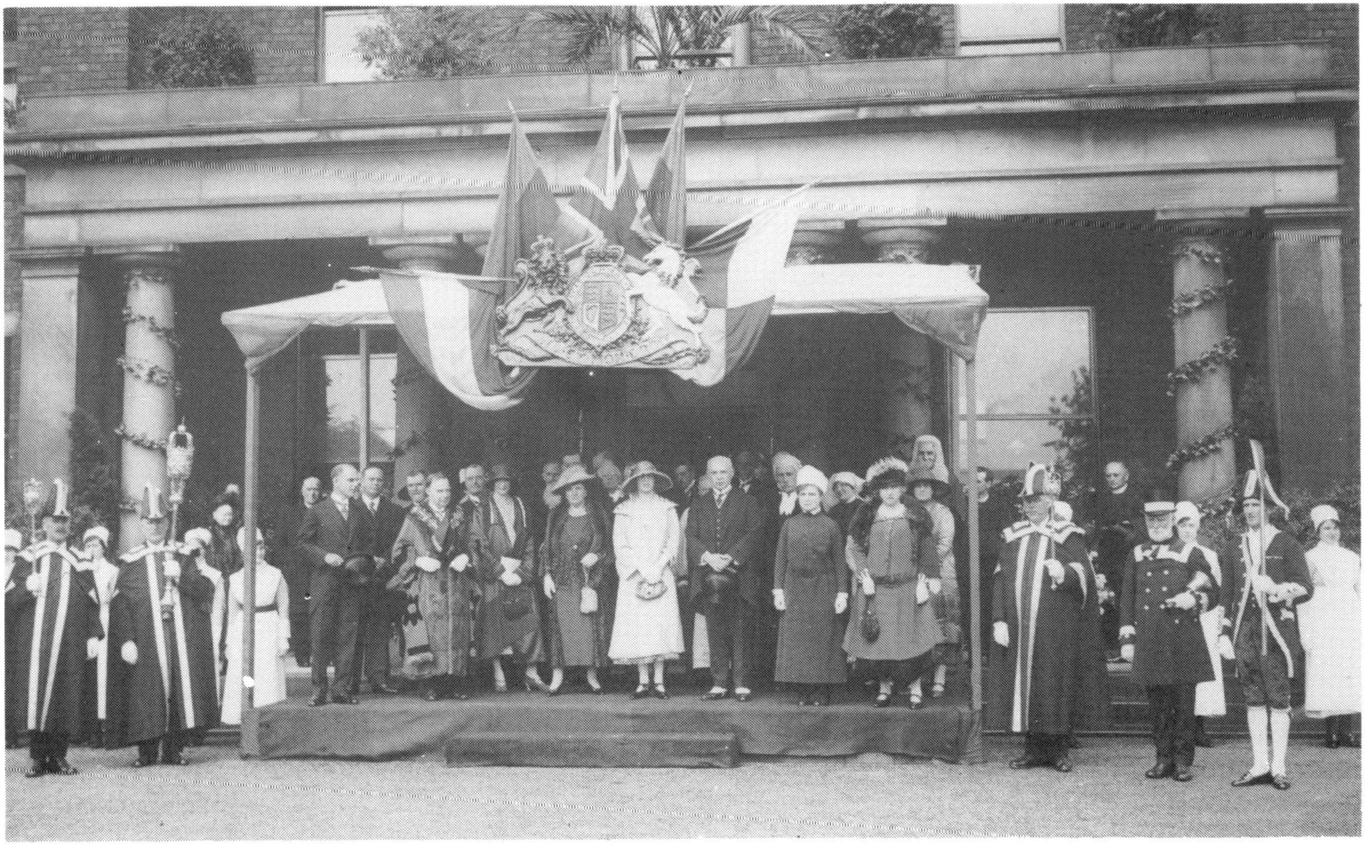

At the Infirmary Entrance. HRH Princess Mary outside the hospital in August 1925.

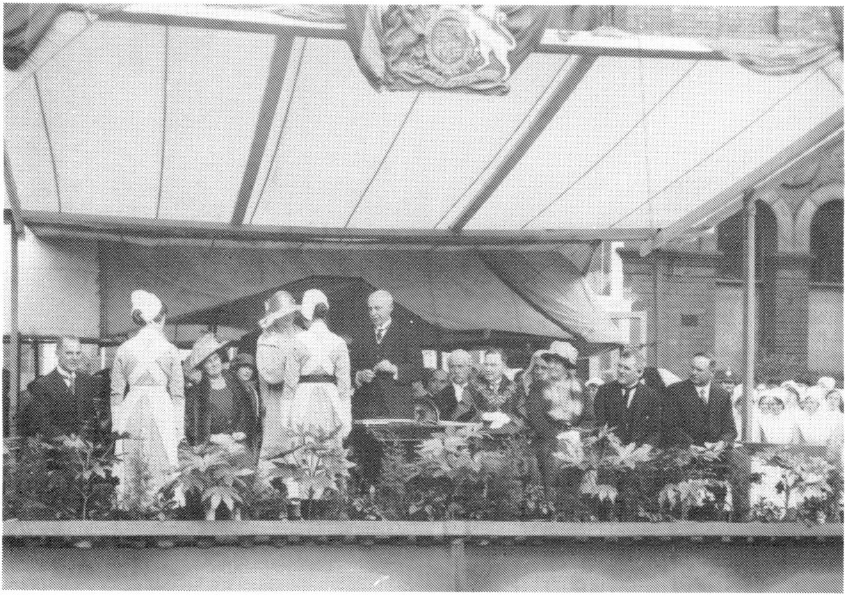

She presents the Foster gold and silver medals to Nurses Hadaway and Phillips and (below) lays the foundation stone of the Princes Mary Wing.

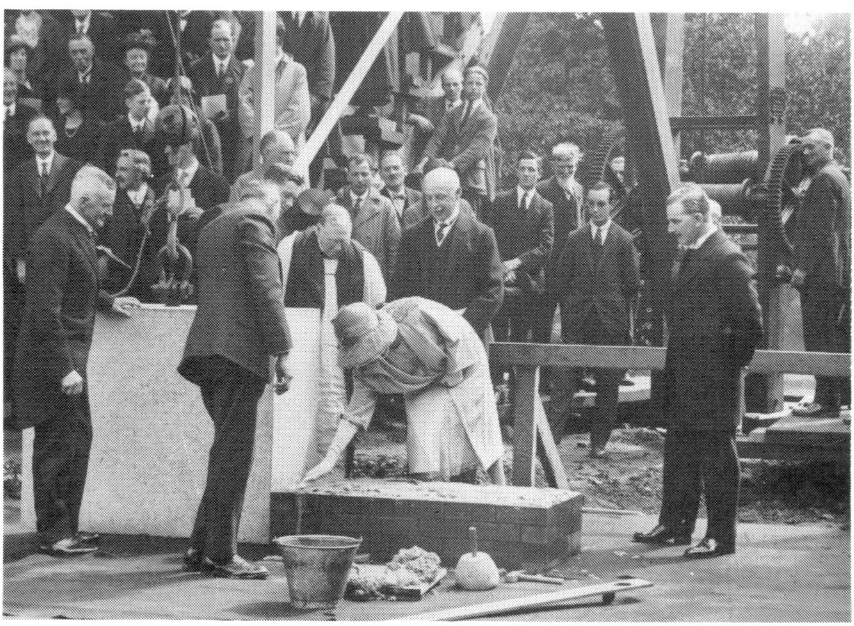

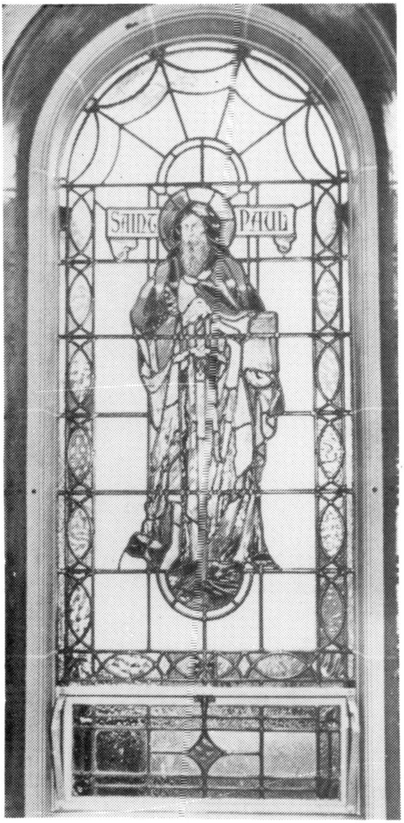

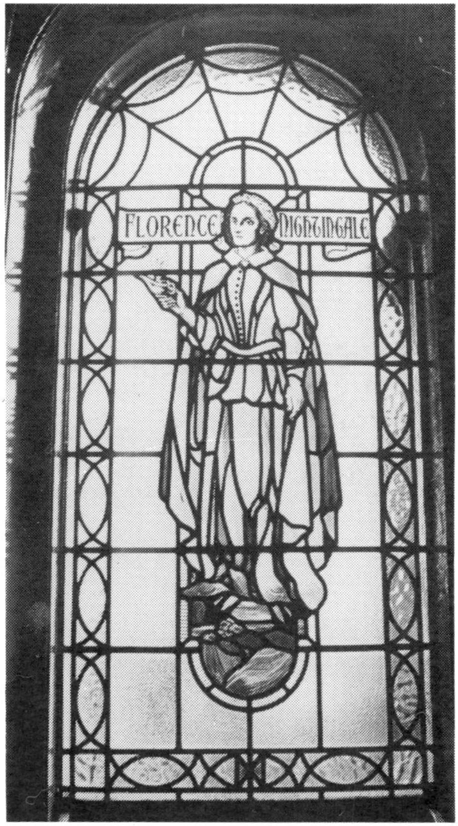

Stained glass windows of Saint Paul and Florence Nightingale, dedicated, respectively, to F. R. Collinson, Senior Surgeon and Vice-President of PRI and to William Galloway, member of the HMC and one of the hospital's benefactors.

Photograph courtesy of Lancashire Evening Post.

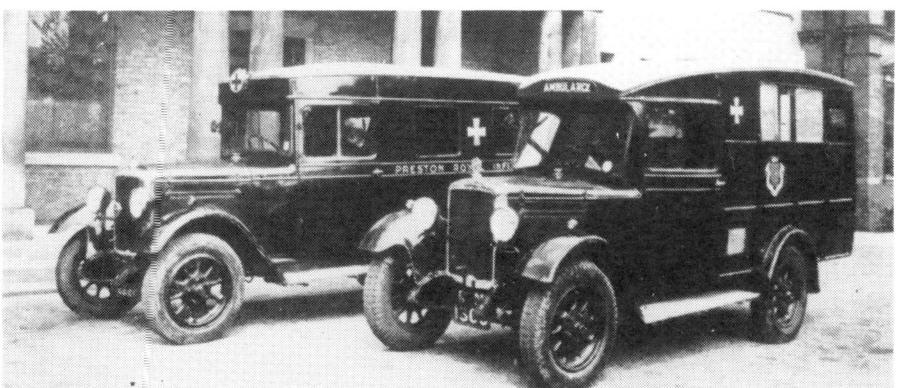

PRI ambulances in the old style.

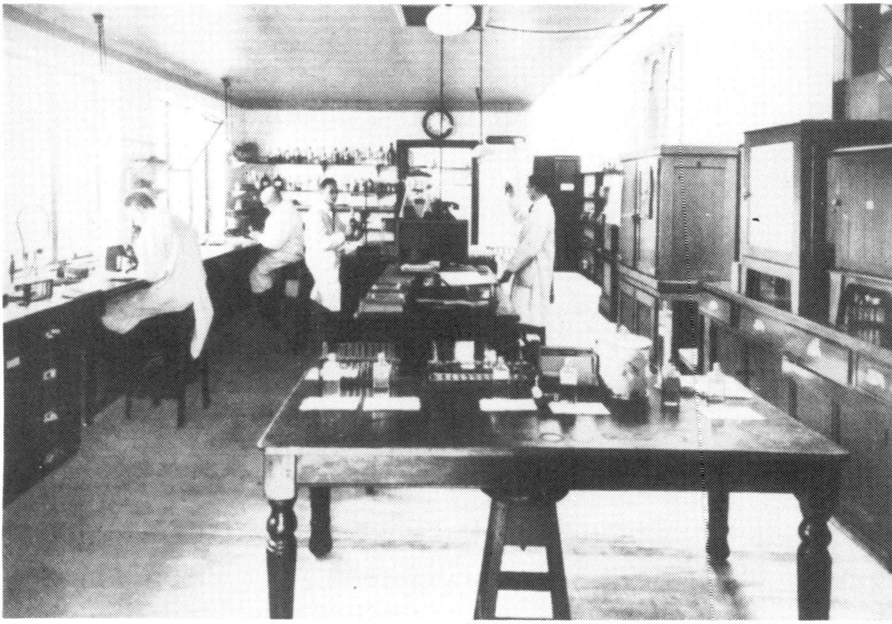

The laboratory in 1935.

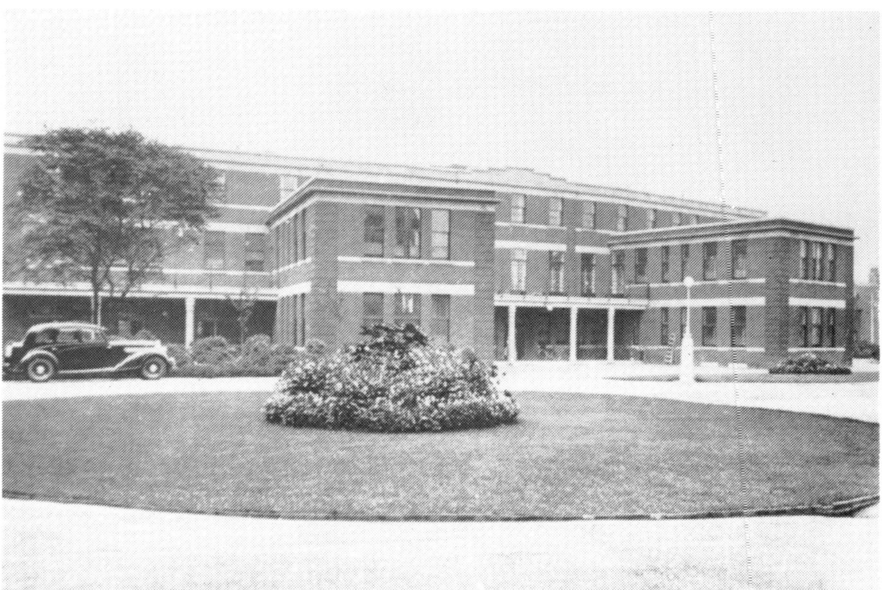

The Maternity Hospital in 1936.
Photograph courtesy of Lancashire Evening Post.

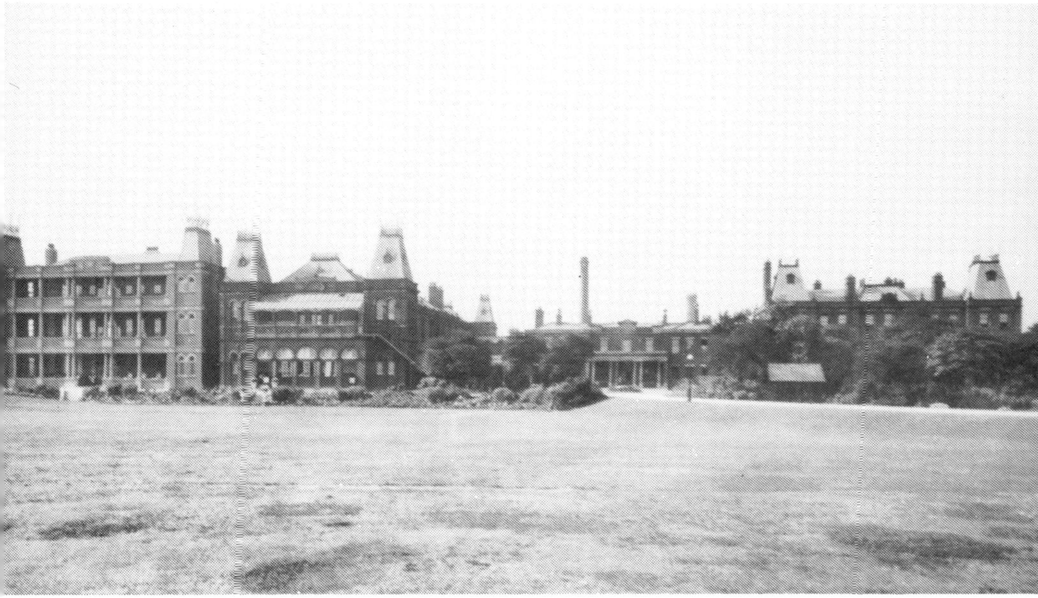

A general view of the Infirmary in 1929.

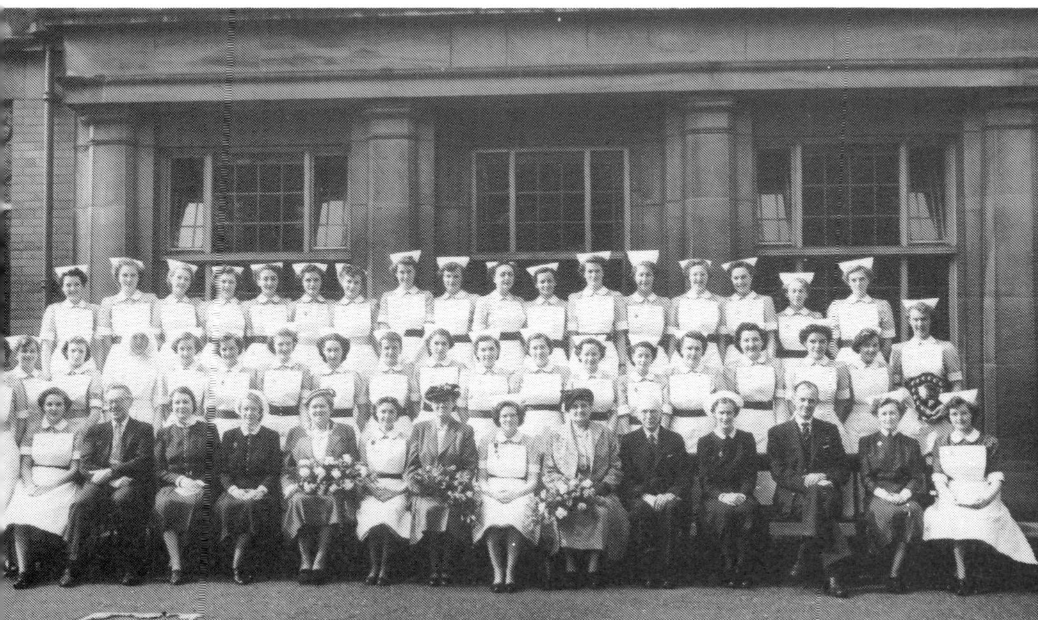

Nurses gathered, probably for the annual nurses badge day.

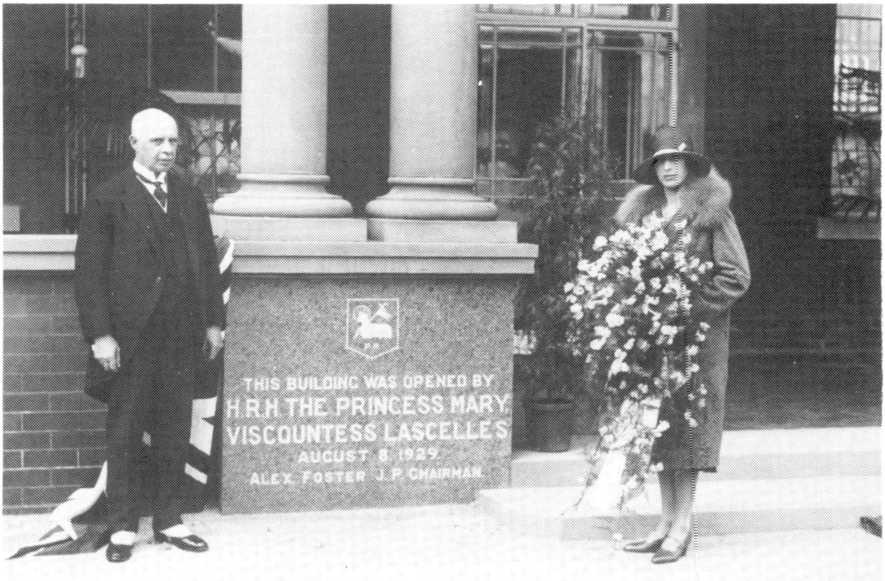
THIS BUILDING WAS OPENED BY
H.R.H. THE PRINCESS MARY
VISCOUNTESS LASCELLES
AUGUST 8 1929
ALEX. FOSTER J.P. CHAIRMAN.

Opening the new Patients Wing in August 1929.

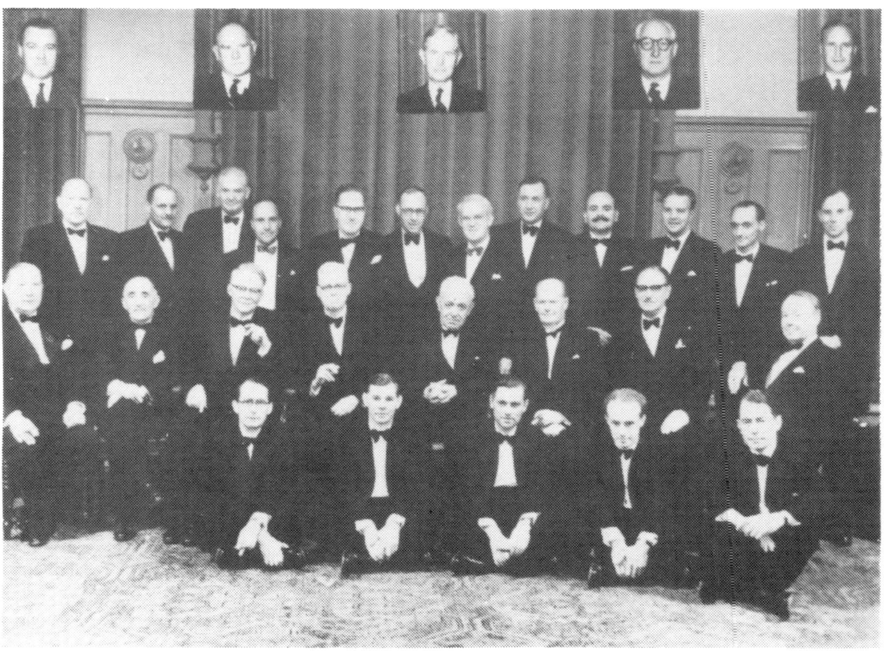

Many well known faces are gathered here in a group photograph of the medical staff in around 1958.

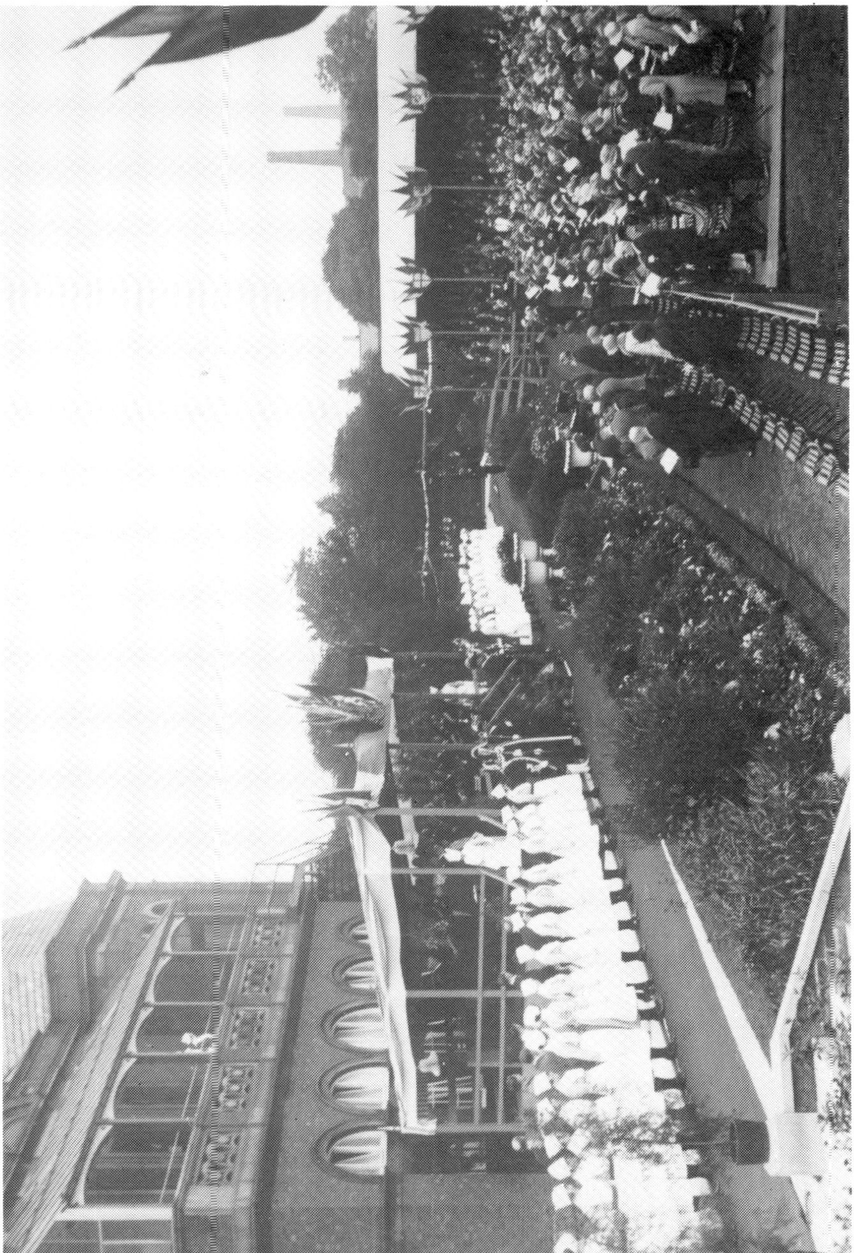

Ceremonies were often done in the grand style . . . this picture dates from 1929.

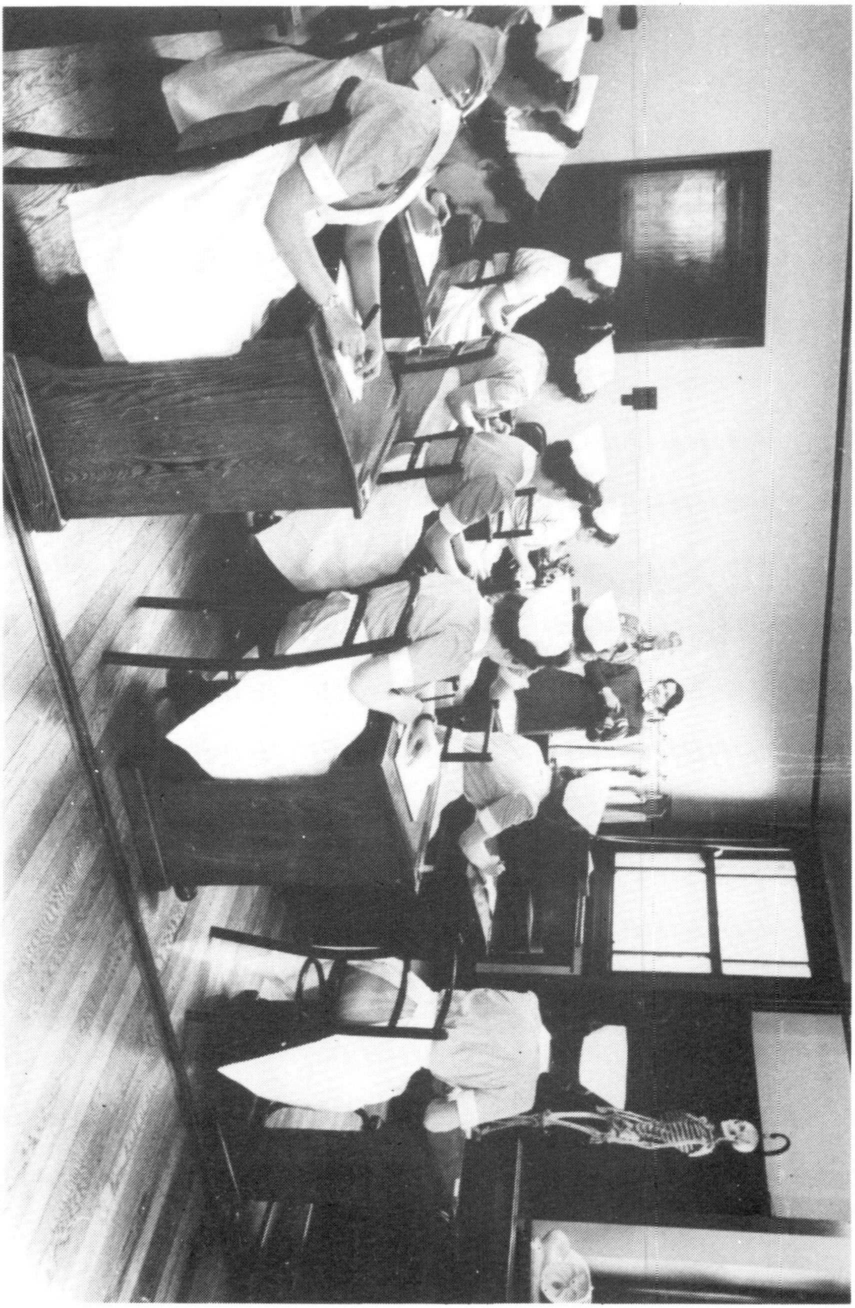

The lecture room in full swing with, at the front, Miss Ogleby, well remembered by hundreds of student nurses over the years.

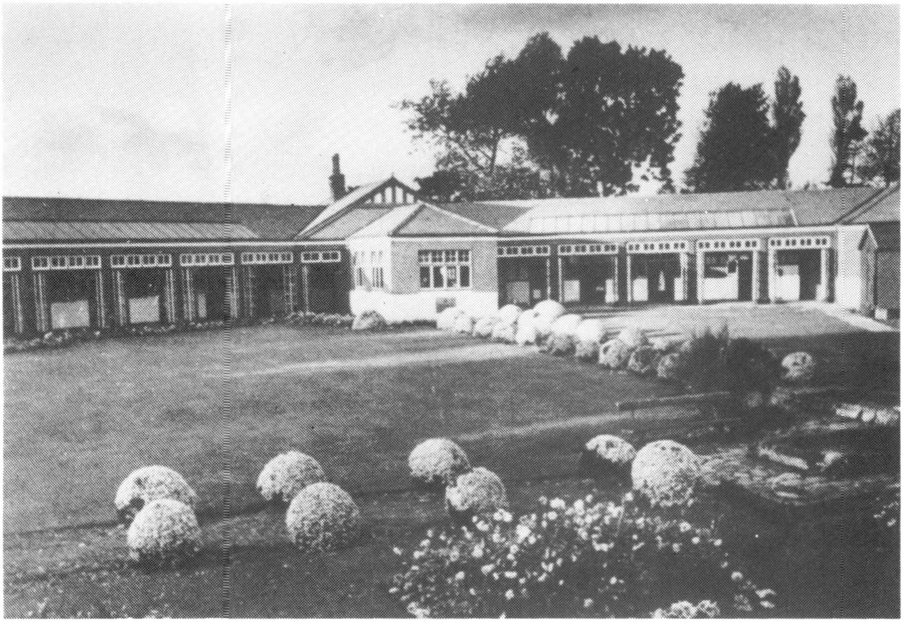

Chestnuts Sanatorium, Ribbleton, later Ribbleton Hospital, in around 1950.

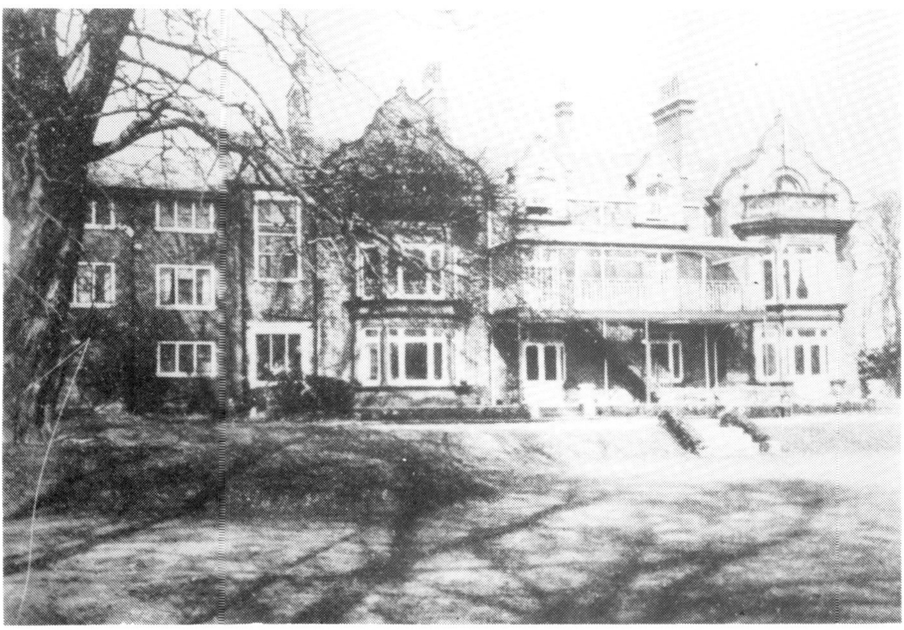

Lostock Hall Continuation Hospital in 1935.

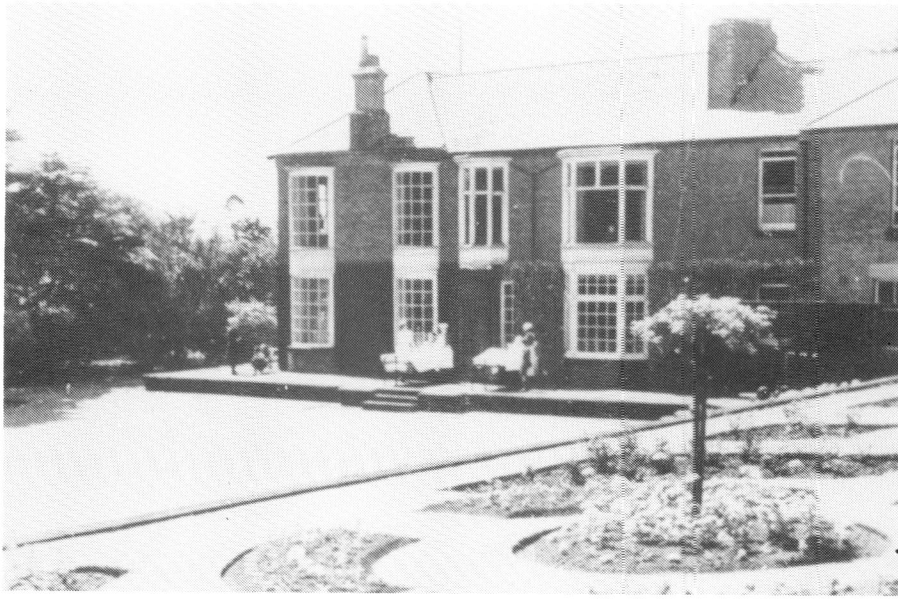

The Willows, Ashton.

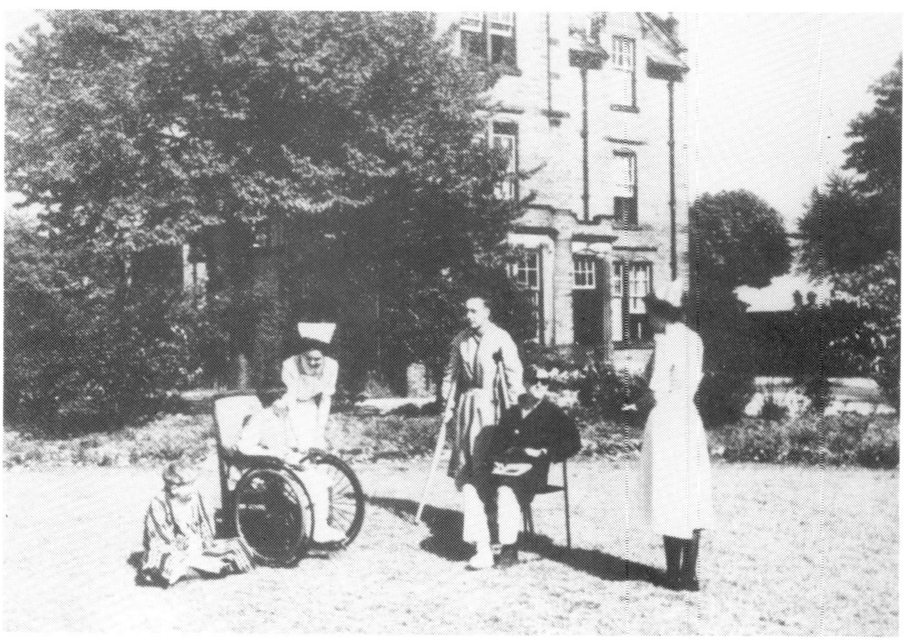

Fulwood Continuation Hospital, Longsands Lane, 1950.

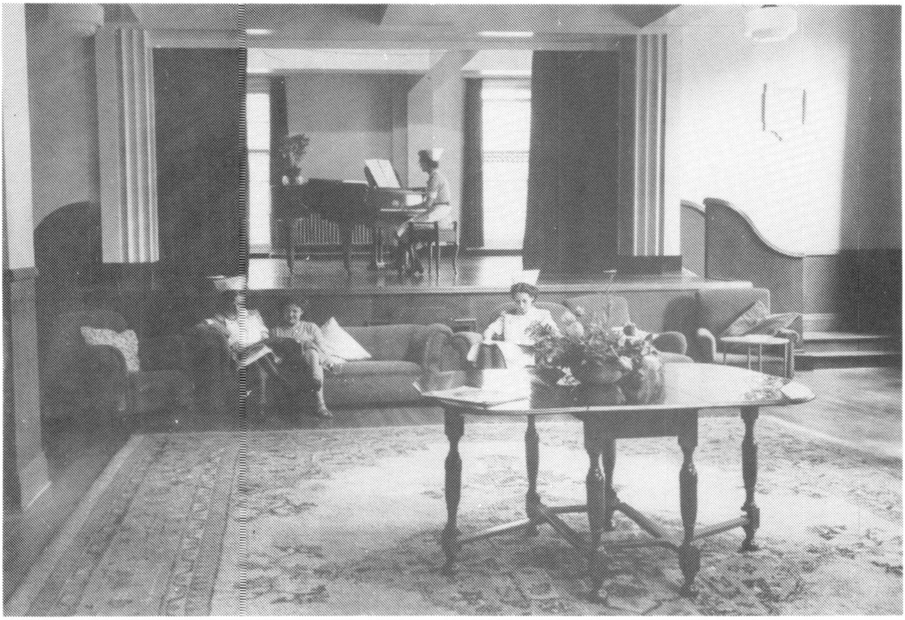

The Nurses Sitting Room; note the stage, which was used for concerts, pantomimes etc.

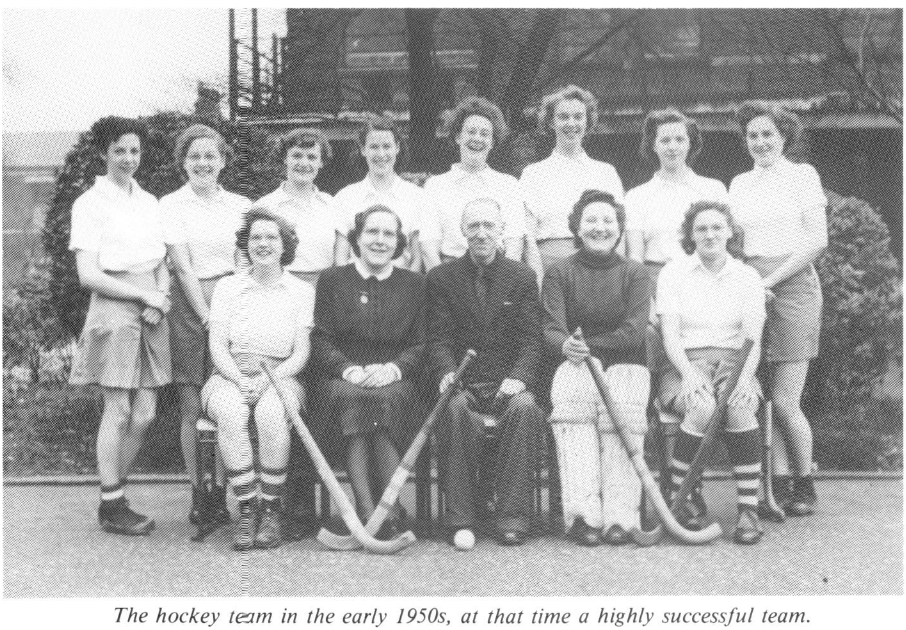

The hockey team in the early 1950s, at that time a highly successful team.

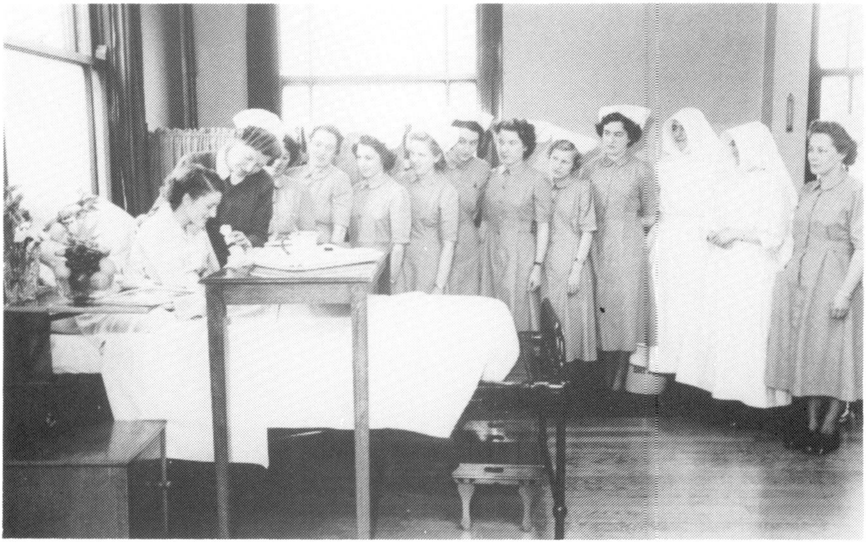

Student nurse training takes a practical turn at the bedside. Many nuns were trained at Preston, often returning afterwards to serve in convents.

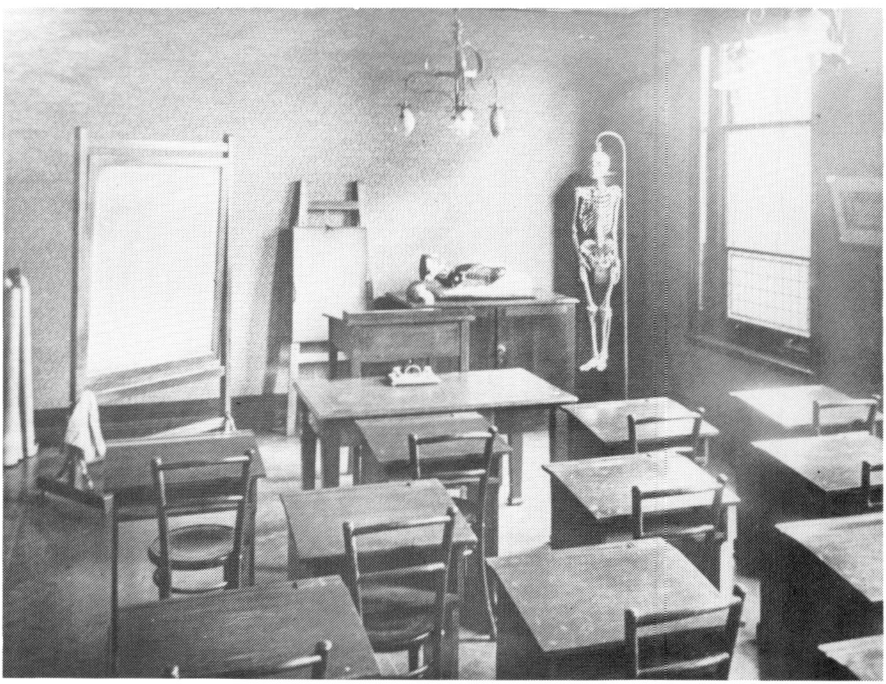

One of the classrooms of the Nurses Training School.

Photograph courtesy of Lancashire Evening Post.

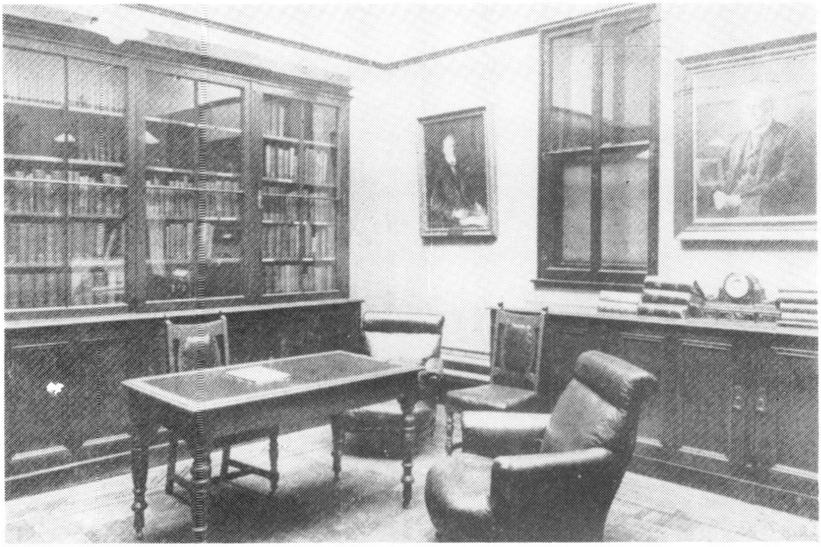

The Brackenbury Library, given by Miss Brackenbury in 1870. The room was later used as the Consultants' Dining Room.

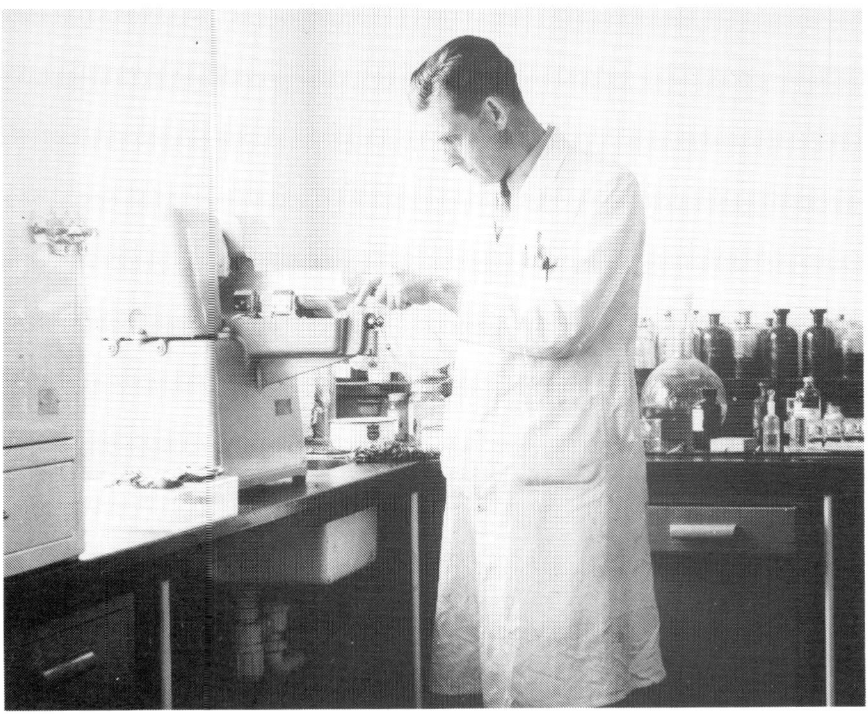

The author, John Wilkinson, working in the Laboratory in 1958.

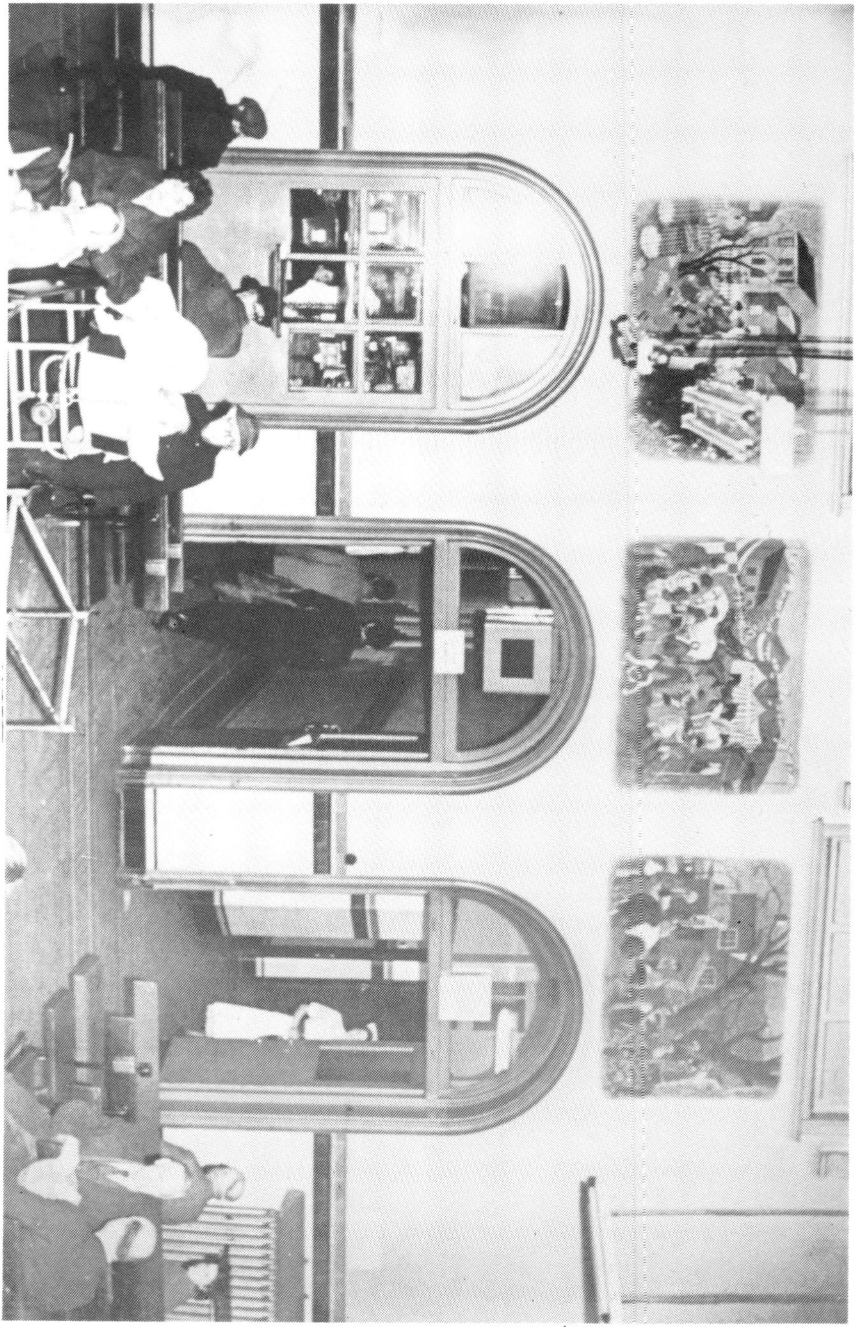

The Out-Patients Department as many will remember it. Note the murals which were painted above the doors by students from Preston Polytechnic in an attempt to brighten the outlook.

Photograph courtesy of Lancashire Evening Post.

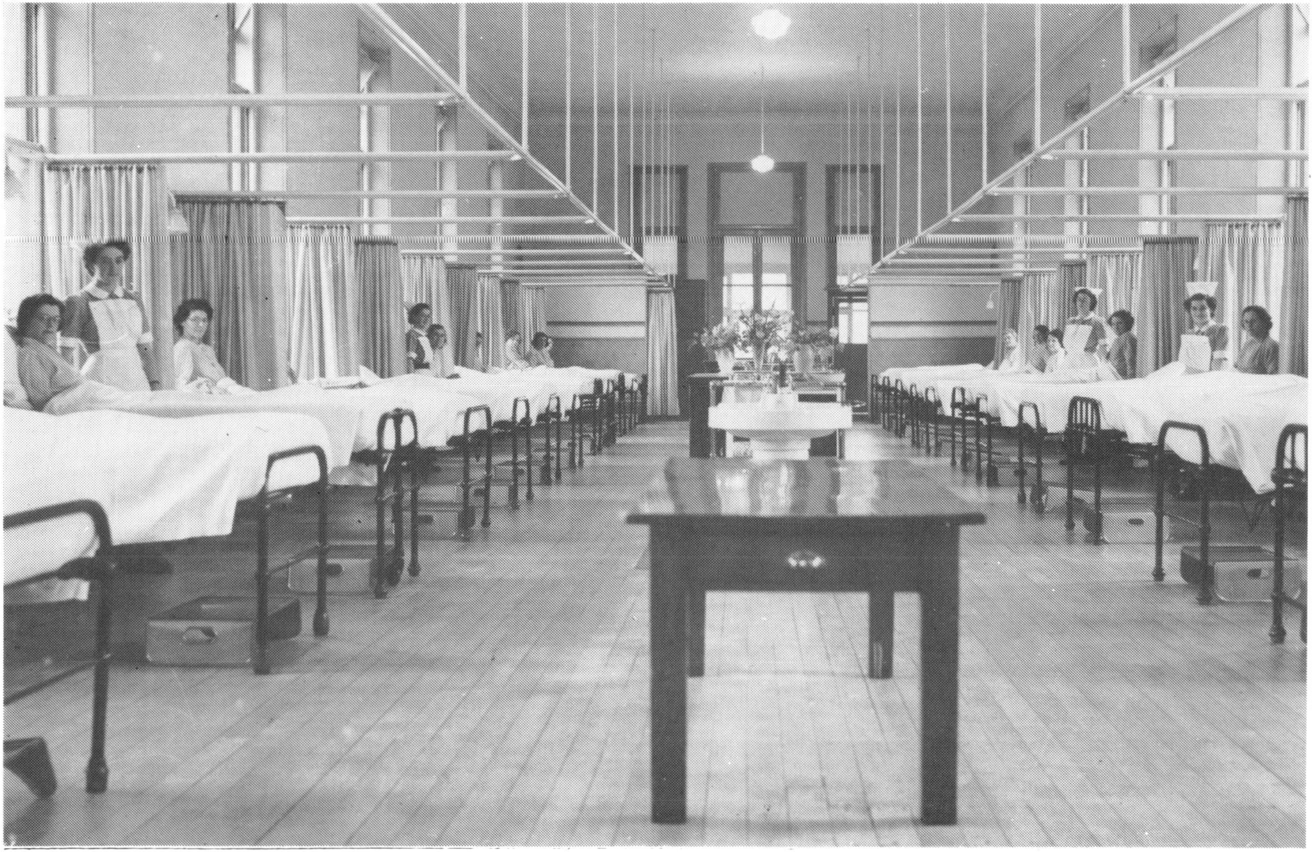

Alice Ward in full swing, awaiting Matron's daily round.

Photograph courtesy of Lancashire Evening Post.

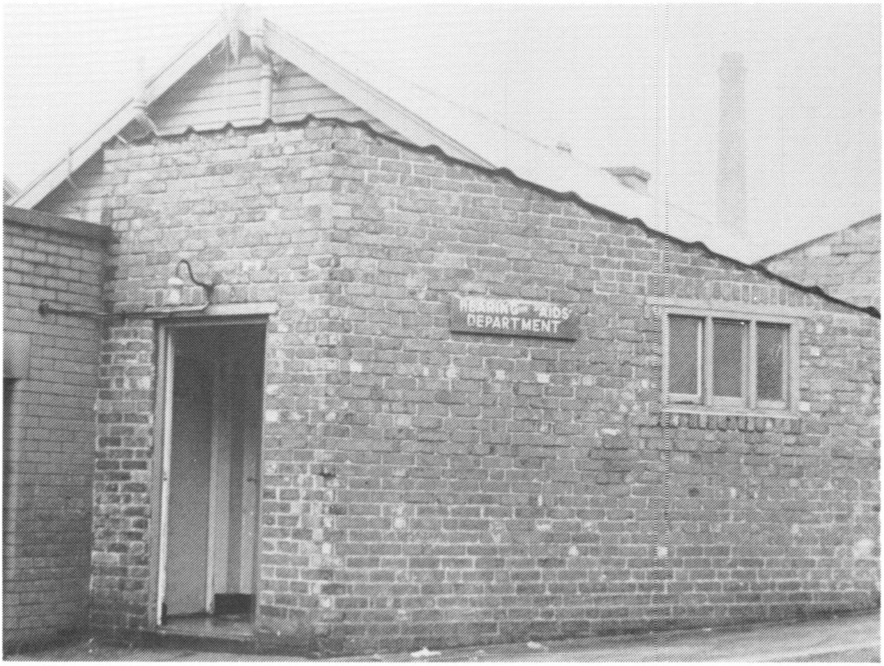

The original Hearing Aids Department, opened in the early 1950s in Stanleyfield Road.
Photograph courtesy of Lancashire Evening Post.

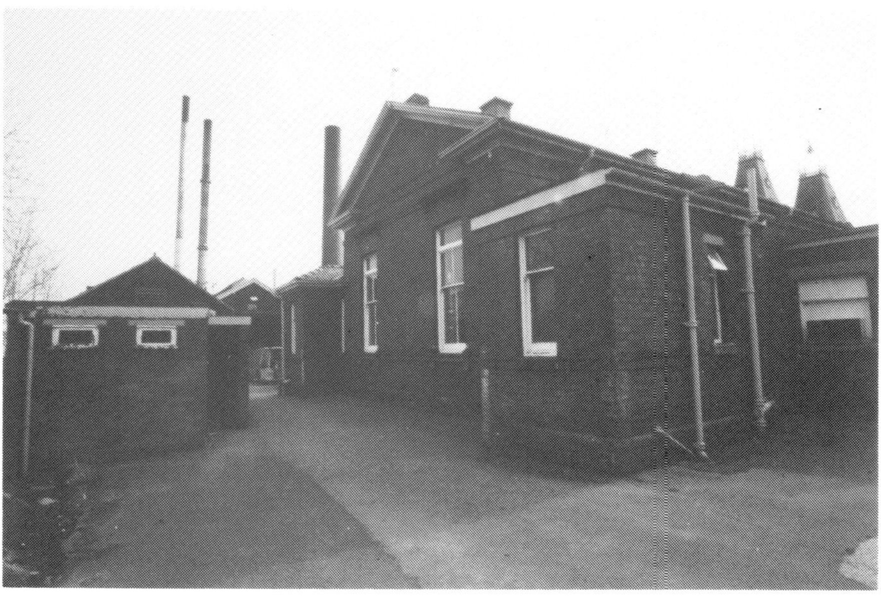

One of the three original Fever Wards. There is an inscription to this effect on the side wall.

the celebrations of Preston Guild 1972. Their success is shown in the following figures for donations to the H.M.C. received *viz.*

To the end of March 1972	£2,690
To the end of March 1973	£5,966
To the end of March 1974	£4,269

In January 1972 a great deal of discussion was taking place regarding the proposed reorganisation of the N.H.S. and the decision was taken to hold seminars and courses on the proposals in order to prepare the senior staff for the wider responsibilities they would have to face in the proposed integration of the Health Service. At the same time arising out of the current policy of the Department of Health and Social Security in attempting to improve the psychiatric services and establish closer links with the general hospital services and the community, discussions had begun regarding an amalgamation of the hospitals in the Preston and Chorley and Whittingham Groups. While agreeing in principle with the amalgamation, the Hospital Management Committee did not agree with the proposed reduction in numbers of both the Preston and Chorley and Whittingham H.M.C.s and in their reply to the R.H.B. they said 'it would seem desirable in the run-up to the restructuring of the National Health Service in 1974 that from a public relations point of view, as many active Committee members as possible should be retained'. In their reply the R.H.B. named the re-appointed members of the H.M.C., reducing the number to 15 with their service to commence from 1st April 1972. Meetings were arranged in April between staff representatives and officers of the R.H.B. to discuss the proposed amalgamation and its implications and agreement was reached to ask the D.H.S.S. to approve the amalgamation in the Autumn of 1972.

Later in the year the findings of the R.H.B. were made known following discussion with the Secretary of State regarding the future membership of the Preston and Chorley H.M.C. after the amalgamation and the subsequent reorganisation of the National Health Service. The Board appointed Mr. W. Bennett J.P., the chairman of the Whittingham H.M.C., to become chairman of the Preston and Chorley H.M.C. from 26th September 1972. Mr. J. Billington, Miss P. C. L. Gould and Alderman T. Jackson of the Preston H.M.C., were appointed to membership of the Whittingham H.M.C. and some of their members were similarly appointed to the Preston and Chorley H.M.C., *viz.* Mr. J. J. Abram (to 31st March 1973) Mr. E. D. H. Hoyle J.P. (to 31st March 1974) and Dr. S. Smith M.D., F.R.C.P., F.R.C. (Psych) D.P.P. (to 31st March 1975). It was anticipated, however, that when the reorganisation of the N.H.S. was implemented from April 1974 these two hospital management committees would cease to exist.

The Hospital Management Committee were stunned in June 1972 by the news of the sudden death of its chairman Mr. J. Tomlinson whilst on holiday. In the same month the former hospital secretary Mr. John Gibson died at the age of 84 and on 9th March 1972 Mr. W. A. H. McKerrow, surgeon at Preston Royal Infirmary for many years before his retirement just after the war, died at the age of 87. Another death recorded at that time was that of Dr. Tom Cank, one of the 'characters' associated with the Infirmary over the years. Dr. Cank, formerly casualty officer for some 15 years, was a true eccentric who was not averse to interviewing his patients on the benches in the out-patients hall when the casualty area was busy.

Dr. Hall, the current casualty officer, was congratulated for a paper he had prepared and presented to the conference of the Royal Society of Health entitled 'non-accidental injuries in children' and which was acknowledged to be a considerable national contribution in this field.

A new policy document issued by the R.H.B. proposing the non-appointment of locums for registrars during holiday periods was dismissed by the Hospital Management Committee. The Medical Executive Committee slated the proposal stating that it was unrealistic to expect a registrar in one speciality to cover for another registrar in another, even for short periods; he would have neither the time nor the knowledge to do it, and it was not feasible to expect a registrar in one hospital to cover for another registrar in another hospital even in the same speciality. The whole exercise was considered to be dangerous both for the in-patient and for emergency patients and would result in the necessity to cut down or cancel out-patient clinics because of a lack of adequately trained staff. The H.M.C. replied to the R.H.B. in this vein stating 'it was an ill conceived economy and a menace to the patient and if it involved extra duty payments could result with the disadvantage of overworked, tired and less trained Junior Medical Staff'.

Toward the end of 1972 discussions on the overspending in nursing salaries were held and it was agreed that this could be covered at that time by underspending in other areas, such as the closure of some wards for upgrading and modernisation but it was pointed out that this would not always be available as a solution to the problem of overspending. The R.H.B. issued a revision of the revenue allocation for the Preston and Chorley H.M.C. for 1972/73 to the sum of £4,696,928 and this was later revised again early in 1973 to the sum of £4,715,177.

With the resignation of the deputy group secretary, Mr. J. W. Roe, a meeting of the H.M.C. was convened on 2nd March 1973 at which five candidates were interviewed for Mr. Roe's post. Mr. B. Calverly was appointed deputy group secretary from 1st May 1973. This was a period of uncertainty with reorganisation in the offing and this was reflected nationally with unrest and industrial action by the hospital ancillary staffs. The Infirmary and other hospitals in the Preston Group were not affected to any degree, however, due to the decision made locally by all concerned that patients must not be affected by the action.

Congratulations were recorded to Miss Wilkinson, the first public relations officer for the Group, on the publication early in 1973 of the first issue of the new group news publication, the *Echo,* which has proved to the present day an ideal vehicle for the exchange of information for both management and staff alike throughout the health authority. The name *Echo* was derived from Preston and Chorley thus:

PR**E**STON
and **C**
H
O
R
L
E
Y

Earlier, in late 1970, an attempt had been made to augment this facility with the publication of some excellent magazines which were well received by the staff. These were edited and produced by Mr. D. Woods, a member of the finance department and unfortunately ceased after he left the Preston district.

A meeting arranged for 11th April 1973 by the Appointments Committee to appoint a consultant in plastic surgery was cancelled as only one application for the post had been received.

Forms were issued early in May 1973 to each member of the H.M.C. for completion and return to the secretary by those wishing to apply for membership of the area health authority. The applications which had to be returned by 26th May 1973 were later submitted by twelve members.

Assurance was sought from the R.H.B. regarding the existing endowment funds available to the hospital management committees and the effect that reorganisation would have on these. In its reply the R.H.B. stated that advice on this subject was to be issued by the D.H.S.S. in due course.

Early in May 1973 it was reported that a tender had been received for the building of the new Preston hospital and this had been submitted to the Manchester R.H.B. On 30th July 1973 a special meeting of the H.M.C. was called primarily to give members an update on the results of a meeting held between the Secretary of State for Health, Sir Keith Joseph, officers of the Manchester R.H.B. and Mr. W. Bennett, chairman of the Preston and Chorley H.M.C. This followed an announcement made by the Secretary of State that he had decided not to approve the lowest tender of approximately £12 million for the building of the new hospital as he felt that a lower tender than the one already received was possible and he wanted to put the project back for tender. He indicated, however, that he had no intention of cutting back in the provision of the services planned and he firmly believed that completion could be achieved by 1978. The Hospital Management Committee called for a meeting between themselves, the Regional Hospital Board and the Secretary of State and it was eventually arranged for Sir Keith Joseph to visit Preston on 24th October 1973. Another visit to the Infirmary was arranged for 3rd October by the local M.P.s, Mr. A. Green and Mrs. Connie Monks, instigated by the medical staff.

In the weeks before Sir Keith Joseph's visit a campaign began against his decision regarding Preston's new hospital generated by the local press and the consultant staff who produced a document denigrating the Infirmary in an attempt to change his views on the matter. The situation was changed following a general election with a new administration at central government and the decision to proceed with the new Preston hospital by phasing the programme of construction. The Regional Hospital Board arranged a meeting on 30th November 1973 to discuss the phasing programme.

This, however, was not the end of the matter as far as the Hospital Management Committee were concerned for at its final meeting on 27th March 1974 members were advised of information concerning the new hospital supplied to a member of the H.M.C. and which had been the subject of recent press articles. Members viewed with alarm the information attributable to the North Western Regional Health Authority that a major capital scheme other than the new Preston hospital was to be given a higher priority in the region's building programme. The last act in the drama of the H.M.C. before disbanding was to register their protest to the R.H.B., the newly formed Lancashire Area Health Authority and the local MPs, following repeated promises of several Secretaries of State in recent years.

Throughout this, however, the work of the Infirmary carried on and at a special meeting held on 30th July 1973, Mr. W. A. Robson, the consultant obstetrician and gynaecologist drew attention to the disruption that would arise at Preston Royal Infirmary during the installation of the new lift shaft and alterations to the antenatal clinic in the maternity department, work on which was expected to commence on 16th September 1973 extending over a period of some four months. It would, he explained, be necessary during this period either to transfer confinements booked at P.R.I. to Sharoe Green Hospital or, if possible, to be confined at home. A system of 48 hour discharges for normal confinements was to be introduced. The building work associated with the new lift shaft was completed, however, late in September 1973 allowing for the re-admission of patients.

In September 1973 there was a call to change the H.M.C. policy regarding the admission of members of the press to its meetings, especially in view of the special importance of reorganisation. The H.M.C. decided they would not change their policy although full press statements would continue to be issued. The R.H.B. gave approval for the appointment of a locum consultant or medical assistant post in general medicine pending Dr. Temperley taking up his appointment as consultant physician to the Preston Group.

The purchase, as a matter of urgency of a replacement blood gas analyser for the group accident research unit at a cost of £1,430 was agreed by the H.M.C. on 1st October 1973 and early in November, increases were levied on meal charges following a recommendation from the D.H.S.S. and a report was requested on the cost of provisions at Preston Royal Infirmary which was to include an examination of the kitchen's facilities.

The resignation was announced from 31st December 1973 of the Rev. W. Elliott, chaplain to P.R.I. The secretary reported that it was not possible to offer the vacancy for this post on a full-time basis and with the concurrence of the Bishop of Lancaster it was recommended that the Rev. R. E. Meredith would fill the part-time appointment commencing from 1st January 1974.

The Hospital Management Committee, early in December 1973 decided that Fulwood U.D.C. should be charged the normal fee payable for their use of the mortuary facilities at P.R.I. In the new year H.M. Coroner expressed his interest and in February 1974 informed the H.M.C. that Fulwood U.D.C. would be prepared to pay with effect from 1st April 1973. A great deal of publicity in the *Lancashire Evening Post* had been issued on this subject and the H.M.C. felt that a further amount of £163 was also due to them in respect of the facilities used during the period January 1972 to March 1973.

In a routine visit to Preston Royal Infirmary and the Stanleyfield Road properties by members of the H.M.C., their report centred around the inadequacies of storage, bathroom and toilet facilities on many of the wards and to the restricted accommodation available to the treasurer's department staffs. They also commented upon the temporary theatre accommodation in the accident and emergencies department which had been made available as a result of the temporary closure of the small and twin theatres. An assurance was given that the accommodation being used as a theatre would revert back to its former use on completion of the work in the twin theatres but the other comments made in their report were only noted.

A recommendation was made by the group catering manager for increases in charges for certain items of food provided in staff restaurants due to increases in the price of commodities. The request was passed for discussion by the Joint Consultative Committee for their views before implementation.

The annual hospitals dances were held in Preston's Guild Hall on Friday 14th December and Saturday 15th December 1973; this venue eliminated the problem in 1972 when a number of people were disappointed through lack of tickets.

On 10th December 1973 Sister Annie Hewitt retired after more than 20 years service in Preston's hospitals, 14 years in the accident and emergency department at Preston Royal Infirmary.

There was a query in February 1974 regarding the accommodation at the Infirmary which was being used as offices by the Group headquarters staffs and whether they would revert to their original use as medical staff accommodation, if and when the Group staff vacated them. It was stated that this matter would be taken into consideration at the appropriate time but it was anticipated that it would be many months before other accommodation became available for district management team and H.Q. staffs. It was emphasised however, that the problem at P.R.I. was not for single but rather for married medical staff accommodation.

Early in February 1974 the Hospital Management Committee accepted the formal resignation of Mr. H. Hill and Mr. J. Hindle consequent to their appointments as district administrator and district finance officer respectively of the new Preston District Authority with effect from 1st February 1974, and from that same date the appointment of Mr. B. Calverly as acting Group secretary and Mr. S. J. Yorston as acting Group treasurer were also confirmed. Nominations were called for membership of Community Health Councils and 8 nominations were put forward. Dr. L. Robertson, director of the public health laboratory at Preston was appointed chairman of the Medical Executive Committee in succession to Dr. B. F. Brearley.

February 24th 1974 saw the re-opening of the maternity department at P.R.I. following extensive upgrading throughout, including the new lift shaft built to accommodate a modern lift later in the year. Bathroom facilities were extended and changing accommodation improved. The labour suite was supplied with C.S.S.D. and one of the delivery rooms had been enlarged but the upgrading of the antenatal clinic was still in progress and was not finally completed until August 1974. A further innovation was the installation of ultrasound equipment and a senior radiographer, Mrs. C. Barnes, had already been appointed for this unit.

Changes in nursing administration saw the resignation of Miss B. Blackstock, chief nursing officer, with effect from 22nd February 1974 and the appointment of Miss Thompson as acting chief nursing officer with immediate effect. Miss Doris Salisbury became the first district nursing officer for the Preston and Chorley District Management Team and together with Miss Thompson attended the first meeting of the D.M.T. on 4th March 1974.

In a foreword to the White Paper on reorganisation on the N.H.S., the Secretary of State wrote that the reorganisation was about administration, not about treatment and care. He amplified the statement by quoting an example 'that the future allocation of resources towards improvements for the service to the mentally ill and handicapped, and to the elderly and disabled would be carried out through a more integrated administrative machine'.

Thus the first reorganisation of the National Health Service since 1948 heralded a time of change, with the formation of a new tier of administration in Area Health Authorities and the replacement of hospital management committees, which would cease to function on 31st March 1974, by district management teams.

Chapter Seven

Improvements 1974-1975

THE District Management Team of the newly formed Preston District of the Lancashire Area Health Authority wasted little time by arranging their first meeting in Preston Royal Infirmary on the first day of the new administration, Monday 1st April 1974, the routine work of the hospitals in the new District carrying on as normal as if no change had taken place.

The first item to be discussed was a directive from the Area Health Authority which called for a scheme to be prepared to convert the east wing of the Civic Hostel at Fulwood to provide office accommodation for the district management team and its supporting staffs. At that time the Civic Hostel was let to the Preston Corporation social services department but they were using only the upper floors and were expected to vacate the east wing in the near future. In view of the decision by the Area Health Authority to terminate the lease of the premises occupied by the former health department of Preston Corporation, the need to provide alternative accommodation was urgent. It was anticipated that the whole scheme would take about 2 years to complete at a cost of up to £100,000 and it was not clear if this finance would be forthcoming from the Area Health Authority.

It was thought that the ground floor of the east wing of the Civic Hostel, being a three storey construction, could be occupied by the finance department with a staff of 57. The first floor would house the nursing staff and some medical services with the remainder of the medical service together with administration and its associated functions on the second floor. The actual number of nursing and administrative staffs to be accommodated was not known at that time with the reorganisation proving to be a period of rapid expansion.

Miss Salisbury, the district nursing officer, advised the D.M.T. that in addition to the senior nursing staffs with their clerical assistants, office space would be needed to be found for 20 health visitors and 40 district nursing sisters who were at that time occupying central accommodation in the offices of the Corporation health department. The possibility of providing accommodation elsewhere for these staffs at reasonable cost was considered unlikely and the alternative suggestion of allowing nursing sisters to be based in their own homes was not pursued as the cost of installing telephones would cost initially £1,600 with an annual charge of some £1,000 rental. Later it was found that the need for accommodation for the district's nursing sisters in the Civic Hostel scheme was unlikely as the problem resolved itself when they became attached to health centres and clinics through which they could be contacted at any time. It was felt that as long as there was a duty room available there would be no necessity to provide telephones in their homes.

The Medical Executive Committee expressed their concern at the provision of patient accommodation at Preston Royal Infirmary and felt that 'there was a need for an intensive care unit, additional beds and improved staff facilities to enable the hospital to carry out its functions over the next five years'. It was pointed out, however, that the North West Regional Health Authority had already determined its priorities for Preston District and was proceeding with the provision of a new hospital and major improvements in facilities for psychiatric and geriatric care at Sharoe Green Hospital. Under these circumstances the possibility of money being made available for further extensions at Preston Royal Infirmary was very remote. The M.E.C. suggested that in order to relieve pressure on beds at P.R.I. perhaps one speciality needed to evacuate to other accommodation and, following wide-ranging discussion on the utilization of beds and the identification of spare capacity in the Health District generally, an approach was made to the division of surgery to consider a more flexible use of empty surgical beds at Sharoe Green Hospital.

In May 1974 the alterations to the top floor of maternity to accommodate the ultrasound equipment had been completed and the upgrading of the antenatal clinic was scheduled to be completed by mid-June. New floor coverings were laid in the out-patient department and also the ground floor ward in maternity and work was completed on the installation of an emergency generator for the Infirmary. The building schedule for the Infirmary for the years 1974/75 were issued in May 1974.

	Estimated Cost
External Decoration	£4,558
Internal painting, wall washing in Boiler House	£594
Pointing, roof and window repairs in Children's Ward	£900
Floor covering in Alice & Orthopaedic Wards & Typing Pool	£1,189
Improvements and adaptations to Physiotherapy & Boiler House	£1,560
Electrical renewal and rewiring in Twin Theatre, Basement corridor and the Finance Department	£950

Restructuring was proposed for the finance department which showed two principal sections, one for financial management and the other for financial services, together with a small audit department to supplement the services provided. The estimated cost of this new structure was £140,680, an increase of some £24,000 over the cost of the former finance administration but this was not considered unreasonable in that the new department was taking over the services formerly provided by the local authority's treasurer's department. However, the problem still remained of the lack of accommodation for the finance department, crammed as it was in the small former dwelling houses opposite the out-patient department in Stanleyfield Road.

It was anticipated that the accommodation at the Civic Hostel would be delayed for two years before it became ready for occupancy. This caused the D.M.T. problems regarding where to put the staff of community division 'A' as there was insufficient accommodation in the Blackpool Road premises formerly occupied by the Preston Executive Council and further problems would arise with the closure in September 1974 of the Market Street premises. The Area Health Authority was pressed to make finance available for the provision of temporary accommodation for the Preston District Management Team and arrangements were made to purchase a property in St. Paul's Road, Preston, for conversion into temporary office units.

There was a further call by the Medical Executive Committee for improvements to the residential accommodation in the Infirmary for medical staff. There was an urgent need to make it more attractive and convenient which was, they claimed, a major factor in attracting suitable applicants for posts. The introduction of extended cover in the medical records department at P.R.I. to enable the department to be opened until 8 p.m. had resulted in the supervisory staff having to work considerably longer hours so the decision was taken to upgrade a clerical assistant on a temporary basis to the grade of higher clerical officer.

The Ladies Comforts League held their annual meeting at P.R.I. on 30th April 1974. Founded in 1912, their collections in 1973 had raised £500 which was used to replace cubicle curtains on the wards in the Infirmary.

April 1974 saw the retirement of Mr. J. Maddocks, area supplies officer since 1971. He had commenced his service in the supplies department at P.R.I. in 1948 as deputy to Mr. Beggs, succeeding him in 1963 as Group supplies officer. A new appointment was announced of Dr. G. Holt as the district community physician for the Preston district.

Plans were approved for the provision of an intensive care unit at P.R.I. and sent to the A.H.A. for final approval. The scheme issued in June 1974 proposed the provision of 5 or 6 intensive care beds adjacent to the accident and emergency department which would utilize the multiple injuries unit, the old hearing aid department and the courtyard between the multiple injuries unit and West Ward. This meant moving the hearing aid department to a new site on a vacant plot of land on Stanleyfield Road. It was also proposed to provide alternative accommodation for social workers on a site adjacent to the physiotherapy department which, while not being an ideal site, did provide an *en bloc* social work area which would be accessible to out-patients and would enable office accommodation to be utilized by accident and emergency senior staff in the space made available by the move. Additional accommodation for the medical ward was also proposed in the scheme, the total cost of which was estimated to be £57,000 and it was hoped to phase the work starting in August 1974 so allowing for the budget cost to be extended over two years, 1974/75 and 1975/76.

The additional accommodation proposed for the medical ward would relieve the overcrowded facilities by providing an E.C.G. room for treatment and storage of equipment, a waiting area for relatives of seriously ill patients and a treatment/examination room. The anticipated time for these alterations was some three or four months but the intensive care unit would take at least twelve months to complete and it might be necessary during part of that time to close both West Ward and the multiple injuries unit.

The Medical Executive Committee early in June 1974 expressed concern at the closure of the private patients ward at Preston Royal Infirmary, urging that it should be reopened as soon as possible. Several times during the next few months this was raised and each time the answer was given that repeated advertisements for nursing vacancies on the ward had resulted in no application being received. The M.E.C. eventually wrote to the British Medical Association in September 1974 asking them to take the issue up with the Department of Health but the private wards at P.R.I. remained closed and were never reopened.

Details were issued in June 1974 of projects currently in progress, including roof repairs to the theatre (£101.20), office accommodation alterations in the physiotherapy department (£242.39), work on the neuro unit (£142.89), repairs and renewal of air vents and the steam trap in the laundry (£150) and renewal of the feed pumps in the boiler house (£630).

A donation of more than £250 toward the cost of a microwave heat treatment machine for the Infirmary's physiotherapy department was presented to Mr. R. S. Garden, senior orthopaedic consultant, by the ladies section of the Garstang National Farmers Union.

Miss Jane Duxbury, a member of the catering staff at Preston Royal Infirmary for 34 years retired in June 1974, the majority of her service being spent catering to the Infirmary's night staffs. Mrs. Elizabeth Wearden, employed in the sewing room for many years, died suddenly on 11th June 1974 while on a cruising holiday in the Mediterranean; she was buried at sea. The death was also announced of Student Nurse Janet Preston who died following an accident on her scooter going home after duty in the Infirmary and her parents later donated a bookcase for sister's office in her memory.

The Hospital Welfare Society presented a cheque for £350 at the end of May 1974 toward the cost of the day room on Alice Ward and they also donated two television sets and two telephone trolleys. Industrial action nationally by nurses was having minimal disruption to the normal working pattern of the hospitals in the Group and so too did the industrial action from 6th July by radiographers following a dispute over their pay. The cost per person per week in the Infirmary's beds was announced as follows, September 1973 - £3.39, December 1973 - £3.38, January 1974 - £3.34 and March 1974 - £3.31.

Early in July it was announced that there would be no money available for the Civic Hostel scheme in the current year. Three months later, on 3rd October 1974, the Regional Health Authority visited Preston to consider future capital programmes and it was agreed then that top priority should be given to the conversion of the Civic Hostel to provide D.M.T. offices at an estimated cost of £170,000, an increase of £60,000 over the estimated figure of the previous April when the scheme was first announced. A host of other projects, some 25 in all, were also given top priority throughout the health district.

An urgent application was made to the N.W.R.H.B. for the appointment of additional consultants in microbiology and morbid anatomy. These posts were approved by the D.H.S.S. in July 1974 but owing to the financial position it was decided that it was not possible for the D.M.T. to proceed with them but that they would be advertised when sufficient finance became available.

The retirement was announced of Mr. W. H. Todd, senior consultant obstetrician and gynaecologist in Preston since October 1946, who had specialised mainly at Sharoe Green Hospital. The same month saw the retirement of Mr. H. Gillet, group catering officer after 28 years service at Preston Royal Infirmary; he too had arrived in Preston in 1946. Another departure at that time was Mr. G. A. Sandham, a porter at P.R.I. for 20 years who retired due to ill health early in 1974. Miss Mabel Brooks retired after 20 years service in the Infirmary's pharmacy unfortunately dying suddenly early in 1977; the death was announced of Mrs. Riddell of Scorton who had been president of the Ladies Comfort League from 1934-1970.

Further industrial action, this time by audiology technicians, arose, the action taking the form of refusing to participate in new procedures or attending any courses connected with new procedures or equipment, aimed, it was presumed, at disrupting the introduction of a new hearing aid. Services continued to be restricted by radiographers in their dispute over pay levels on July 19th, 23rd, 24th and 25th and August 1st, 6th, 14th, 23rd and 28th. On these dates they would only deal with urgent cases under the same conditions they would operate on statutory public holidays.

Under a scheme for the retraining of married lady doctors, Dr. (Mrs.) B. Taylor was appointed as supernumary senior registrar in medicine to undertake duties in the Infirmary and at Sharoe Green Hospital for five sessions a week.

It was announced early in July 1974 that the Regional Health Authority had invited tenders from 7 firms for Phase 1 of the new Preston hospital, the closing date for receipt of these being 19th September 1974. Approval was received early in August from N.W.R.H.A. for the demolition of farm buildings on the site purchased for the new hospital at a total cost of £910 made up as follows:

(a) Demolition of buildings associated with Manor House Farm	£650
(b) Demolition of buildings of Blackhurst Farm & Cottage	£230
(c) Removal by NORWEB of redundant electricity services	£30

Accommodation was found for the medical illustrations department in the grounds of Ribbleton Hospital and the District Management Team sent a request to the Area Health Authority for an increase in staff for the ultrasonic scan department in the maternity department pending the appointment of an additional consultant radiologist. There was a request by the surgical division to improve and expand the plaster room facilities at P.R.I. They also recommended changes they considered necessary in the accident and emergency department, i.e. the installation of plastic type swing doors at the entrance to casualty from the main hall to minimise noise and dust and to maintain privacy; that an area be set aside in the dressing room for two trolleys so that it could be used also as an admission block and they wanted the provision of additional clerical staff so that a 24 hour service could be provided for the documentation of patients. The first request was agreed by the D.M.T. as a matter of urgency but the other recommendations were to be considered more fully, eventually all the changes being accomplished.

The minor capital programme for 1974/75, issued early in August 1974, included the installation of autoclaves in the small theatre at a cost of £1,500, the supply of an operating lamp into the ophthalmic operating theatre (£1,750) and an automatic coal feed system in the boiler house at a cost of £7,000; this item was later deferred until the 1975/76 programme. The building supervisor reported that during July and August 1974 building work had been completed in the upgrading of the antenatal clinic, the Preston Royal Infirmary workshops had been repainted, the rear road of the Infirmary had been concreted and the laboratory footpath had also been reconcreted. The fixtures and fittings in the neuro unit were almost completed.

The R.H.A. indicated support for the acquisition of a plot of land between Stanleyfield Road and St. Paul's Road and while this was achieved any plans for its ultimate use never came to fruition; it was used as a car park for the Infirmary.

The finance officer drew attention to a deficit in the trading account for the out-patient buffet during the year ending 31st March 1974. It was noted that charges for refreshments had remained unaltered since 1971 so an immediate increase in the price of a cup of tea to 3p was agreed with further increases in other charges to follow after investigations.

The financial situation for the Preston District for the months of April, May and June indicated an overall net overspending of £24,941 which practically absorbed the reserve held, *viz* £25,976. It was reported that stricter control needed to be exercised for the remainder of the current financial period, especially in those departments showing the higher expenditure trends, namely:

(a) Provisions	£16,910
(b) Medical appliances and equipment	£13,000
(c) General services	£23,000
(d) Buildings	£29,000
(e) Domestic repairs	£23,000

These overspendings were chiefly in the hospital sectors of the District together with provisions at Whittingham Hospital. An example was given of the tremendous impact of the rise in the price of oil during 1973 where the main boiler plant at Sharoe Green Hospital consumed 630,000 gallons during the year 1973/74 at a cost of £45,000, the cost for the current year being £90,000, exactly double, and this did not take into account any further price rises occurring later in the year.

Two members of the D.M.T., County Councillor Mrs. Horam and Mr. Cannon, made an obligatory visit to inspect the Infirmary and in their report recorded certain 'black spots'. On the storage of medical records they commented 'on the fire risk in the basement area where records were stored' and also pointed out 'the tiny size' (8′ × 7′) of the office used by the medical records officer. The kitchen was too small to cater for the 600-700 meals provided daily. The floor was slippery and more guards needed to be provided for the equipment used. The provision of just one small cold store for perishable goods was insufficient and the smell in the potato peeling area of the kitchen was, they reported, appalling. The air conditioning system was so antiquated it refused to function at all and it was not surprising that there were serious staffing problems. They recommended that the Area Health Authority should consider the need to appoint a safety officer. The casualty department too was criticised, the members being appalled to find that this major accident hospital for the Preston District had only three cubicles in which to receive patients and there appeared to be insufficient seating facilities in the waiting area. They readily supported the proposals for the provision of an intensive care unit. The children's clinic and waiting room they found completely inadequate, being very inaccessible to mothers with young children. The pathology department, built as recently as 1958, they found chronically overcrowded and in their opinion dangerous. They reported a need for the display of a fire exit sign in the nurses home, even though the means of exit was by way of one of the sister's flats and their condemnation of the boiler house was devastating. Mrs. Horman and Mr. Cannon reiterated, however, that they were reporting on the poorer services of Preston Royal Infirmary and they wished to stress in their report that many of the facilities they had visited, such as physiotherapy and hydrotherapy, urology, the maternity departments, the nurses home and in particular the day room and overnight stay facilities erected by voluntary efforts were extremely good. They also made note of:

> the fact that the Private Patients Wards remained padlocked and recommended that a decision needed to be made whether this was a permanent arrangement and if so whether alternative use might be made of the accommodation.

With the growth of the transport department in the summer of 1974 it was decided to replace the petrol pump situated on the back road of the Infirmary at a cost of £352, as the old one had nearly rusted away with age. It was agreed to convert rooms on the maternity ground floor to provide teaching accommodation at a cost of £775 and in his report for August/September 1974 the building supervisor reported that work on this scheme had already begun. An alternative scheme at a cost of £2,500 was suggested for the genito-urinary theatre which would include the provision of a W.C. and changing cubicle in addition to a new corridor and entrance. The purpose of the corridor was to enable G.U. out-patients to gain direct access (via the Holden Ward/laboratory corridor and the proposed new corridor) to the second theatre position in the G.U. theatre without having to pass through the first theatre. This would permit fuller and more flexible use of the G.U. theatre generally and was the scheme that was eventually adopted.

The Medical Executive Committee raised the question of the increasing difficulty being experienced by medical staff in finding car parking spaces at the Infirmary and a sub-committee consisting of Miss Salisbury, Mr. B. Calverley and Dr. L. Robertson was set up to investigate and report back to the D.M.T. Dr. W. R. Swinburn was appointed to the post of consultant in rheumatology and rehabilitation to the Preston District and Wrightington Hospital from 1st January 1975. The four rheumatology beds at Sharoe Green Hospital were transferred to the Infirmary in beds released by Dr. Temperley who was to use the vacated beds at S.G.H. for gastro-intestinal endoscopy examinations.

The decision was taken to continue the policy of 48 hour discharge which came into force as a result of the temporary closure of the maternity department and from 1st October 1974 S.G.H. would operate the same policy in the light of the trend toward 100% hospital confinements. It was believed that this would lead to considerable integration between the staff in the hospital and the community.

Following re-organisation in the Preston District, the second in line posts were announced as follows:

> Mr. Brian Calverley as general administrator in operational management. Mr. Richard Pearson as general administrator in planning.

A progress report issued in September 1974 on the projects undertaken in the Infirmary included alterations in the maternity department, internal decorating of rooms in the nurses home, redecoration in the children's ward including the fitting of new window frames in various rooms, redecoration of the dental department and the children's clinic. Redecoration of the orthoptic department in Stanleyfield Road had also been completed and at no. 36 Stanleyfield Road a serious structural fault had been revealed making it necessary to replace the curtain joists and rebuild part of the rear elevation brickwork. There was also work in progress on Green Ward, involving the replacement of the west elevation windows which had been damaged during a storm. Expenditure had also been necessary for roof repairs along the West Ward corridor (£42.59) and repairs to some plasterwork in the pathology department (£42.16). In October 1974 a proposal was made to rearrange the dining rooms in P.R.I. by converting the staff dining room into a snack/sandwich bar (later christened 'The Bistro') and to integrate all staff except medical staff into the nurses dining room for hot meals.

The Medical Executive Committee in November 1974 was asked to consider their policy for the retention of medical records owing to increasing problems with storage accommodation for these records in P.R.I. A number of options were considered, including microfilming and the destruction of records after a set period of time. The balance of opinion was that records should not be destroyed and the process of microfilming was considered unsatisfactory and at that time expensive. It was felt therefore that steps should be taken to increase the storage accommodation available and before any final decision was taken on the matter a comparison on the relative cost of each course of action needed to be made.

It was reported that fifty applications had been received in reply to the advertisements for the post of registrar in general surgery at Preston Royal Infirmary. Six candidates were called for interview on Wednesday 7th November 1974 and an appointment made to commence on the 13th November.

On 2nd October 1974 four hundred people gathered in the Charter Theatre of Preston's Guild Hall to witness the handing over of certificates and prizes to over 100 nurses and mid-wives. This was the first prize giving ceremony held since the re-organisation and also the first combined ceremony for both nurses and mid-wives. It was also the fiftieth anniversary of the awarding of gold and silver medals in Preston.

The report of the Halsbury Committee of Inquiry into the pay and conditions of service of nurses and mid-wives had been received, as had communications giving guidance on the implementation of the awards made to nurses and mid-wives. Difficulties, however, arose in implementing them due in no small part to the increase in the number of staff necessary to do so, the alternative being the temporary closure of some of the departments over the Christmas holiday period. Discussions were arranged between the senior nursing staff and members of the finance and administration departments to determine a District policy on the interpretation and subsequent implementation of the Halsbury awards. The Medical Executive Committee approved arrangements that were made for the closure of wards at Sharoe Green Hospital to enable the nursing staff to take the additional holidays awarded under the Halsbury Report but no alterations were made to the ward situation in the Infirmary. The situation came into force on 23rd December 1974 and was to be reviewed monthly but it was anticipated that the service would revert to normal as from April 1975, by which time the nursing staff would have taken their additional holidays. The medical staff, however, were concerned not only that the arrangements were well publicised but that the reasons for the action were made clear and they also stressed the probable consequence of the increases in waiting lists which would result.

Notification was received in November 1974 from the N.W.R.H.A. that purchase of the plot of land adjoining Stanleyfield Road for the proposed new hearing aid department, had been completed. In December the medical executive committee raised the question of the bed situation in the Preston District and the particular problem of finding beds for additional consultants, also the unsuitability of some beds for the specialities to which they were allocated. It was reported that a recent meeting with the social services department representatives had highlighted the fact that there was little hope of alleviating the bed shortage by the discharge of patients to social service accommodation because no such facility was available.

The District Management Team were also appraised that recent meetings had been held between the R.H.A. and the Area Health Authority which made it clear that funds would not be forthcoming for the conversion of the Civic Hostel to provide offices for the District Management Team headquarters. In view of this it was agreed to make enquiries regarding the renting of office accommodation in the Preston town centre and obtain approval from the A.H.A. for this course of action as a matter of urgency. They re-emphasised the fact that it was essential to move headquarters staff from the Preston Royal Infirmary, not only to improve administrative efficiency but to enable improvements to be made to the environment of the patients and the staff of the Infirmary.

Early in January 1975 the D.M.T. discussed the position in the Health District resulting from the introduction of 'sanctions' by the consultant medical staff; any disruption had been limited at that time but it was expected that the effect could be intensified if the action continued.

A move by the N.W.R.H.A. to close the Infirmary's laundry, under a scheme to rationalise the laundry arrangements with the District, resulted in no decision being made until the D.M.T. had been given the results of a works study programme being carried out by the Regional Hospital Authority on both the laundry and transport services in the Preston District prior to the introduction of incentive bonus schemes.

Early in 1975 Miss Alice Corbishley, a member of the Infirmary's sewing room staff for 32 years, retired, as did David Sharples, technician in the E.N.T. theatre for 20 of his 28 years service in P.R.I., his retirement unfortunately lasting only until February 1977 when Mr. Sharples died. Another member of the Infirmary staff died around this time, Cyril Kershaw, who was employed at Preston Royal Infirmary for over 40 years and remembered mainly as the porter in the maternity department. In February 1975 Mr. Stephen Davies was appointed to the post of district personnel officer being among the many changes to the administrative structure in P.R.I. at this period; Mr. S. Rawlinson being appointed principal administrative assistant and Mr. N. Sutcliffe, principal administrative assistant (salaries and wages) in the finance department with effect from 28th January 1975.

Acute problems due to the lack of office accommodation for the finance department, split into two units at this stage in P.R.I. and Whittingham Hospital, was restricting the effective working and integration of the department. It was claimed that because of the cramped conditions in the finance department, housed in Stanleyfield Road, sickness among the staff was at a high level, with some 330 days having been lost through absence, with 26 members of staff out of a total of 35 having been ill for periods varying from one day to others as high as 77, 46 and 39 days.

Once again the urgent necessity to find alternative accommodation was raised. The situation regarding the conversion of the Civic Hostel at this time was that permission had been received from the N.W.R.H.A. for the work to commence and a sum of £9,819 had already been used for the purchase of building materials and carpets. Work on the conversion was expected to commence on the 14th April 1975 but the question still remained of finance; in August the A.H.A. allowed a sum of £20,000 toward the conversion which made it necessary to control the expenditure on the upgrading very carefully.

A meeting was held in the Infirmary on 31st January 1975, called following representations made on behalf of the nursing staff over fears regarding the risks involved while working in the multiple injuries unit. The main concern was the recent introduction of haemodialysis in the unit and the possibility of infection from hepatitis. Dr. D. N. Hutchinson reassured the meeting, although he did express the view that the unit opening directly onto the main throroughfare of the Infirmary's accident and emergency department did create major problems for the control of cross infection. A code of practice for use by all staff working in the multiple injuries unit was drawn by Dr. D. A. L. Watt and a recommendation was made by Miss Salisbury that 4 nursing sisters be appointed to staff the unit, so making it unnecessary to rely on the nursing staff of the accident and emergency department; the unit could also call on the nursing bank for further staff as required.

The nursing bank was proposed by the district nursing officer in February 1975, its purpose being to have a pool of part time trained staff willing to work for short periods of time at little notice. The aim was twofold: to provide increased nurse cover and to provide an opportunity for trained nurses to keep in touch with modern trends during a period when family commitments prevented permanent employment. Obviously aimed at trained S.R.N. and S.E.N. nurses with young families, it was hoped to employ some 20 nurses in the first instance. The district nursing officer issued a report she had received from the North West Regional Nurse Training Committee following their visit to the Preston School of Nursing on the 18th April 1975. Concern was expressed regarding the conditions under which students and pupils were being trained at Preston Royal Infirmary and they stated that there was no evidence of any real improvements having been carried out since their last visit to P.R.I. in October 1973. The D.M.T. was asked to regard the improvements and safeguards recommended as a top priority in 1975.

The District Management Team recorded its approval and pleasure at the decision of the D.H.S.S. to proceed with Phase 1 of the new Preston hospital in May 1975; later, in July, the N.W.R.H.B. accepted a tender for Phase 1 at a cost of:

Building and Engineering	£6,728,487
Furniture and equipment (including X-Ray)	£801,007
Fees	£928,829
	£8,458,323

The contract was for 36 months and work was expected to begin on 1st August 1975.

The question of the private ward was again raised by the M.E.C. in a letter to the Area Health Authority. They were once again informed that the ward had been closed due to staff shortages which was unconnected with the national situation which had subsequently developed regarding private beds. A meeting between the consultants and representatives of the trades unions was suggested in an attempt to resolve what they considered to be a waste of valuable resources. Such a meeting, however, did not take place and the private ward at Preston Royal Infirmary never re-opened again in that capacity. It was noted that the number of out-patients awaiting appointments at P.R.I. on the 1st May was 2,399 and Miss Salisbury drew attention to the problems experienced by the nursing staff as a result of the shortage of beds for emergency cases at P.R.I.

Chapter Eight

The new hospital takes shape 1975-1979

AMONG the comings and goings early in 1975 were the appointment of Mr. M. R. Wharton, formerly senior registrar as consultant in orthopaedics to replace Mr. Garden from 1st April 1975 and Dr. N. K. Siakia, consultant in dermatology from the same date.

In February 1975 Mr. R. S. Garden M.B., M.Ch. Orth., F.R.C.S., F.R.C.S. (Edin), senior consultant orthopaedic surgeon retired. Having qualified in Aberdeen in 1934, he came to Preston Royal Infirmary as a house surgeon and, following war service as a Lieutenant Colonel in the R.A.M.C., he returned to Preston where his work brought the name of P.R.I. as a progressive orthopaedic centre to the notice of orthopaedic surgeons throughout the world. I consider it an honour and a privilege to have assisted Mr. Garden with some aspects of his research work during our years at Preston Royal Infirmary.

Mr. Roland Beare left the service having served in the supplies department since April 1949. Sister Marjorie Oakley who had been associated with P.R.I. for more than 20 years, latterly as sister on East Ward, retired to become a relief district nursing officer. There were many appointments made during this period to the district administrative team, including Mr. R. E. Oxburgh, finance, from the 30th June 1975, Miss C. M. Forster, personnel department, from 7th July 1975 and Mr. J. F. Calderbank, District Headquarters (planning) from 1st July 1975, these few appointments illustrating the expansion of the National Health Service taking place as a result of re-organisation. Another aspect of the re-organisation became apparent early in 1976 when a directive was issued to all staff members throughout the Preston District making them conscious of the need to exercise economy due to financial restraints.

The Department of Health and Social Security called for 'restraint in costings' and proposed a standstill, i.e. the full year cost of management staff in all disciplines on the payroll in March 1976 should not be exceeded during the financial year 1976/77. They later issued a document entitled *Review of the National Health Service Management Costs,* a scheme advising cuts of 5% and 10% in management budgets and indicating further re-organisation of the service with proposals for the abolition of some health districts by merger.

Another D.H.S.S. document issued entitled *The Way Forward* quoted:

> while the Government has ensured that there will continue to be at least a modest rate of increase in resources for these services in the country as a whole, I appreciate that we cannot hope to make significant and rapid changes in the desired directions without a more rapid growth of resources. I am convinced that there is scope for making faster progress in the desired directions by making better use of the resources which we have already. In some Districts, long sought improvements will be further delayed. Some Hospitals will have to continue to manage with facilities which are outdated or inadequate. The expectations both of the professions and of users will not be satisfied. In other places where services are not under the same pressure, the provision of new facilities which are expensive will have to be postponed . . . But the further restraint required implies increased rationalization, closure of some units, curtailment of some Services in some places and more effective use of staff and facilities.

This, then, was 'The Way Forward' following the re-organisation of the National Health Service only two years before.

In May 1976 the Government set up a Royal Commission on the National Health Service to consider, in the interests of the patients and those who work in the N.H.S., the best use and management of the financial and manpower resources of the National Health Service. Its report, issued in July 1979, considered the objectives of the N.H.S. should be:

(1) to encourage and assist individuals to remain healthy.
(2) to provide equality of entitlement to health services.
(3) to provide a broad range of services of a high standard.
(4) to provide equality of access to these services.
(5) to provide a service free at the time of use.
(6) to satisfy the reasonable expectations of its users.
(7) to remain nationally responsive to local needs.

When presenting the report of the Royal Commission to Parliament, the Secretary of State indicated that the report 'merited careful study' but he drew attention in particular to the recommendation 'that the administration of the Health Service should be simplified by eliminating, in most cases, one tier of management' and the recognition by the Commission 'that management decisions should be taken at the lowest effective level'. The Secretary of State indicated that he would be issuing a document on the major issues of structure and management, giving the first indication of a further re-organisation of the N.H.S., admitting the failure of the 1974 re-organisation structure.

The Medical Executive Committee continued to express its concern at what they considered the inadequate facilities available at Preston Royal Infirmary and in June 1975 outlined the urgent remedial action they considered essential to allow the Infirmary to carry out its function as the main acute hospital for the Preston district. They stressed the point that it was essential for the action to be taken to enable the Infirmary to continue this function for the next ten years until the completion of Phase 2 of the new hospital.

Their suggestions included the utilization of the newly acquired site adjoining Stanleyfield Road to provide car parking, so relieving the congestion in the Infirmary's forecourt, accommodation for medical records and x-ray storage, a new hearing aid department and accommodation for medical social workers. They raised yet again the provision of an intensive therapy unit, suggesting it should be built on the Infirmary's tennis courts and for which plans were under consideration for the purchase of three portakabins. They proposed the transfer of the pharmacy into the accommodation vacated by the multiple injuries unit, with a pharmacy store to be built adjacent to the main store which would allow the expansion of the accident and emergency and the x-ray departments into the accommodation vacated by the pharmacy. Extensions to the department of pathology by the provision of portakabins were also proposed along with an upgrading of the houses in Stanleyfield Road to provide staff residences when these premises were finally vacated by the District H.Q. staffs.

It was agreed that these proposals for development at P.R.I. should be put to the area and regional officers and that a case should be made for an additional allocation of funds to be made available in the current financial year to enable the work to commence as soon as possible. A further meeting was held on Wednesday 3rd September 1975, attended by all those most concerned in the provision of an intensive care unit, to discuss at length all aspects of the situation. The major problem was of course the availability of space for such a unit and the possible sites were agreed to be:

(1) The tennis court.
(2) Conversion of West Ward.
(3) A conversion of the day room recently provided by the Welfare Society.
(4) The recently acquired land in Stanleyfield Road.

It was finally agreed that the most suitable site was the first mentioned, the tennis court, and it was agreed that the scheme would be linked with an extension of the laboratory and in view of this proposed laboratory extensions would have to be postponed. The whole scheme including the cost of a comprehensive care unit was to be submitted to the Area Health Authority as a top priority for the 1976/77 programme.

During this period the multiple injuries unit at P.R.I. remained closed for many months due to a lack of trained staff and facilities. An internal adaptation to provide a 3-bed intensive care unit at a cost of some £3,500, subject to suitable arrangements being made for medical and nursing staff cover, was proposed in November 1975 but in March 1976 further proposals were made for re-opening the unit and a request was made for yet another meeting to discuss this very vexing subject.

In June 1975 there was a proposal to install an E.M.I. body scanner into the Infirmary with the full agreement of the regional scientific officer but this too resulted in protracted delay so that in March 1976 the Medical Executive Committee expressed its concern at the delay in installation and in April 1976 it was reported that the scanner, still not installed, had become out of date and a further £50,000 would be needed to update it. In January the E.M.I. scanner was put out to tender and was finally installed in December 1976. In January 1977, however, the District Management Team received a letter from the Area Health Authority advising that the updating of the scanner would probably take place some months after the machine had been put into operation. The updating itself would take some five to seven weeks to complete, during which time the scanner would be out of action; the cost of the update would be met by the D.H.S.S. The estimated running cost of the scanner was £31,000 per annum and staffing costs would probably be £17,000.

Mr. S. Farrar arrived at the Infirmary on 30th June 1975 to commence his duties as administrator and Mr. J. Flaherty was appointed to the post of deputy group secretary on 9th July 1975. It was a sign of the times when in June 1975 a decision was taken to replace the black and white television sets on the wards to colour television sets as and when the old sets needed replacing.

Among the many changes taking place in the Infirmary the most spectacular were some of the structural alterations made to accommodate further expansion of services. By March 1975 the scheme was completed to upgrade the genito-urinary theatre and install new x-ray equipment, the alterations to the dining room were completed and made available to staff members other than nurses. The occupational therapy department was extended to provide a practice room and double glazing was fitted to the balconies of the medical ward, the children's ward, Brown and Green Wards and to the orthopaedic ward. Repairs were carried out on the roof of the small theatre and both Holden Ward and the records department offices were redecorated. The eye ward too was decorated and access made to attached portakabins to extend the ward's cramped accommodation and vending machines were placed into the new snack bar christened 'The Bistro'. In the main kitchen, including the vegetable preparation room, during June and July 1975, tiles were laid to both floors and walls in a general upgrading of the Infirmary's basement area and in August at the request of the A.H.A. a list of ten schemes was submitted for consideration in the 1976/77 small capital schemes programme. Top priority was given to the following schemes for the Infirmary:

Priority I	An upgrading of the E.N.T. theatre at a cost of £60,000.
Priority II	Provision of a medical records office, occupational therapy, a car park and hearing aid department at a cost of £200,000 (utilizing the new site in Stanleyfield Road).
Priority III	Complete rewiring of the nurses home at a cost of £25,000.
Priority IV	A replacement lift for Alice/Albert Wards (£20,000).
Priority V	New boilers for the boiler house (£175,000).
Priority VI	Improve the lighting in maternity and rewire the ground floor (£20,000); also ventilation to the labour suite (£10,000).
Priority VII	Upgrade the kitchens (£75,000).
Priority VIII	To supply accommodation associated with the new E.M.I. body scanner (£20,000). A request was also made for the provision of an intensive care unit, upgrading and resiting of the pharmacy and extensions to the children's clinic.

Looking further ahead to 1977/78, also in discussion in August 1975, major extensions to the pathology department at an estimated cost of £80,000 and an upgrading of the children's ward estimated at £75,000 and a renewal of the air conditioning plant in the x-ray department (£10,000) were envisaged. Top priority was given also to the need for a consultants office in the accident and emergency department at a cost of some £3,000 but this and the children's clinic extensions were later deleted from the programme, so saving some £10,000. Alterations to the laboratory animal house and the virology department together with a 3,000 foot extension to relieve the congestion in this rapidly expanding department began in September 1975 and was completed in March 1976. Work was in progress during this period to rehabilitate the plaster room which was too small to accommodate the volume of work passing through the department.

In September 1975 painting was carried out externally on the medical ward and the balcony was decorated and had a new floor laid; louvre windows were fitted in the children's ward at a cost of £204.47. Orthopaedic ward also had a new floor covering laid with the ward being redecorated.

It was announced on 20th August 1975 that the contractor had taken over the site of the new Preston hospital in Fulwood and work had commenced in clearing the site, and in October the formation of the District Commissioning Team to oversee the proceedings of the new hospital was first suggested, later to be fully implemented.

A further example of robbing Peter to pay Paul occurred in December 1975 when it was announced that underspending in various departments made it possible for the District Management Team to provide portakabins at P.R.I. for office accommodation (£8,000), cash registers (£2,600), the purchase of two new vehicles for the transport department (£4,300) and an automatic barrier for the new car park in Stanleyfield Road (£2,000). New floor covering was laid in the Infirmary's main corridor and a new lamp installed in the ophthalmic theatre.

During 1975 trouble arose nationally over the position of junior medical staff and the long hours of duty expected of them for little recompense. Sanctions were introduced by the consultant medical staff in January 1975 which at first showed limited disruption but as the action progressed it intensified when the junior medical staff at Sharoe Green Hospital on October 15th took industrial action for 24 hours. They dealt with emergency cases and some routine services only and the action escalated when the junior medical staff at P.R.I. also took action with effect from 9 a.m. on 22nd October 1975, the whole episode lasting some three months, October to December 1975. Steps were taken to clarify the position regarding hours of duty as a matter of urgency to enable new contracts of employment to be prepared and when this was finalised early in 1976 the cost to the service showed an increase of £113,000 per annum.

As far back as August 1971 a crisis had arisen which brought the Infirmary's accident and emergency department to near breaking point due to a shortage of casualty medical staff. This was brought about by the reluctance of young doctors to work in casualty departments as they felt their dedication was abused by patients who attended with trivial injuries and conditions about which they should have consulted their own GPs. The strain was particularly apparent at bank holidays and weekends and the lack of staff caused casualty staff to work 24 hours or longer without a break in order to keep the service going. In the Preston District the situation arose where GPs in Chorley were called upon to staff the casualty department at Chorley Hospital because of the lack of casualty officers and there was a fear that the department might have to be closed completely. This generated a great deal of comment from local government authorities and other sources in Chorley and resulted eventually in the formation of a pressure group whose aim was to separate Chorley from the Preston group of hospitals entirely to allow Chorley to have its own health authority, an aim finally achieved some 10 years later, in 1981.

Banking services provided by the National Westminster Bank were made available for the first time when they opened a branch office in the Infirmary from Thursday 4th December 1975. Opening hours were each Thursday between 11.30 a.m. and 2.30 p.m., the office being situated in a room off the nurses home corridor.

The death was announced of Mr. S. Sumner D.O., F.R.C.S., former consultant ophthalmologist at Preston Royal Infirmary for many years. He died on 22nd September 1975 in South Africa, having retired there in 1965.

The chairman of the Lancashire Health Authority, Mr. Wm. Bennett, received the C.B.E. in the new year honours list and work began on the east wing of the Civic Hostel to provide accommodation for the vastly expanding District H.Q.'s staff and community services which were stretching the Infirmary's accommodation to its limit.

Early in 1976 a competition was announced for a new badge design for nurses. There were two badges at that time, the Preston and Chorley School badge and the Whittingham badge, and staff members were invited to submit designs for a new single badge. Judging of the new badge designs was completed before Christmas 1976, the winning design being submitted by Miss Janet Wallis, a physiotherapist at P.R.I. who was awarded a prize of £25. In January 1977 it was agreed that the D.M.T. would purchase 500 of the newly designed badges at a cost of approximately £4,000.

New extensions to the hospital staff social club in the grounds of Deepdale Hospital were opened on Monday 26th January 1976. The extension, which incorporated Radio Deepdale, cost £15,000, the District Management Team donating £1,500 and the Hospital Welfare Society also contributed, the remainder being raised through functions held and profits from the bar.

On 26th January 1976 the Medical Executive Committee made its first request to the D.M.T. to name the new hospital Preston Royal Infirmary; they continued throughout the year to press for a decision without success.

Staff dances were held at Whittingham Hospital on December 4th 1975, January 16th 1976, January 30th and February 13th, indicating yet again how the numbers of staff members had grown since re-organisation and also the popularity of these annual functions.

Two trees on the Deepdale Road boundary of the Infirmary were blown down, damaging the fence, as a result of a violent storm early in January 1976. The small theatre roof was damaged and the roof sheeting on the x-ray department was ripped off in the gales. Damage was sustained to most of the hospitals throughout the District, mainly chimneys being blown down.

A coronary care unit to provide better management of acute emergencies was opened late in 1976. The female medical ward was converted into two areas over a period of one month at a cost of £6,000 which included the provision of new equipment. A former patient of the medical ward, Mr. John Smith, donated £500 toward the scheme and this was used to provide the piped oxygen points in the unit which would accommodate 8 patients.

The new hearing aid department which had first been suggested in 1974 finally opened in August 1977. The highly technical examinations in the specially constructed sound proofed room were carried out by the two consultant otologists, Mr. H. Wickham and Mr. F. B. Duff, with audiometry being carried out by the four technical staff under the guidance of their chief, Mr. George Poulton. The total cost of the unit on completion was £28,500.

The number of out-patient attendances at P.R.I. during 1976 was given as 94,884, with attendances in the accident and emergency department being 56,369. Work commenced early in 1977 on upgrading the multiple injuries unit into a five bed intensive care unit at an estimated cost of £15,719.20. Dr. P. D. Salpekar, a pioneer in this field, was promoted to consultant clinical physiologist (intensive care) and placed in charge of the new unit when it became ready for opening during October 1977. The District Management Team had raised the question of staffing the new unit on several occasions, principally the need for four senior house officers, and in June 1977 a meeting of medical and senior nursing staffs was arranged to agree the operational policy for the unit when it finally opened. The Medical Executive Committee were not happy with the layout of the unit, however, and believed that alterations were needed before the unit would be suitable for patients. At the end of June the M.E.C. would not accept plans for the temporary use of the intensive care unit as a neurosurgical theatre and they insisted that the unit should open for intensive care purposes as soon as possible after 1st August 1977. Meanwhile, it was announced that an air chilling unit for the intensive care unit, to enable it to be used temporarily for neurosurgery, had already been purchased at a cost of £375. The M.E.C.'s objections caused problems when the small theatre closed on 11th July for the installation of air conditioning, making it necessary to transfer the neurosurgical lists to the main operating theatres on Wednesdays and Fridays.

In December 1977 meetings were held in the Infirmary to discuss with all relevant staff the question of the intensive care unit and the difficulties being experienced in running the unit. It was revealed that the I.C.U. had closed because of a shortage of adequately trained nursing staff experienced in intensive care, due, it was stated, to an abnormally high number of leavers and subsequent recruitment difficulties. Seconding staff to the unit from the wards was having adverse repercussions on the wards so that this arrangement had been discontinued. The medical staff 'were unanimous that the Intensive Care Unit should be given higher staffing priority over all other needs in the hospital and that the unit must be reopened as soon as possible'. In January 1978 it was stated that the unit was available for use but a remedy for the staffing problem on a permanent basis was still being sought.

The retirement was announced in November 1976 of Miss Amy Gratrix after 34 years at Preston Royal Infirmary. She was recruited during the war years into the nursing service but decided eventually to spend most of her service at what she described as the heart of the hospital, the switchboard. Miss Muriel Meek, seamstress at P.R.I. for 46 years, also retired. She had commenced in the sewing room at the Infirmary when she was 14 years of age at a time when electric sewing machines were not in evidence, hand sewing was the order of the day for the mending of sheets, towels etc., and the art of embroidering the Infirmary's initials on every garment and piece of linen was taught. Jim Bolton, who started as a trainee engineer on 11th May 1928 when the Infirmary had no plumbers, joiners or electricians, and the works staff consisted of Mr. Sumner the engineer, Mr. H. Norris, assistant engineer and Jim, retired on 24th December 1976.

Approval was given early in 1977 for Phase II of the new District general hospital which it was hoped would begin building in March and would take some three years to complete at an estimated cost of over £7 million. This phase was to contain the ward and theatre block for ophthalmic, E.N.T., surgery, neurosurgery, plastic surgery and burns unit, linked to a seven storey block with the theatre suite on the ground floor. Twelve theatres with an emergency theatre and plaster room were planned with a service area on the floor above containing plant rooms, relatives' overnight accommodation and medical staff on-call rooms. The next floor was to have the paediatric unit with accommodation for 103 beds and cots with facilities to allow for mothers also to be accommodated. Above this there were to be a further four floors, each consisting of 4 general wards, each containing 30 beds, although at this stage the final allocation to specialities had not been decided. The estimated cost at this stage was some £6,991,868.

The wards were designed on a 'race track' principle with 6 bed and 4 bed bays and single bedrooms set out around service rooms. Later it was hoped that separate schemes would provide for residential accommodation, pharmacy and pathology facilities, also a 120 bed mental illness unit and a 56 bed elderly sick mental illness unit, both with day hospital facilities. The first stage of building at the new hospital site was just beginning and it was anticipated that some of the service areas would be ready for handing over to the District Management Team by the contractors in the summer of 1977. There was, however, some anxiety being expressed at the uncertainty of the whole scheme, created by changes in policy concerning the new hospital.

The commissioning officer, Stephen Davies, issued a programme early in January 1977 highlighting the expected dates of handover on the completion of building of each block; in May, the boiler house, the mortuary, garages and workshops and chapel; in June, the kitchen, dining room, stores and in July the additional Phase I accommodation. The isolation unit should be handed over in August with the x-ray department in October 1977. In April 1978, physiotherapy, occupational therapy, medical illustration, with accident and emergency, medical records and out-patients to be handed over in March of 1978.

The artificial limb centre, the property of the D.H.S.S., itself was due for handover to the D.H.S.S. in September 1977, opening for patients in late October 1977.

The fluctuating cost of Phase I of the new hospital was announced early in 1977; it had gone up in March 1977 to £8,477,356, the previous figures having been £6,728,487 in July 1975 and in October 1976 it was £8,242,767. The commissioning team for the hospital consisted of Dr. Gordon Hesling, representing the medical staff, Eric Carleton, project administrator, Geoff Callon, hospital engineer, Geoff Unsworth, commissioning nurse and Stephen Davies the commissioning officer. On 2nd May 1977 they moved into temporary accommodation in the new District Headquarters in the Civic Hostel which was not fully ready to accommodate all the District Headquarters staffs until August 1977.

The District finance staffs were to be accommodated on the ground floor where there was also to be a reception area, a post room, telephone operator and duplicating and photocopying facilities. The first floor would accommodate the district nursing officer, district community physician, the chairman of the Medical Executive Committee, the district supplies officer, district domestic services manager, district catering manager, district transport manager, fire prevention officer and other associated staffs. The top floor was reserved for the district administrator, the district personnel officer, district works officer, community administration, planning officer, patients services officer and their staffs and also the board room.

This was a time of sweeping changes in the affairs of Preston Royal Infirmary with the transfer of many staff into the new District Headquarters and further changes were imminent with the movement of staff and services into the new District general hospital which was rapidly becoming a reality after so much speculation in recent years.

It was accepted that the transfer of the D.H.Q. to the Civic Hostel would relieve the Infirmary's telephone switchboard of a substantial load but it was agreed to investigate the adequacy of the switchboard at Sharoe Green Hospital for the traffic it would be asked to carry in the future. This did prove a problem in the early days of the newly transferred administration. The Medical Executive Committee requested an improved and extended telephone switchboard for the Infirmary at that time quoting the delay and frustration felt by general practitioners trying to contact the Infirmary. They also requested that a 'no smoking' sign and an extractor fan should be provided for the public telephone box situated outside the consultant's room at Preston Royal Infirmary at the base of the board room staircase, a touch of pique perhaps!

The finance officer requested permission to write off certain financial losses which included a quantity of influenza vaccine value £50.40 which had been stolen from one of the hospital's vehicles on 27th October 1976, a 50p coin which had been lost under the floorboards in the Infirmary's general office on 21st April 1977 and also stock to the value of £68.21 which had been lost due to a flood which occurred in the cellar of the pharmacy on 4th April 1977.

In October 1975 schemes were considered for an early inclusion of a pharmacy (£350,000) and pathology department (£350,000) into the programme for the new hospital. These were originally in the first phase of the hospital but were later removed, though how it was expected to operate a 1,000 bed District general hospital efficiently without them was inconceivable. They were both later included in the building programme for 1978/79, although the pathology department was a single phase of a much larger plan.

Priority was given for rewiring the nurses home (£30,000) and for replacement of the Albert/Alice Ward lift. This was given high engineering priority due to the increasing possibility of a permanent breakdown and the recently issued, highly critical reports of lift inspectors. The scheme would involve complete replacement of the cab and mechanism and also fireproofing of the lift shaft. This would involve the closure of the lift for several weeks, posing problems regarding the use of Alice Ward during the closure and alternative means of access for food trolleys from the basement would need to be found. In September 1977 it was found that the lift could not be installed because the equipment could not be delivered in time for payment to be made in the current financial year. It was later decided to carry out the work over a period of 18 weeks in the summer and autumn of 1978; the question of access from the basement was solved by the use of the lift in the nurses home.

A tender of £18,865 for the upgrading of the ear, nose and throat theatre was accepted in October 1976, although the final figure on completion of the work early in 1977 was £28,127. In the same period an approach was made to the R.H.B. regarding the running costs for an electron microscope which had been purchased by the public health laboratory. Accommodation was found to instal the instrument in a room off the corridor connecting the laboratory to the Infirmary, opposite Holden Ward and the microscope became operational in April 1977.

The question of a name for the new hospital was raised once again in July 1977 when the District Management Team suggested the 'Preston General Hospital' should be submitted to the Area Health Authority and the Regional Board. The Medical Executive Committee suggestion of 'Preston Royal Infirmary' was not acceptable to the D.M.T. but the M.E.C. countered by suggesting that Buckingham Palace be approached to obtain Her Majesty's permission to call the new hospital 'The Queen Elizabeth Hospital', but this too was rejected. A decision was needed by October 1977 so the suggestion was made that local opinion should be sought for a name. On 26th October 1977 the Medical Executive Committee once again raised the question of a name and pressed for a direct approach to be made to invite Royal patronage. They were informed by the D.M.T. that the decision rested with the Area Health Authority. The next move came early in 1978 when the Community Health Council wrote suggesting a competition to name the hospital but they wished to choose the winning name themselves. A meeting was arranged at the end of February 1978 attended by regional and area chairmen and administrators in contact with the Lord Lieutenant of Lancashire to discuss and agree on a Royal title. The District Management Team stated that if Royal approval could be obtained they would prefer 'The Royal Preston Hospital' and that finally was the title agreed upon.

The Ladies Comforts League in June 1977, on the occasion of the annual general meeting held in the Infirmary, presented a cheque for £500. A sum of £1,550 was raised to purchase special photographic equipment for use in South Theatre during exploratory work inside the bladder. This money had been accumulating since 1974 from donations by the Kirkham Young Farmers Club, Leyland Truck and Bus hourly paid workers, the W.R.V.S. and two children from Fulwood, Cheryl Parkinson and Ian Burgess, who raised more than £12 carrying out odd jobs.

Plans were formulated to convert the former District Headquarters accommodation in Stanleyfield Road and on the main Infirmary site to provide additional improved accommodation for residential medical staff and also a number of departments, some £20,000 being spent. Conversion of the group stores to a records department and record store was also envisaged at a cost of £10,000 to replace storage in the Albert Ward basement and to relieve the overcrowding in the records department. Additional laboratory space for the haematology department at an estimated cost of £20,000 with other alterations to the laboratory itself to relieve pressure and enable improvements to be made to the decontamination and washing-up area in the department of microbiology and to allow a fire escape to be installed. Less priority however was given to other projects planned at that time, e.g. a scheme to instal air conditioning into medical ward was deferred pending a general upgrading of the ward following the completion of Phase I of the new District general hospital. The same reason was given to an upgrading of all electrical services in the maternity block, at a cost of some £30,000. This was regarded as of low priority in view of the limited life of the department generally. The question of a central linen room for P.R.I. was also held in abeyance to await the outcome of discussions on the future policy for laundry services in the Preston District.

Among the schemes carried out in P.R.I. during 1977/78 were the installation of a neuro-centrix in the x-ray department, work on which commenced in June 1977 and was finally completed in February 1978; the maternity lift shaft conversion was completed in November 1977, as was the air conditioning in the operating theatre, and throughout 1977 rewiring of the nurses home progressed, being finally completed in March 1978.

The estates management budget during 1977 was so overspent that instructions had to be issued to cease all work on maintenance schedules for the remainder of the financial year with only day to day maintenance being allowed. It was noted that 'during the four power cuts affecting the Infirmary during the National Power Workers Industrial Action, the emergency generator restored power on an average of 3 to 9 minutes'.

Among the many long serving members of the Infirmary's staff leaving the service at that time were Mrs. C. B. Howard (Sister Orr) who retired as nursing officer in the accident and emergency department after 40 years at Preston Royal Infirmary. With her long experience and knowledge in this field she had advised on the planning of the intensive care unit and she also helped with the planning of the accident and emergency department in the new hospital. Sister Irene McNeil of the light department retired in July 1977 after 31 years service. Miss Julie Jolly, who had been secretary to Miss Livesey, Miss Watt and Miss Dixon, spanning more than 20 years, retired, and also two members of the transport department, Tom Bretherton with 27 years and George Quick, 24 years service. Another familiar figure in the wards and departments of the Infirmary, Mrs. D. Lovelady (known to everyone as Miss Briggs) retired, after more than 20 years service, on 30th June 1977. She was known as the lady almoner, although her official title was principal medical social worker. Mrs. Fox, domestic supervisor, also retired, after 29 years at Preston Royal Infirmary; she began as a domestic on Alice Ward, then spent 20 years as an orderly before returning to the domestic staff, becoming supervisor in 1973. Mrs. L. Singleton, a domestic on Holden Ward at Preston Royal Infirmary for over 12 years, died on the ward shortly after her admission. Mrs. Irene Fosbrook, sister of Albert Ward, died in February 1978 and Miss Isa Withers died on 3rd February 1978; she was the lady almoner of the Infirmary and ran the records department for many years and had retired in 1954 after more than 30 years service. The death was announced of Mr. R. Cunliffe Shaw, consultant surgeon at Preston Royal Infirmary since the 1920s until he retired on 31st March 1964; he died at his home in the Isle of Man.

Mr. Ian Brownrigg arrived in Preston as district personnel officer from 1st May 1977 and Mr. John W. Roe, formerly deputy group secretary for five years up to March 1973 when he moved to Ormskirk, was appointed area administrator to the Lancashire Area Health Authority. Changes in the consultant staffs included Dr. Michael Geake, consultant chest physician for 25 years, who left to take a new position in a private hospital in Sussex and Mr. A. Robson, consultant gynaecologist at P.R.I. for more than 25 years, who retired in February 1978 and Mr. N. Covell, consultant orthopaedic surgeon who left in the summer of 1977.

The Medical Executive Committee in June 1977 referred the District Management Team to the shortage of residential accommodation for doctors required to stay overnight in the Infirmary and they expressed the opinion that a fully equipped and permanently manned blood transfusion service was a pre-requisite to the opening of the accident and emergency service at the new District general hospital. They also requested improved facilities for photocopying at the Infirmary.

It was announced in August that the D.H.S.S. had placed an order for equipment to upgrade the E.M.I. scanner to be delivered in September 1978, eighteen months after the scanner had been installed.

In September 1977 the D.M.T. was informed by the district nursing officer that an expansion of the Nurse Training School was essential to increase substantially the intake of pupil nurses to meet the future staffing needs of the Health District. The west wing of the District Headquarters was quoted as ideal accommodation. In October, the district nursing officer's report to the D.M.T. drew attention to 'the unhappy state of affairs which exists in Brown Ward at the present time and which, if not eased in some way, could cause a breakdown in Orthopaedic Services'.

A report to the D.M.T. in May 1977, compiled by the orthopaedic surgeons and a group of nurses highlighting the high patient dependency on the ward, recommended the transferring of beds to Sharoe Green Hospital from Brown Ward and the orthopaedic wards and also the provision of sitting areas on both the wards in the Infirmary. This had not been acceptable to the M.E.C., who persuaded the D.M.T. that the situation should remain as it was for the next three years until the accommodation in the new hospital became available. The district nursing officer pointed out that 'the situation had worsened in the previous 6 months, the morale of the nursing staff was at its lowest ebb, with one Sister resigning and another Sister with many years experience on Brown Ward applying for other posts'. Two staff nurses had also asked for a transfer due to pressure of work and it was the opinion of the D.N.O. that unless the number of beds on Brown Ward was reduced immediately, by mid November the ward would have to close due to unsatisfactory levels of staffing. Four beds in Brown Ward were eventually closed and a meeting was arranged between the orthopaedic surgeons, the geriatricians and the social services representatives to consider ways of alleviating the problems caused by the blockage of orthopaedic beds. Urgent discussions were arranged between the senior nursing staff and the surgeons to review the situation fully and the opportunity was taken to explain the personnel aspects of planning for the new hospital and the relation of staffing levels to the nursing budget.

The District Management Team approved expenditure on several items totalling £80,908 in October 1977, later increased to £87,062. These schemes were only permitted if the work could be completed before 31st March 1978 as the funds being allocated would then have to be returned to the Regional Hospitals Board. Among the items of expenditure for P.R.I. were £5,000 to provide an office for the consultant of the accident and emergency department; £9,000 to provide fire escapes from the nurses home; £2,000 for signposting; £2,500 for security within the Infirmary and £6,500 for a replacement washing machine for the laundry. The £2,000 allocated for signposting in the Infirmary was later withdrawn 'due to lack of funds' and because it was felt that the new hospital was too near completion and such expenditure would be a waste. It had been suggested that the signs would eventually be transferred to the new hospital when the wards and departments moved but arrangements had already been made for new signs at the new hospital.

The £2,500 allocated for security for the Infirmary's premises was to include controlled entry under closed circuit television to the accident entrance via the accident department, a similar system for the entrance by the clock card hut and at the main door from the priority car park via the switchboard. Concern had always been expressed regarding the Infirmary's security, more especially following a tragic case at Blackpool Victoria Hospital where children had lost their lives and staff members had been seriously injured by a mentally disturbed member of the medical staff. The Infirmary had grown out of all proportion to its original intention and over the years had acquired many entrances. For years the main corridor had been used by many people whose only justification was to gain access to and from the town centre and attempts to remedy this situation had met with little success. The installation of closed circuit television cameras at all entrances to the Infirmary in the cause of security, especially at night, proved unsuccessful when the night staff, early in 1979, refused to operate the equipment. This was no doubt understandable, for a lack of portering staff made the coverage inadequate from 5 p.m. - 10 p.m. Monday to Friday and after 1 o'clock on Saturday until the porter's shift began on Monday mornings. The question of security in the Infirmary continued to be a problem over the years and, with the appointment of a security officer for the Preston Health District in 1984, this became one of his main tasks as the problem had now become magnified by the decreasing numbers of departments and staff on the Infirmary site.

A pilot scheme for a twilight community nursing service in the Preston Royal Infirmary sector of the District commenced in October 1977 as part of the District's plan for services for the elderly. Nursing would be available between 7 and 11 p.m., seven days a week, with the nurses being based in P.R.I.. If the scheme proved successful it was hoped to extend it throughout the Health District.

In December 1977 a tender of £22,999.47 for the new laboratory extension of the department of haemotology was accepted. Discussions were held in the same month on extraordinary expenditure programmes, money or finances arising from the carry over from current and previous underspending and how they should be utilized. Arising from this, £2,000 was allocated for alterations to the P.R.I. general office for added security as a pay office, but again with the proviso that the work had to be completed before 31st March 1978. At this time permission was granted by the D.M.T. to write off the loss of brass candlesticks from the Infirmary's chapel, their value estimated to be £25.

Since the dissolution of the Brackenbury Library, now being used as the consultants' dining room, a request was made 'on the desirability of access to books likely to be of benefit to members of staff in their working capacity irrespective of their duties'. It was decided that as far as the staff were concerned the supply of reprints in a rest room would perhaps be more beneficial than a library. As part of the re-allocation of accommodation plan for the Infirmary following the transfer of the D.H.Q. staffs to the Civic Hostel, the doctors' mess on the ground floor corridor was expected to move upstairs and it was considered that this would be the ideal site for a staff rest room. These plans never materialised, however, and the staff rest room remained a dream.

As part of the Christmas celebrations, dances were arranged for the staff of the Infirmary sector in the nurses dining room early in 1978. The dance held on 17th February was the first held for many years and was enjoyed by all who attended; due to lack of support, however, the other two proposed dances had to be cancelled.

On Sunday 5th March 1978, an N.C.O. in the King's Own Royal Border Regiment was admitted into Preston Royal Infirmary suffering from the 'bends' following his diving activities earlier in the day. Mr. S. Farrar, the Infirmary's administrator, arranged for the transfer of the patient by ambulance to a decompression chamber at *H.M.S. Neptune,* near Glasgow. Mr. Farrar and the Infirmary's staff were later thanked by the commanding officer, Lt. Col. R. J. Hodges M.B.E.

Miss Mary Thompson, treasurer of the Ladies Comforts League for more than 40 years, presented £800 on behalf of the League members, the money being used to supply window and cubicle curtains in Alice and West Wards.

Dr. D. L. H. Goddard, consultant chest physician, retired in May 1978 after 15 years and Mr. J. B. Clarke was appointed consultant obstetrician and gynaecologist as a replacement for Mr. W. A. Robson.

The new hospital had reached the stage where the structural frame of the main ward block had been completed in July 1978. A traditional 'topping out' ceremony had been held where the Regional Health Authority chairman, Mr. Sydney Hamburger, donned a safety helmet and trundled a wheelbarrow of cement along the roof of the 22 million pound hospital to help complete the last cement section of the seven-storey Phase II. The outside appearance of the hospital gave the impression that the building was nearer completion than it actually was, arousing rumour and speculation among staff members that wards and hospitals at P.R.I. were to be closed imminently. These fears were allayed to some degree however by an announcement from the personnel officer, Mr. Ian Brownrigg, that no transfer to the new hospital would take place for at least 18 months and, in the case of wards, for some 2-2½ years. Full consultation was promised with all staff interests at every stage. Phase II of the building was proceeding according to programme, it was reported, but there would still be a ten-month gap between the completion of Phase I in May 1979 and Phase II in March 1980, with patient services being operational 6 months after the completion dates.

In February 1978 the D.M.T. noted that the E.M.I. body scanner was not in the capital programme issued, as it was hoped to obtain a new whole body scanner. It was also noted that there would be inadequate provision of residential accommodation on the new hospital site so a request was made to the N.W.R.H.B. suggesting the purchase of 10 houses on the housing estate adjacent to the hospital in Sharoe Green Lane.

An upgrading of the Infirmary's telephone exchange, with four additional exchange lines and switching equipment, took place in October 1978 in an attempt to ease the congestion and at a cost of £5,373. A scheme was submitted to the Regional Board to replace completely the telephone installation which had been in constant use for 17 years. This was considered by the D.M.T. to be the basic requirement for maintaining reasonable service for the Infirmary's remaining years of service. At the same time approval was sought for a system 85 ultrasound scanner for P.R.I. at a total cost of £15,119.81 plus VAT, the installation costs being £1,500.

The environmental health officer was asked by the D.M.T. to inspect and report upon the Infirmary's kitchens in December 1978 and once again the D.M.T. requested funding from the Regional Hospital Board for a major upgrading of the Infirmary's kitchens. A quotation for cleaning the kitchens was accepted in January 1979 in the sum of £1,750, although the estimated cost of work required to upgrade the kitchens completely was £11,482. A temporary kitchen was formed in the waitress service area, and redecoration and cleaning of all kitchen equipment commenced on Monday 22nd January 1979 and was completed by 21st February. Repairs to the floor in the eye theatre were carried out early in 1979, a new incinerator was installed and a chimney erected. Drainage and lighting of the car park in Sedgewick Street were completed and tenders invited for the installation of a stand-by generator. Work on the conversion of the stores in Stanleyfield Road was in progress and in February 1979 the ultrasonic scan unit in maternity was relocated.

The district nursing officer, Miss Salisbury, agreed when asked to investigate the effect of a cutback of £250,000 in the nursing budget for 1979/80 and the same exercise was carried out in catering and the works department. Later, in March, Miss Salisbury stated that, on investigation, to keep within the cash limits of the proposed nursing budget, two general wards would have to be closed for 12 months. The situation was also complicated by the need to increase the numbers of trained staff in specialities for the new hospital. The finance officer reported in March that further complications had arisen following the industrial action by ancillary staffs and the award of back-dated incentive bonus scheme payments which had to be paid, so adding further to the deficit at the end of the financial year. Later in the year, in August, a special meeting of the D.M.T. was held to discuss restrictions in services as a result of the general financial position.

They decided on greater control on the replacement of staff, with vacancies being filled only where absolutely necessary; no new equipment, furniture or fittings were to be ordered without D.M.T. approval; greater controls over catering were to be introduced and it was decided that 3 cold meals a week and continental breakfasts would be served to patients. They also proposed the closure of Lostock Hall Continuation Hospital and the Willows Hospital on a temporary basis.

Early in 1979 an expansion in consultant posts in general medicine, neurosurgery, haematology, immuno-pathology and radiology was granted by the N.W.R.H.B.. Posts in geriatrics, histopathology, medical microbiology and chemical pathology were not granted. The Medical Excutive Committee suggested that, as it had always been their policy not to appoint consultants who might put a greater strain on the anaesthetics and radiology services, the post for neurosurgery should not be filled. To compensate for this they hoped that permission might be given to appoint a further consultant paediatrician instead.

Chapter Nine

The end of an era 1979-1980

THE retirements were announced on 31st March 1979 of Dr. A. F. Ollerenshaw, consultant pathologist and Dr. James Mackay who had been appointed as consultant venereologist to the Infirmary in 1950. Among the many comings and goings from Preston Royal Infirmary in this period were Mr. G. K. Tutton, consultant neurosurgeon at P.R.I. since 1955 who retired in July 1978, Mr. K. J. Keogh being later appointed to succeed him. Dr. Alec Burton was appointed to replace Dr. Goddard as consultant chest physician. Mr. Leslie Lee, charge-hand plumber for 30 years at the Infirmary, retired and also Mr. George Armstrong, the district pharmacist. Miss E. Blacklidge, head of the occupational therapy department for many years, retired and also Mrs. Lily Melling who had looked after the consultants' dining room for more than 20 years and in October, Mrs. Betty Collinson retired having served for many years as orderly on West Ward and latterly as a domestic, taking care of the patients' day room and relatives' accommodation.

Miss Lorna Mercer, sister on the ophthalmic ward and editor of the Preston Royal Infirmary Nurses League *Journal,* retired at the end of 1978, the following year, 1979, being the fiftieth anniversary of the founding of the League by Miss Marks in 1929.

A change occurred in the administration of the Infirmary when Mr. S. Farrar who had arrived in June 1975 resigned to be succeeded by Mr. Peter Fearn who commenced in his post in September 1978. There were a number of deaths also recorded in this period of members of staff associated with the Infirmary over the years. Mr. A. McDowall, former consultant plastic surgeon at Preston Royal who had retired in 1968 died in September 1978, remembered as a considerate and charming gentleman. Mr. R. R. Brown, affectionately known as 'Brown of Inventories', which was the term he gave himself when introducing himself to members of staff on his appointment, died at the end of 1978. 'Jock' was held in high esteeem by everyone with whom he came into contact and tributes were paid to his kind and efficient manner. The death was reported of Tom Moulding, for many years the hospital's barber, one of the old fashioned kind who could be seen 'stropping' his cut throat razor before starting his daily rounds of the wards. A great lover of poetry and an active member of the Preston Poetry Circle, Tom had won several prizes for his efforts.

Dr. Philip Rigg died at the age of 78 on February 20th 1979. A Preston born doctor who worked in the town for 50 years from being a consultant physician at Preston Royal Infirmary before the war, a commission as Major in the R.A.M.C. serving in North Africa and returning to Preston as a general practitioner, he retained his links with the Infirmary until his retirement in 1971.

Dr. A. A. Miller, formerly director of the pathology department at Preston Royal Infirmary, died on 5th October 1978 at the age of 76. Dr. Miller arrived at Preston Royal Infirmary following the retirement of Dr. F. B. Smith in 1948, when the laboratory was confined to three rooms above the out-patient department. He stimulated a rapid development of the service which culminated in the planning and commissioning of the new laboratory in Meadow Street in 1958, which became one of the leading centres for the training of doctors and medical laboratory scientific officers.

In December 1978 the death was announced of Dr. D. A. Anderson at the age of 70. Dr. Anderson came to Preston Royal Infirmary on leaving the R.A.F. in which he had served during the war, facing like many others the upheaval, the changes in practice, administration and attitudes occasioned by the inception of the National Health Service. He was a match to this challenge and under his benevolent but firm leadership the hospital medical services in Preston and district burgeoned and flourished. In the latter years of his working life he became increasingly aware of the importance of the exchange of ideas and experiences between doctors of all disciplines, mundanely referred to as post graduate education. Preston, he decided, must have a post graduate medical centre second to none, so he applied himself to this project with remarkable singlemindedness and, in 1969, the centre was finally opened. It is the envy of speakers and visitors from all parts of the country and is of inestimable value to doctors working in Preston. Dr. Anderson would have been the last to claim that he was solely responsible for its existence but he was the initiator of and the driving force behind the project and for as long as the post graduate medical centre remains it will keep Dr. Anderson's name alive.

The District Management Team decided to raise the retirement gift value for long serving members of staff from £30 to £35 with effect from 1st January 1979.

Mr. C. H. Beard, the consultant plastic surgeon stated that 'because of pressure of work on burns, trauma etc., he had only admitted 2 patients from his waiting list since the end of October 1978. His list was now some 2,000 patients to which approximately 10 more were added each week.' The only way to cope with this situation was to stop treating burns etc., and he urgently needed more assistance in the form of extra junior staff, extra beds and operating time.

The first sections of the new hospital building were formally handed over to the District Management Team on 29th March 1979. These consisted of the dining rooms and kitchens, stores, linen handling unit, the mortuary and workshops, followed a week later by the boiler house, although the boiler house had been manned for several weeks previously.

Donations to the value of £655 were received from the St. Ambrose Old Time Dancing Club by Mr. Taylor, the consultant eye surgeon, in April 1979, the money being used to purchase two diamond lance knives each costing £375; the additional £95 was funded from a previous donation of £100. In May 1979 a legacy was bequeathed to the Infirmary by the late Lorna Lucy Cartmell, to be used for patient comforts and a donation from the Clare Davis Fund of £700 was also received in the same month and placed into the endowment fund for future use in the Infirmary's children's ward. A further donation was received in June of £450 from the estate of the late Rev. John Jolly and £373.75 of this was used to purchase a 26″ colour television set for Brown Ward.

Schemes for 1979/80 on the question of fire precautions were announced in May 1979 and the programme for Preston Royal Infirmary was as follows:

1. Replacement of the fire alarm System	£25,000
2. Provision of a fire escape from Medical Ward ICU	£10,000
3. Provision of means of escape from Pathology	£2,200
4. Modification of fire exit and replacement of fire escape, Alice Wd	£3,500
5. Provision of smoke detector in Baby Care Unit	£500
6. Provision of CO^2 extinguisher system, deep fat fryer	£3,500
7. Installation and upgrading of fire doors and screens	£2,500
8. Placing fire doors on magnetic release	£5,000

These schemes were quickly brought to the fore when fire broke out in the basement record store under Albert Ward just before midnight on Friday July 13th 1979, apparently caused by an electrical fault, the sprinkler system coming into operation. The fire damaged the main electricity cables causing a mains failure, completely blacking out the hospital. Mr. T. Riley, the senior nursing officer for the Infirmary, who was present when the alarm went off initiated the necessary action which included bringing into operation the major accident plan. Albert and Alice Wards were evacuated and in quick succession South, Holden and the children's wards and part of Green Ward were evacuated and at one stage consideration was given to the maternity department. The accident and emergency department was closed and patients referred to Blackpool Victoria Hospital and Blackburn Royal Infirmary. Forty five patients were evacuated to Sharoe Green Hospital and 6 patients to the children's unit at Chorley. The evacuation had been dealt with swiftly and capably mainly due to the effort and organisation of Mr. Riley. Some medical records and films were destroyed by the fire and the extent of the damage to the fabric of the building and services was estimated to be of the order of £15,000-£20,000.

The repercussions from the fire were many and varied. It highlighted a lack of consultation existing between medical and nursing staffs. Storm lamps were issued throughout the Infirmary's wards and departments for use in such an emergency. A special meeting was convened on Tuesday 21st August 1979 to discuss the fire, identify the faults and use the experience to formulate precise plans to deal with major incidents for each of the hospitals in the Health District. The meeting was attended by all the relevant senior members of staff from the District administration, nursing and works staff, together with representatives from the Lancashire County Council Fire Brigade and the Area Health

Authorities' fire prevention officer. Many recommendations were made to the D.M.T. by the meeting which would require a considerable amount of money. The D.M.T. on 19th September received the report and agreed to consider the priority recommendations later.

Work commenced on the replacement of the Albert/Alice Ward lift and the fire-damaged floor of Albert Ward on 13th August 1979. West Ward was to be used for mixed surgical and medical male patients and female medical patients were to move to the male medical ward but no patients were transferred to Sharoe Green Hospital which had at one stage been suggested. It was decided that all non-urgent admissions would stop until Albert Ward was returned to use and all GPs were circularised on the situation and their co-operation requested. Things returned more to normal when Albert Ward re-opened on 27th August 1979.

Phase IV of rewiring the nurses home at P.R.I. was included in the regional engineer's programme for 1979/80 at a cost of £20,000. This phase would include the pupil Nurse Training School for which temporary accommodation would have to be provided. No accommodation was available at P.R.I. so it was agreed that the school could be re-housed on the first floor of the centre block of district headquarters which could be made available at minimal cost from early August when the rewiring exercise was due to start. Urgent repairs were necessary to the lift in the nurses home at a cost of £5,081 in August and the lift in the pathology laboratory also needed attention, the cost of this in August being estimated at £4,566; later in October this had increased to £5,303.

The finance officer explained how £180,000 had been overspent in the first three months of 1979/80 and drew attention to further factors which would exacerbate the situation, which included pay awards to staff, VAT, the increase in the price of oil and inflation generally. He drew attention to the fact that £2.5 million had been omitted from the capital programme required for major adaptations at Preston Royal Infirmary and Sharoe Green Hospital. Overspending was evident in all aspects of expenditure of the health district; for example, in the diagnostic departments, the main reason for the increase was increased on-call commitments in both radiography and pathology, the radiography figure having increased by £171 and the pathology figure by £700 over the figures issued three months before in May 1979. On the increased cost of fuel it was revealed that the health district used 9,078,000 litres of oil a year and that every 1p per litre increase in the price of oil added £90,000 to the fuel bill. The price of oil had increased by 1.86p per litre so far in the current year. The District also used 11,300 tons of coal each year and the price of coal had increased by £3 per ton.

A further complication in the field of finance arose in August with the announcement of a reduction in working hours for nurses to 40 hours per week from 1981. This was not to be funded by the D.H.S.S., the extra cost having to be borne from District funds and the district nursing officer expressed the opinion that a reduction of patient services was a possibility.

This was a period of grave concern nationally regarding the National Health Service. It was reported that:

> it was fast developing into a national scandal with Hospital lists assuming hopeless proportions, more that 600,000 patients awaiting Hospitalisation across the

> Country, in some instances a wait of three years. Doctors and Nurses were becoming increasingly frustrated by delays, lack of resources and the plague of industrial disputes which added to their difficulties.

The Royal College of Nurses in their report to the Secretary of State for Health and Social Services, Mr. David Ennals, stated:

> Nurses are no longer able to cope with workloads to a standard which is compatible with their professional training . . . they are forced to witness and participate in the decline in standards of patient care. Morale is low due to declining standards of care, staff shortages, increased workloads, poor career development facilities and low pay. The incidence of untrained staff, learners and auxiliaries left in charge of patients is believed to be very high and, on top of all this, the number of student nurses fell last year by 17% and many training courses had to be cancelled.

This was the position nationally at the start of 1979. In July the Royal Commission published its report and this was followed by a government order to health authorities to cut £125 million from their budgets before 31st March 1980, setting in motion the hasty drawing up of plans to curb spending. In some instances, where authorities had already exhausted areas of saving such as energy costs, staff recruitment and hospital maintenance, inroads were made into patient services. The newly elected Health Minister, Mr. Patrick Jenkin, expressed his confidence that the savings could be restricted to administration services, thus limiting the effect on patients but it soon became evident that health authorities were having to propose measures in other directions such as temporary or permanent closure of hospitals and clinics, the closure of wards and special units, leaving vacancies for doctors and nurses unfilled, cutting holiday cover for doctors and other staff, reducing cleaning and maintenance programmes, reducing staffing levels and deferring measures which were necessary to ensure that hospitals met the Health and Safety at Work Act standards. There was also a trend to postpone all new developments aimed at improving the National Health Service generally. All these measures would inevitably produce, in time, a deterioration in the services that the N.H.S. could offer to patients.

In the laboratory at P.R.I. it was announced that there would be no emergency on-call services after 17th June 1979 due to a dispute over emergency duty payments. The consultant pathologists agreed to carry on the emergency services during the dispute and in August an on-call rota was re-introduced; by the end of October, however, emergency services were again restricted with no weekend cover as a result of the failure of negotiations at national level over payments.

The question of car parking at Preston Royal Infirmary was raised once again during 1979 with the failure of two consultants, called to the hospital in an emergency, to find parking spaces — spaces at the front of the Infirmary which were reserved for such an eventuality were on that occasion occupied by visitors' cars. There was a call to extend the cover given by the British Legion car park attendant to exclude visitors from parking on the Infirmary's forecourt. It was decided to issue Priority 1 car parking passes to members of the consultant medical staff and official car users who travelled to other N.H.S. premises during their normal course of employment. It was also suggested that the former tennis court, at that time being used for unrestricted parking, could also be used for priority parking. It was pointed out, however, that if all the members of staff mentioned were issued with parking permits, there would still be insufficient spaces available.

At the end of June 1979 plans for the handing over of Phase II of the new hospital to the Health Authority were issued. The handover was to be in seven stages:

1. Level 116 wards 22-25 and Level 113 wards 18-21 including access by lifts and staircases were to be handed over finally on 10th August 1979.
2. Level 106 wards 9-12 and Level 109 wards 14-17 on 14th September.
3. Level 103 children's ward on 19th October 1979.
4. Level 100 ENT plastic & burns wards, plant rooms, medical staff on-call and relatives' accommodation and the burns treatment unit had still to be arranged.
5. Part of Level 96 and part of Level 100 on 5th November 1979.
6. Part of Level 96 on 26th November 1979.
7. The remainder of Level 96, ophthalmic and neurosurgical wards and plant rooms at Level 100, lower basement and external work 17th December 1979.

The Commissioning Team for the new hospital requested that they be allowed to move into the new hospital premises in February 1980, occupying offices on the administrative corridor. This was the earliest date by which telephone communication could be established in the hospital and a telephonist would need to be appointed who would also be required to undertake copy/typing/clerical duties. The switchboard was to be connected to three outside lines with approximately 30 extensions scattered throughout the hospital. It was also considered that February 1980 would coincide with a period of increasing activity within the hospital precinct with staff visits to view the new facilities and the placing of equipment etc. Occupation of the building would of course increase the security to some extent. The chapel and isolation ward from Phase I of the new building were handed over on 4th September 1979, followed the following day by the 4th and 5th floors from Phase II. In the same month recommendations of bed allocations for the new hospital were announced and the appointment of an assistant domestic manager from 3rd September and of a storekeeper from 24th September.

Additional staff were requested for the ultrasound department at Preston Royal Infirmary, approved originally in October 1978 but never implemented. The Medical Executive Committee deplored the decision of the District Management Team not to allow these appointments, needed to cope with the increased workload of the department and in November they requested once more for further staff, the lack of which, they claimed, was restricting the diagnostic work of the department. The M.E.C. stated:

> they were unanimous in their opposition to any cuts in patient services and they pointed out to the D.M.T. that for virtually the past year only acute cases had been admitted to the Hospitals in an attempt to make economies. They did not agree with the proposed closure of Lostock Hall Continuation Hospital or the 'Willows', the purpose of which they saw as an attempt to reduce the throughput of patients at Preston Royal Infirmary and Sharoe Green Hospital and they wanted it made clear to the public that this was not merely the closure of two Convalescent Homes but a direct cut in acute services.

The District Management Team in October 1979 increased the value of the retirement gift to staff leaving after 20 years service to £40 and it was agreed for the first time to include consultant medical staff in the entitlement of a gift, beginning from 1st January 1980.

The fire-damaged floor of Albert Ward was finally completed in September and the work on the Alice/Albert Ward lift replacement was progressing smoothly. Alice Ward had been redecorated and the upgrading of the intensive care unit was in its final stages. The Infirmary was being painted externally and the long process of rewiring the nurses home was still going on, final completion of this being achieved in June 1981.

In October, it was decided to transfer the media room from the laboratory at P.R.I. to Whittingham Hospital, following a visit of the Health and Safety Inspectorate who made the recommendation on health and safety grounds; the media room is that section of the microbiology laboratory which caters for the preparation of suitable media for the growth and well being of micro-organisms — a very important part of the art of bacteriology. In November 1979 it was announced that the cost of the move to Whittingham was approximately £30,000 and the pathology division drew attention to the fact that the laboratory housed the regional sub-disciplines of virology and immunology and the cost of accommodating these disciplines had been borne locally with no finances coming from the Regional Health Authority. Their presence in the laboratory added greatly to the already acute shortage of space, which in turn led to the contravention of the Health and Safety at Work Act. The pathology division asked for financial assistance from the N.W.R.H.A. to implement the move to Whittingham.

It was reported that 37 sheets had been stolen from the Infirmary, a man being charged for the offence; the sheets were later returned to the Infirmary on the conclusion of the case in Preston Crown Court.

The Ladies Comforts League at its annual general meeting held in P.R.I. donated £750 for the purchase of window and cubicle curtains for the eye ward. Following their meeting the Ladies had afternoon tea with Mr. Peter Fearn, the Infirmary's administrator, Mr. T. Riley, the senior nursing officer and Miss Doris Salisbury the district nursing officer.

A kidney cooling unit which helped to maintain kidneys at a constant temperature during operations was presented to the Infirmary by the Preston South Rotary Club; the machine, which cost £720, was accepted on behalf of the Infirmary by Mr. W. J. C. Thomas, from the Rotary president, Mr. Kevin Fletcher.

The retirement was announced of Mr. Wm. Bennett C.B.E., chairman of the Lancashire Area Health Authority, on 31st July 1979. He had held the post since his appointment on re-organisation in 1974, having previously acted as chairman of the Preston and Chorley Hospital Management Committee following the death of Mr. J. Tomlinson. The District Management Team registered its disapproval of the manner in which the D.H.S.S. had handled Mr. Bennett's retirement. Mr. R. E. Hodd, B.Sc., Dip. Ed., a barrister and former director of education for the County Borough of Blackpool, was appointed to succeed Mr. Bennett for a two year period of office. Two new consultant appointments were announced, Mr. T. A. Flaherty, consultant haematologist in the laboratory and Mr. N. R. Gaze, consultant plastic surgeon.

Among the members of staff leaving the service were Miss L. E. Stirzaker, 38 years at Preston Royal Infirmary latterly as nursing officer for the operating theatres. Mr. Roy Duckworth, who began work in P.R.I. in 1942 in the days of Mr. John Gibson, and who had played a valuable part in the growth and development of the finance department for 37 years and Mrs. Mary Halstead who had spent 25 years at Preston Royal Infirmary, the first three years in the nurses home as a domestic and the remainder of her service in the out-patient department. The death was announced of Mary Murray, also a domestic at P.R.I. for 25 years, who had retired just one year previously.

In September 1979 Albert Ward was re-opened for patients and a working party was set up by the D.M.T. consisting of Miss Thompson, Dr. Holt, Mrs. Smith, Dr. Saikia and Mr. Flaherty to make recommendations regarding the arrangements for light therapy at P.R.I. and the new hospital. By the end of November all the projects being carried out in P.R.I. had been completed; these included the Albert/Alice Ward lift replacement, the intensive care unit, external painting, redecoration of the nurses recreation room and rewiring and decoration of the Nurses Training School and preparatory site work had begun for a radio isotope unit.

In the week commencing 19th November 1979 visits began by members of the nursing staff to view the new hospital or those parts of it which had been handed over. Expressions of astonishment and awe at the size of the new structure were common among those seeing the inside of the hospital for the first time. Escorted visits by many groups of staff were organised in the months that followed.

It had been suggested by the D.M.T. in April 1979 that there should be a cut of 2% in all budgets across the board within the Health Authority. The district nursing officer had notified the D.M.T. that it would not be possible to reduce the nursing service to that level of funding within the financial year without a reduction in service which at that time was estimated to be equivalent of two 26-bedded wards. The reduction of 87 nurses in the general/community division over the eighteen months up to October 1979 had brought the total nursing establishment to 35 below the agreed funded establishment for 1978/79. In October, following the 2% cut in the allocated budget, the nursing division showed an over spending of £94,000.

Industrial action by some medical laboratory scientific officers over payments for emergency on-call services continued throughout the latter part of 1979. A reduced service was supplied by the pathologists who provided emergency blood transfusion cross matching and the examination of cerebrospinal fluids. All consultants in the Health Authority were warned that there was a danger of no emergency services being available at all if the demand for laboratory tests out of hours was not severely restricted to true emergencies. The dispute persisted with the pathologists carrying out restricted on-call service until an offer of higher on-call rates was made by the Secretary of State via the D.H.S.S. in February 1980 when once again an on-call rota for emergency duty was established from 26th March 1980.

On the positive side, the Infirmary received a bequest of £1,540 from Mr. F. Keighley to be used to replace the cubicle curtains on Alice Ward and five colour television sets were purchased following a donation of £1,300.65 from the W.R.V.S. These were distributed to the female medical ward, orthopaedic ward, Alice and South Wards and to the first floor of the maternity hospital. The Infirmary also received a legacy of £2,911.54 under the will of the late

Francis John Horsburgh, following the death of his wife on the 22nd June 1976 who had a life interest in the estate.

The decade came to its end with an atmosphere of rumour and conjecture pervading the corridors of Preston Royal Infirmary as to the future. There had been much speculation throughout 1979 regarding a name for the new hospital and it had been anticipated that H.M. The Queen, on her visit to Fulwood Barracks on 10th May for the octocentenary celebrations, would have bestowed Royal patronage on the new hospital. This was not achieved, however, until later in the year and was finalised with the District Management Team passing Resolution 1469/iii in January 1980 agreeing that the 'the Preston Royal Infirmary should in future be re-named the Preston Infirmary'. I hope that the new hospital never forgets that she carries her regal title because it was earned with 150 years of service by countless generations of devoted staff in the red bricked building in Deepdale Road.

Chapter Ten

A new decade and new challenges

MOVING into the eighties at the start of another decade there was the prospect of other widespread changes for the National Health Service in Preston with the advent of yet further re-organisation of the whole structure of the N.H.S. and the removal of the area health authorities set up just six years before.

One of the first items discussed by the D.M.T. at their meeting on 2nd January 1980 was the consultative document *Patients First* issued by the government. On the 27th February, the chairman of the Area Health Authority visited the Preston D.M.T. to discuss with them the considerations which would need to be observed in the setting up of a new health authority for the Preston and Chorley district and the changes in structure and management envisaged in the *Patients First* document.

The Medical Executive Committee in January 1980 expressed their concern at the shortage of nurses which, they claimed, was leading to increases in waiting lists and the prospect of further cuts in nursing budgets anticipated together with a reduction of the working week for nurses to 37½ hours would do little to improve the situation. In the discussions on the nursing service that followed during February, the district nursing officer reported that ward 15 and one theatre at Sharoe Green Hospital were temporarily closed and the children's ward at Chorley District Hospital was also closed while the nursing staff problems were so acute and there had also to be a reduction in staffing levels in the community nursing service. The D.N.O. also reported that routine admissions to the Infirmary's children's ward and the ophthalmology services had been reduced, and stated 'that a further cut in the numbers of nursing staff at Preston Royal Infirmary would have to be implemented to achieve the approved Establishment'.

The concern of the consultants was expressed 'that no specific directive had been given to cut services and the public were not being made aware of the continuing reduction in service'. The D.M.T. agreed that 'the Area Health

Authority be reminded of the need to appraise the public of restrictions in service which was necessary at the present time'. Nevertheless the trend of more patients being treated each year continued.

The district nursing officer drew attention to the effects of the 37½ hour working week for nurses about to be introduced and pointed out that approximately 250 extra staff would be required to offset this. On 18th February 1980, the D.N.O. held a meeting with all senior nursing staff and ward sisters to discuss the eventual move to the Royal Preston Hospital and further meetings were planned during April with staff nurses, state enrolled nurses and nursing auxiliaries.

The Commissioning Team for the Royal Preston Hospital sought the approval of the D.M.T. to commence the installation of major x-ray equipment on 1st April 1980 and they requested that from the same date a superintendent radiographer should be appointed, also a medical records officer. They notified the D.M.T. that the main telephone switchboard installation would be handed over within one month with all the alarm services to the panels on the switchboard connected; this would mean the commissioning of the switchboard during the daytime period notwithstanding the D.M.T.'s refusal to allow the commissioning staff to move on to the new hospital site.

In March 1980 a legacy was bequested to the Infirmary from the estate of the late C. P. Bradley of £50,844.39. The D.M.T. agreed to replace those parts of the Infirmary's broadcasting system in use in the wards scheduled to remain, at a cost of £5,000 using some of the interest accruing from this most generous legacy. A complete overhaul of all the equipment would have cost £11,585 plus V.A.T. A further £5,000 was received from the estate of the late C. P. Bradley for the use of the Infirmary, making the total received from this source by 7th May 1980 £64,987.57. A cheque for £2,500 was received early in June for the Infirmary's use being a one-third share of the estate of the late Rhoda Cath Wright Talbot of Thornton, Cleveleys.

The x-ray and physiotherapy staffs took strike action for one day on Thursday 27th March 1980, withholding their services because of their dissatisfaction at their recent Clegg pay award. Arrangements to provide emergency cover were made but the x-ray staffs refused to undertake non-x-ray duties, i.e. dark room or portering from Monday 24th March. In the summer of 1980 industrial action by the works staff continued to disrupt the affairs of the health authority.

A financial statement issued on 7th May 1980 for the twelve month period to 31st March 1980 indicated an overspending of £125,000. Approval, however, was granted by the D.M.T. for a programme of schemes for the Infirmary which included a replacement of the fire alarm system (£25,000), air conditioning in the twin theatres (£10,000) and improvements within the laboratory on Meadow Street (£10,000). Improvements to the Infirmary's kitchens costing £70,000 were to be funded by the Regional Health Authority.

Problems had also arisen over the implementation of the 37½ hour working week for nurses where the change over of staff was occurring during visiting hours. The question of open visiting was discussed where it was anticipated that the bulk of visiting would take place between 2 p.m. and 8 p.m. Each sister would assess the situation for her ward and indicate the periods when visiting would be permitted; the periods when visiting would not be allowed would be during the consultant's ward rounds in the afternoons. Such schemes were already operating without official backing and the D.M.T. did agree to the policy of open visiting in the nature of a trial before transfer into the Royal Preston Hospital.

Detailed discussions in July 1980 of plans to accommodate geriatric services mentioned several options, one of which was the use of the Infirmary. The disadvantages identified at that time were the poor standard of accommodation, the deficiency of toilet and bathroom provision and the lack of day rooms, but the most restricting factor was the time limit on the Infirmary's life. It was envisaged that cold orthopaedic and gynaecological services would vacate the Infirmary by the end of 1984. There were advantages in the availability of accommodation, the cost effectiveness of concentrating services on one site for the duration of the major works at Sharoe Green Hospital and the ease with which staff could be transferred. It was agreed therefore that the Infirmary offered a reasonable possibility for use by geriatric patients from mid 1981 until the gynaecological services transferred to Sharoe Green Hospital in 1984, by which time accommodation would be available at the Royal Preston Hospital. The District Management Team considered that the medical ward and the eye ward would be most suitable for the purpose of providing 58 beds, using either East Ward, rehabilitation or out-patients as a day hospital with 45 beds being eventually supplied at the Royal Preston Hospital.

The special surgical division asked that a hearing aid department should continue at the Infirmary in the Stanleyfield Road audiology building following the transfer of other out-patient services to the R.P.H. The reasons quoted for this were:

(a) the department would be staffed from R.P.H. so that no additional staff would be required;

(b) the department was required to manufacture its own moulded earpieces and the noise of this work, if undertaken in the audiology workshop ar R.P.H. would disrupt the work in the adjacent consulting rooms;

(c) it would pressure on the E.N.T. consulting suites at the Royal Preston Hospital; and

(d) the Infirmary was considered more convenient for hearing aid users, the majority of whom were elderly.

This policy was adopted by the D.M.T.

Another fire at the Infirmary on Saturday 19th July 1980 caused damage to fixtures and fittings to the sum of £3,142.18 with a further £6,000 being necessary later to make good the damage caused to the room and nearby areas. The doctor's mess president requested assistance from the D.M.T. toward paying the bill for the cost of the rented colour television set damaged in the fire, the bill was for £175 and the mess funds contained just £30.

The breakdown of a deep freeze cabinet resulted in the loss of frozen food to the value of £83.84 and on August 7th the Infirmary's petrol pump was broken into and 32 gallons of petrol stolen. The sum of £36.20 in respect of the petrol and a further £50 to replace the broken locks and fittings were written off together with the £83.84. On 13th August 1980 a 100lb. tumble drying machine was purchased for the Infirmary's laundry at a cost of £3,995 plus VAT. Holden Ward was redecorated and further painting externally was carried out at the

Infirmary. The district transport department based at the Infirmary now numbered 24 members.

Members of the Preston South Ladies Circle presented a gift of £200 to Dr. A. G. Hesling, consultant paediatrician for use with the special care baby unit at the Infirmary and a charity set up in November 1979 by Mrs. Barbara Martindale which was called the Preston Laser Gun Charity aimed to raise in excess of £20,000 to purchase a laser gun for use in the Infirmary. Patients requiring treatment had to travel to Manchester or London as Preston had no such equipment. The laser gun was used to prevent blindness in diabetic patients but was also used for the treatment of other retinal diseases. In November 1980 about half of the £20,000 required had been raised from bequests, donations, raffles and many charitable functions. The fund reached its target of £22,500 in just 14 months and the laser gun was formally presented to the hospital for the use of the eye surgeons, Mr. P. Taylor and Mr. Fitzmaurice. New advances in neurosurgery put the Infirmary into the headlines in the spring of 1983. A new laser instrument called that Cavitron Ultrasonic Aspirator was being used by the neurosurgeons for the removal of hitherto inaccessible brain tumours. The instrument was on loan as the Health Authority was unable to purchase it outright but the *Lancashire Evening Post* launched a highly successful campaign to raise the £75,000 necessary for its purchase. This target was reached in just three weeks, illustrating once again the generosity of the Preston public toward the Infirmary and the work continued to be carried out there regardless of the constant threats of closure and the label of 'Slum of a Hospital' used on occasion by the press in describing the Infirmary. Early in 1986 the *Lancashire Evening Post* launched an appeal to raise sufficient funds by public subscription to provide the Health District with a whole body scanner to commemorate the centenary of the newspaper. Within six months over £250,000 had been raised and the scanner installed in the Royal Preston Hospital. All credit again to the people of Preston.

A call 'for prudence in expenditure during 1980/81 until the adequacy of the Government's cash limits for Preston District were known' was issued to staff members. It was expected that money would still be tight in the new financial year but if everyone maintained the strictest control on waste and continued to economise in every possible way, small improvements might be made possible in areas closest to the patient. It was hoped to prevent the stringent economies which had taken place in the past six months.

Toward the end of 1980 there was much talk of the transfer of staff to the Royal Preston Hospital. There was confusion too by the clash of names as staff still continued to refer to Preston Royal Infirmary as they had always done (and many older members of staff always will do). Discussions were held with staff organisations and meetings were held on 16th September and 31st October 1980 discussing staffing levels, working methods and transfer arrangements among many other topics. A number of the departmental heads had already been appointed and were busily engaged on detailed planning on how their departments would be organised. The physiotherapy department was due to open for out-patients on 5th January 1981 with the out-patient department to open in March 1981 and in-patient services to follow in the late spring and early summer of 1981.

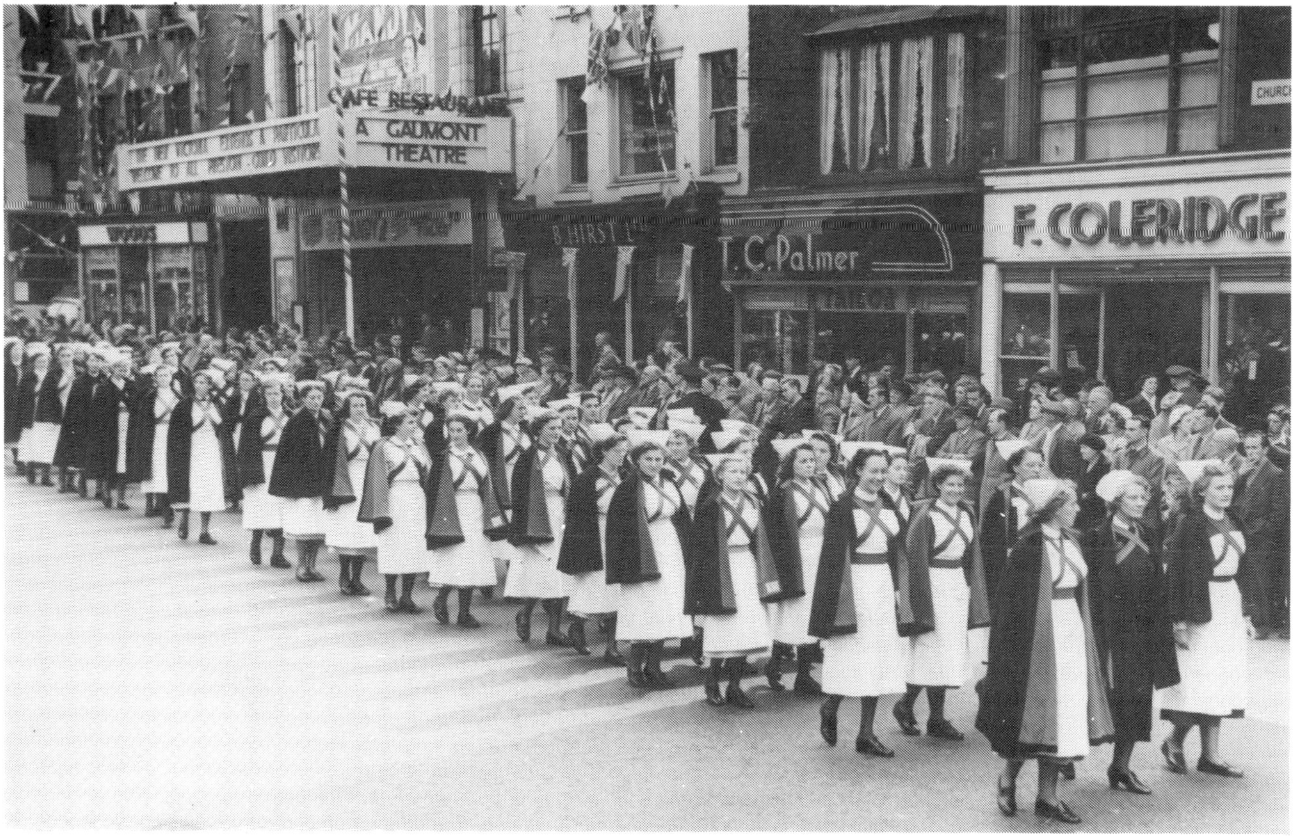

Guild Year, 1952. The parade of PRI nurses in the procession down Fishergate led by Matron, Miss N. Livesey.

Photograph courtesy of Lancashire Evening Post.

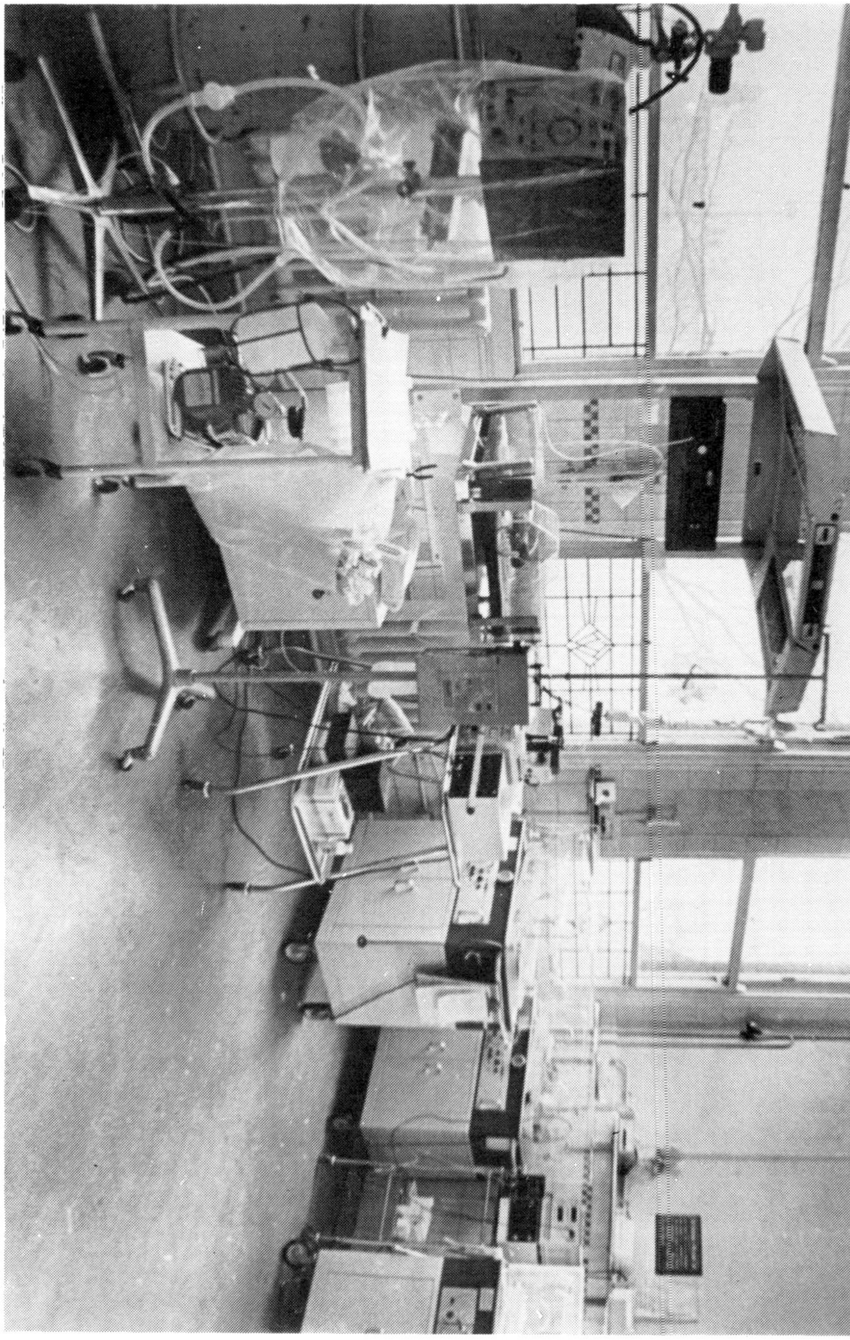

Part of the Maternity Department shortly after closure.

Photograph courtesy of Lancashire Evening Post.

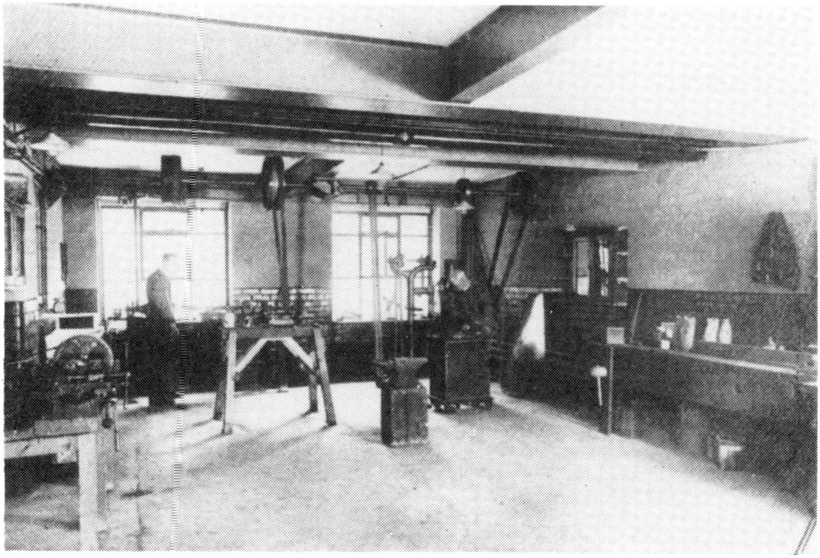

The Engineering Workshops in 1925.

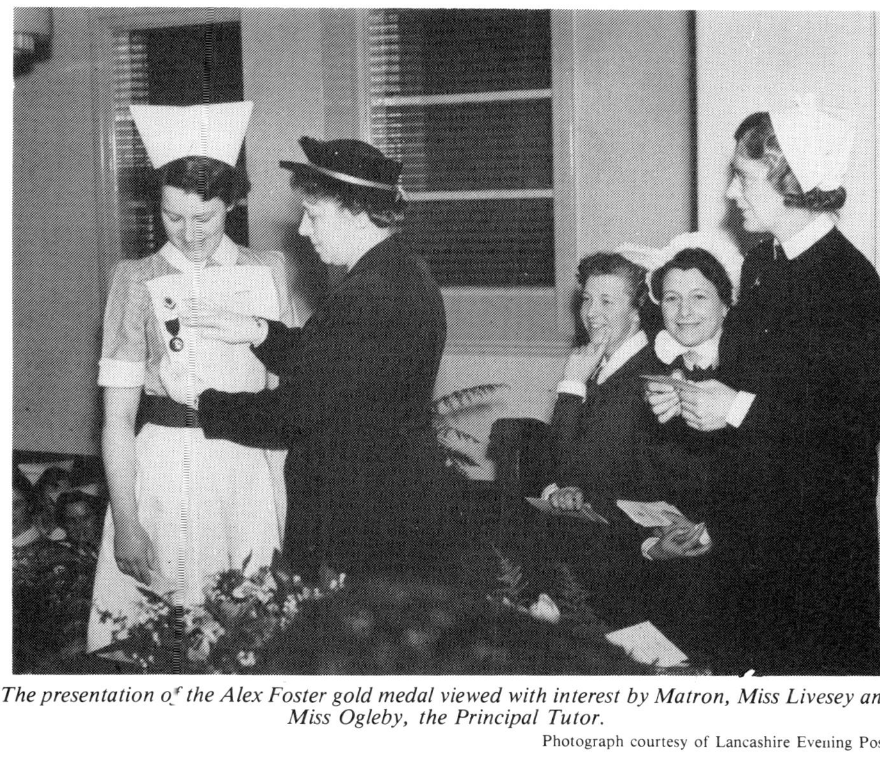

The presentation of the Alex Foster gold medal viewed with interest by Matron, Miss Livesey and Miss Ogleby, the Principal Tutor.

Photograph courtesy of Lancashire Evening Post.

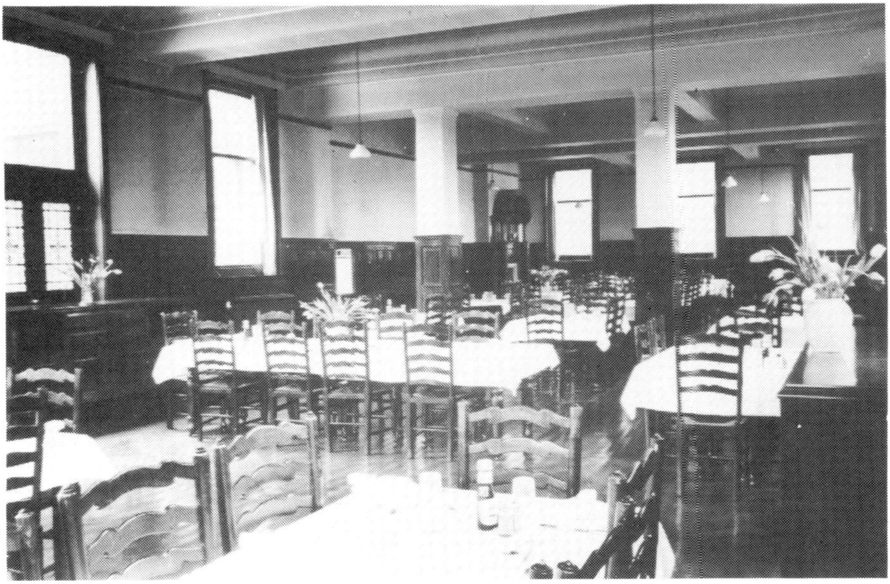

The Nurses' Dining Room.

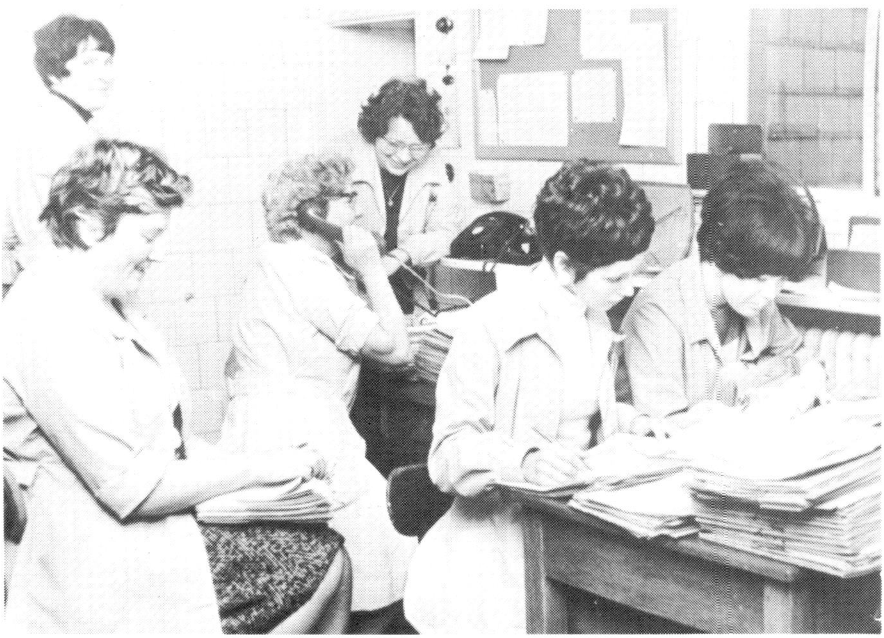

The Records Department always seemed to be cramped for space. It moved to this location when the new laboratory was built in 1958 and remained there until 1981.

Photograph courtesy of Lancashire Evening Post.

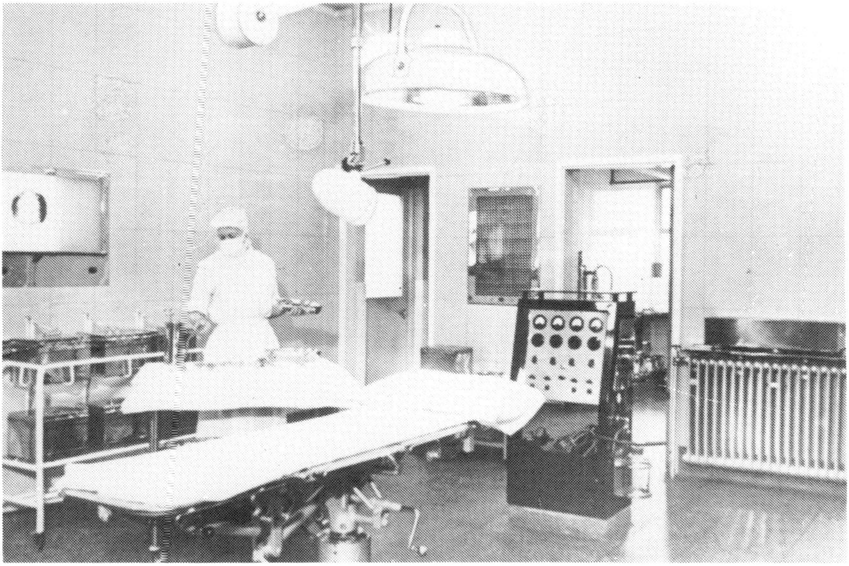

Getting ready . . . the operating theatre.

Photograph courtesy of Lancashire Evening Post.

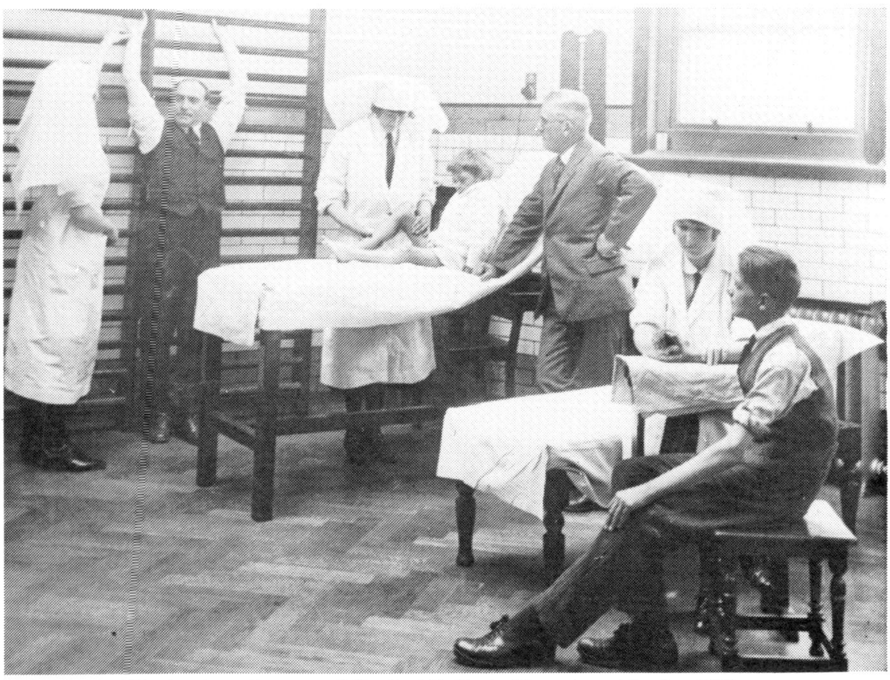

The treatment room of the Out-Patients Department in the 1920s.

Photograph courtesy of Lancashire Evening Post.

All communications to be addressed to the General Manager.

Preston Corporation Transport Department.

Head Offices: Deepdale Road, Preston

H. CLAYTON,
A. M. I. E. E.
GENERAL MANAGER.

TELEPHONE No. 56273.

OUR REF HC/HCM/MS
YOUR REF.

9th July, 1934.

Alec. Foster, Esq.,
Chairman of Board of Directors,
Preston Royal Infirmary,
PRESTON.

Dear Mr. Foster,

Foundation Stone Laying Ceremony.
12th July, 1934.

I beg to acknowledge receipt of your letter of the 9th instant, and in reply beg to say that arrangements will be made for our tramcars to make as little noise as possible when passing the Infirmary on Thursday, the 12th instant, during the above ceremony.

Yours faithfully,

H. Clayton

GENERAL MANAGER.

A delightful relic from the 1930s. We can only presume that the tram wheels were muffled in some way in order to 'make as little noise as possible'.

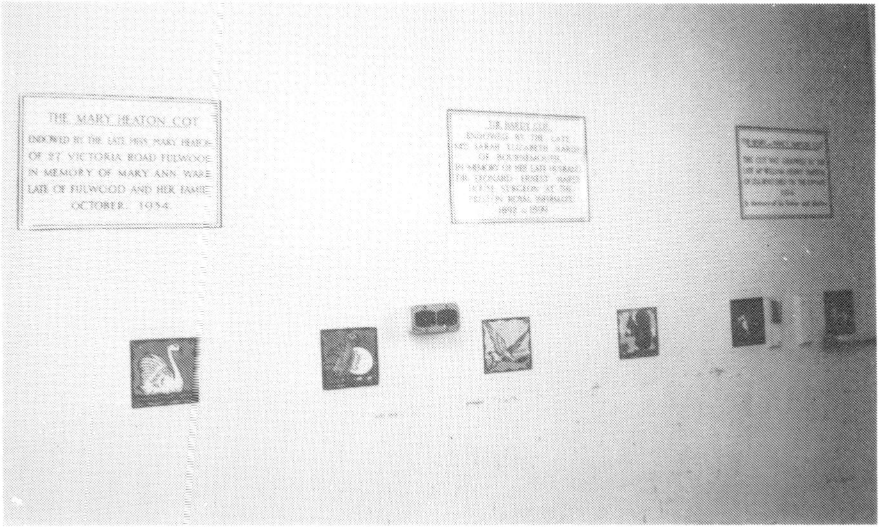
THE MARY HEATON COT
IN MEMORY OF MARY ANN WARE
OCTOBER 1954

Some animal tiles (with a detail of one shown below) in the Children's Ward of PRI. The plaques above them record some of the many private donations made for beds and cots at the Infirmary in its early years.

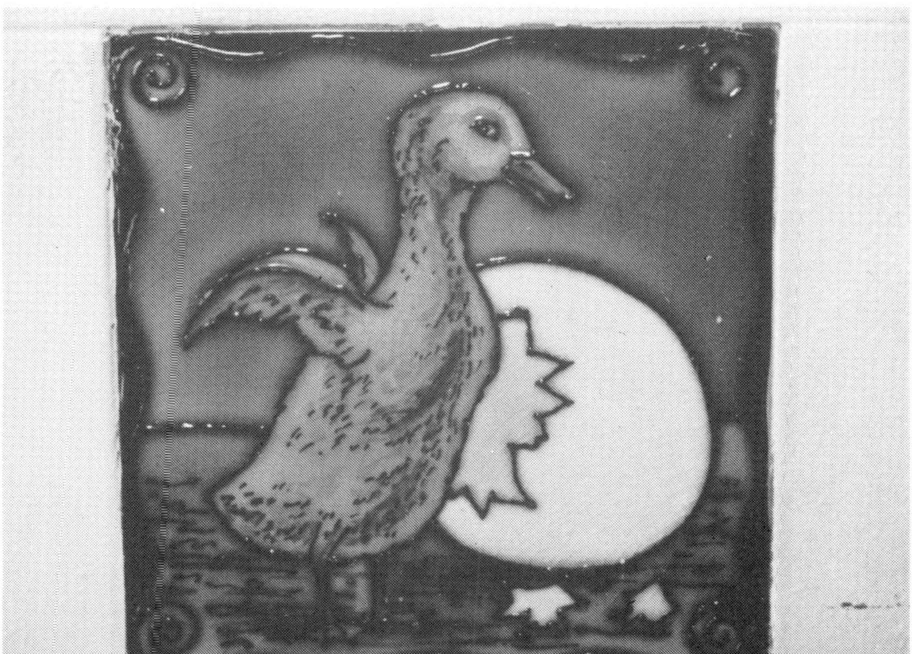

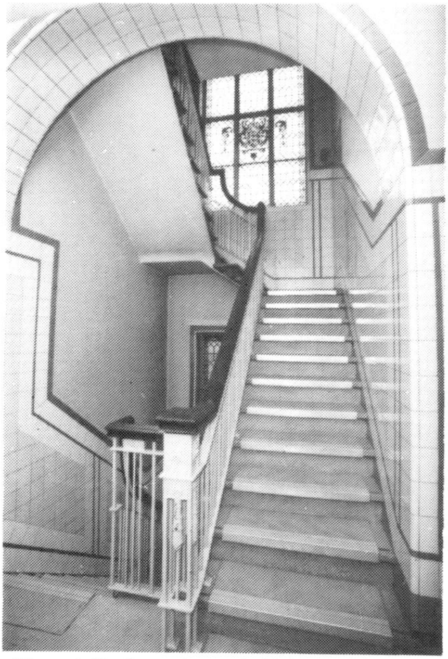

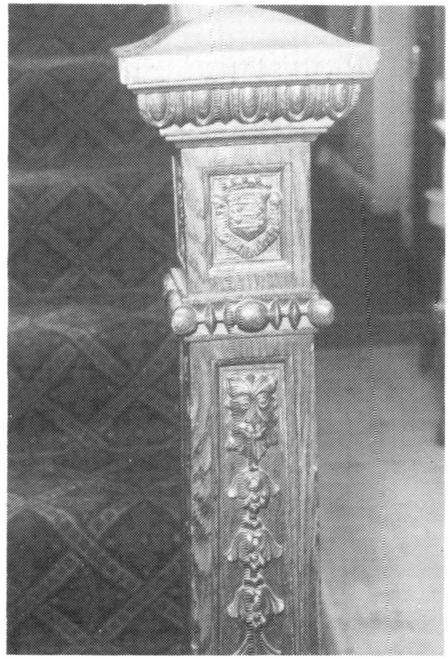

Above left: the staircase in Princess Mary Wing, with the beautiful stained glass window at the top. Above right: a detail from the main staircase which led to the Board Room, with the PRI crest visible.

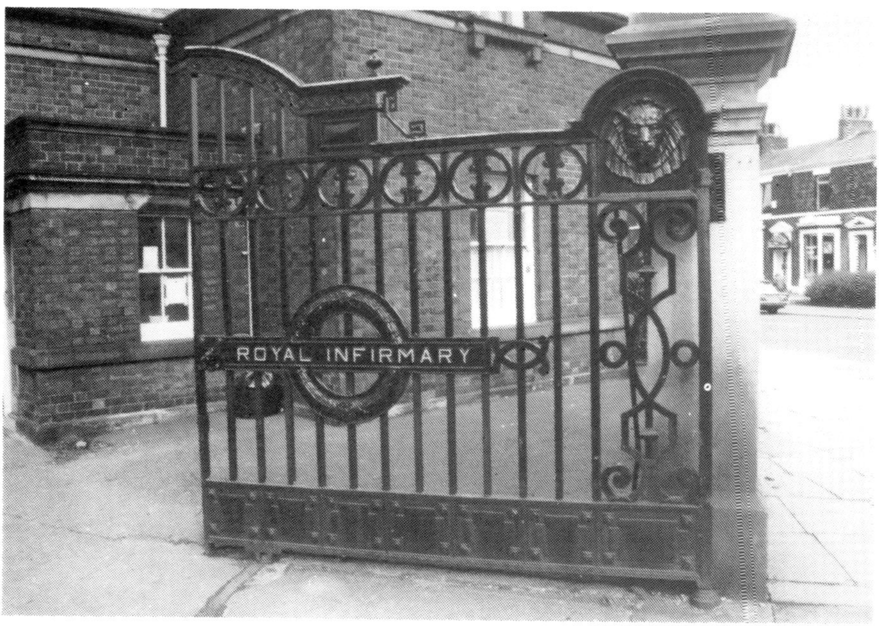

The Infirmary's main gates are of substantial construction and of pleasant design.

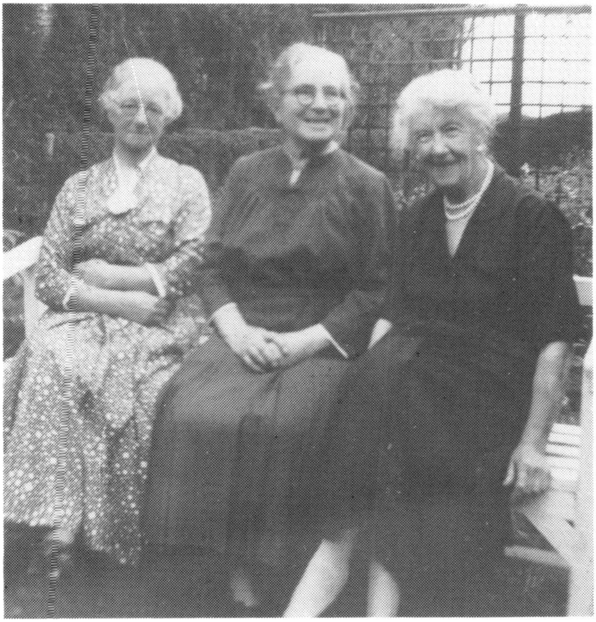

A rare photograph of Miss Marks, Matron (centre) and Miss Rossiter, Assistant Matron of PRI (right). Miss Marks founded the PRI Nurses League in 1929, which still meets on the first Saturday in May each year to reminisce over days gone by.

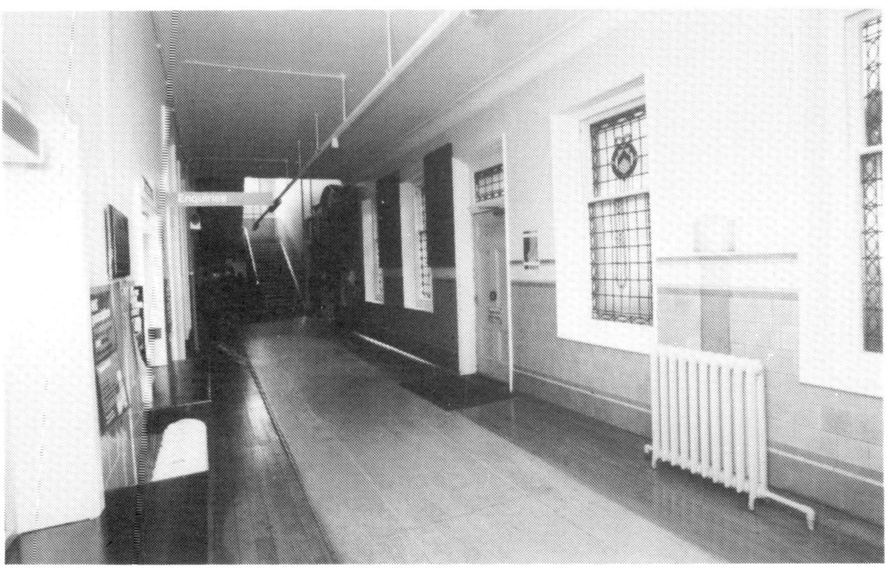

The main corridor of PRI.

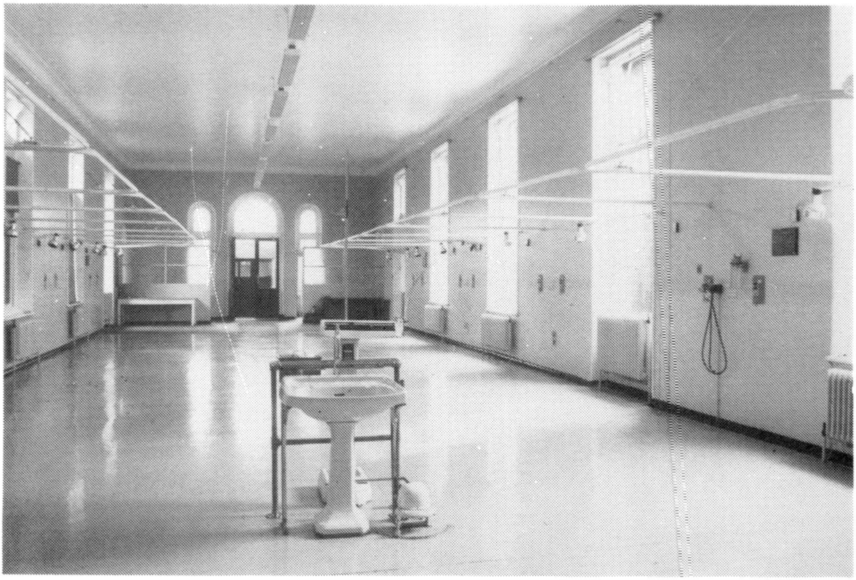

All gone . . . an empty PRI ward in 1986.
Photograph courtesy of Lancashire Evening Post.

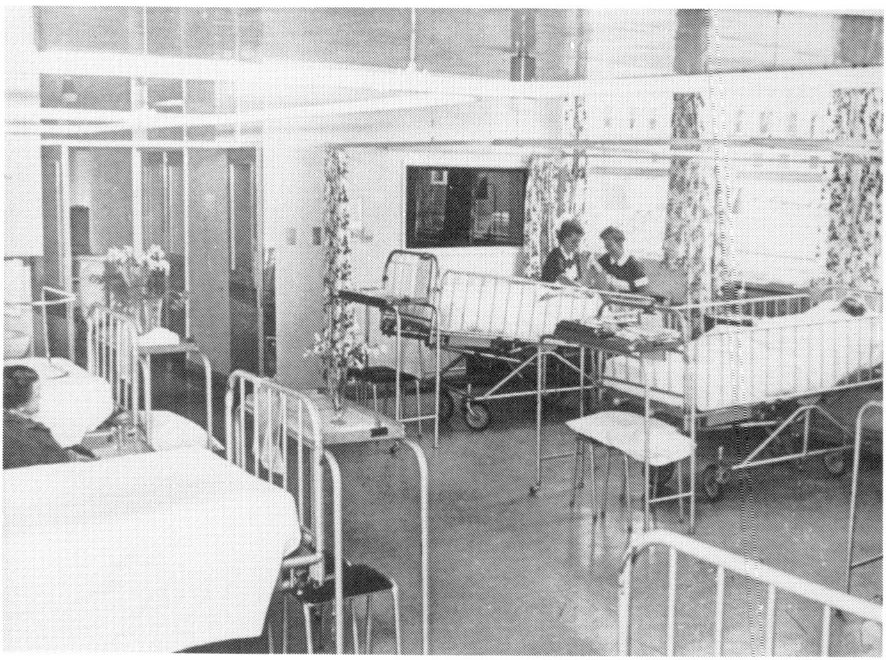

Holden Ward, the Infirmary's neuro-surgical ward.
Photograph courtesy of Lancashire Evening Post.

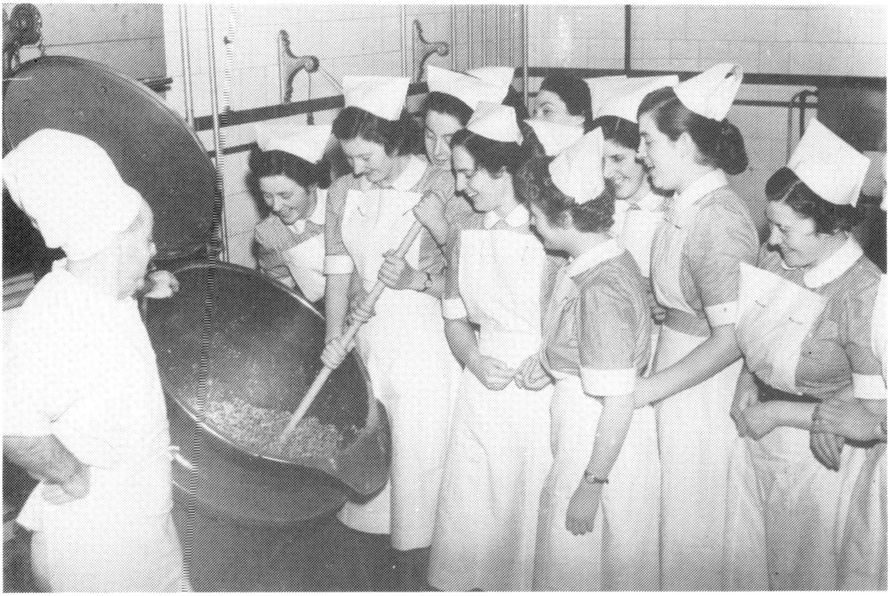

An Infirmary tradition was the stirring of the Christmas pudding mixture for good luck.
Photograph courtesy of Lancashire Evening Post.

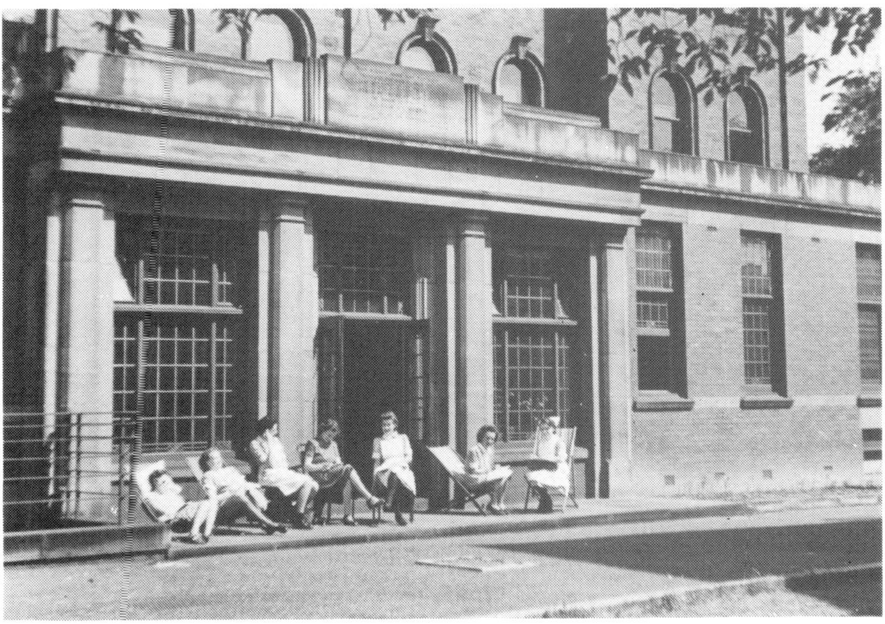

Taking the sun in front of the 1940 nurses extension.

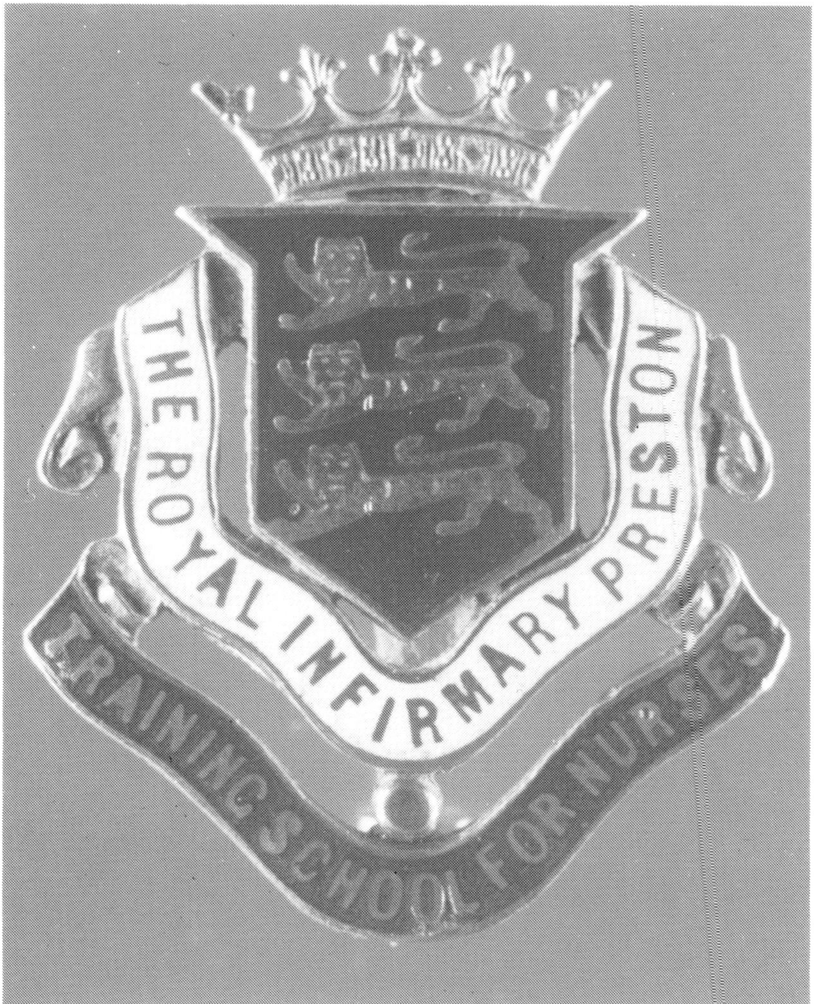

The Infirmary Training School badge, received after qualifying.

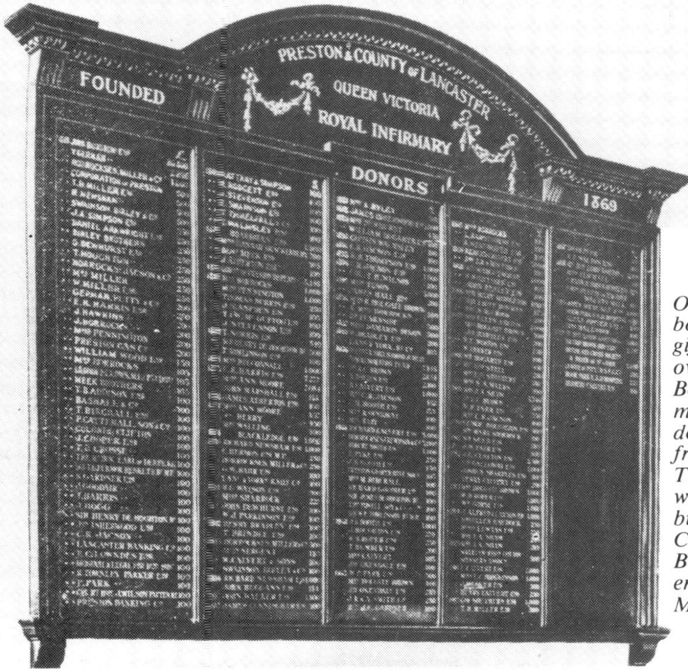
PRESTON & COUNTY OF LANCASTER
QUEEN VICTORIA
ROYAL INFIRMARY
FOUNDED
1869
DONORS

One of the donor boards which records gifts and donations over the years. Below left: the memorial recording the donation of £10,000 from Alderman Thomas Parkinson which enabled the building of the Children's Ward. Below right: the entrance to the 1936 Maternity Hospital.

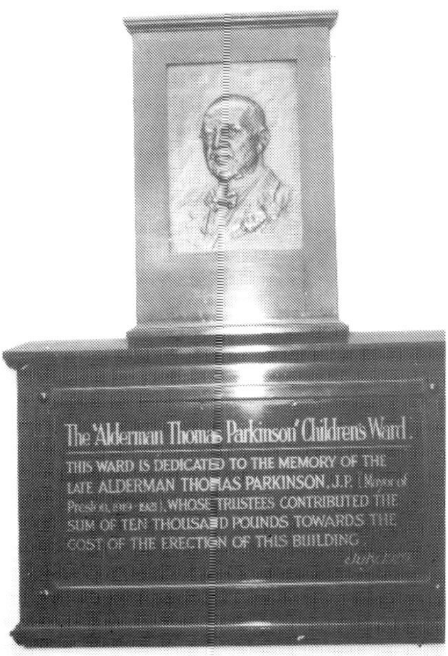
The 'Alderman Thomas Parkinson' Childrens Ward.
THIS WARD IS DEDICATED TO THE MEMORY OF THE
LATE ALDERMAN THOMAS PARKINSON, J.P.
WHOSE TRUSTEES CONTRIBUTED THE
SUM OF TEN THOUSAND POUNDS TOWARDS THE
COST OF THE ERECTION OF THIS BUILDING.

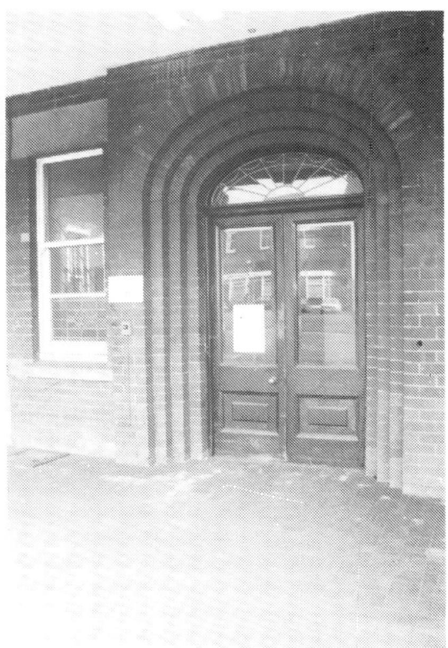

The now famous wall tiles of the Children's Ward. Erected shortly after the Great War, Preston Corporation paid for 6 of these tiles as a memorial to those who fell in the war.

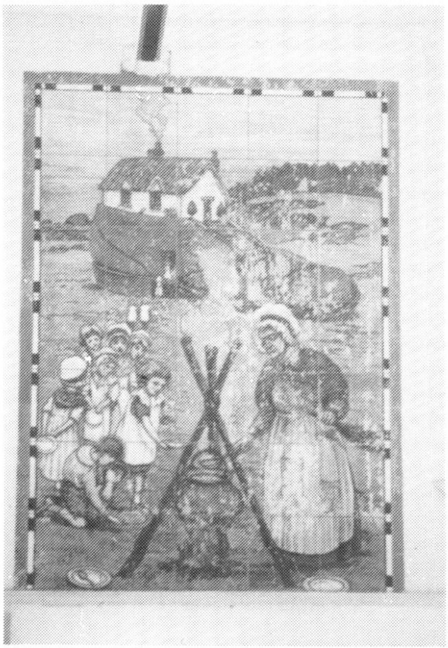

The Old Lady who lived in a shoe.

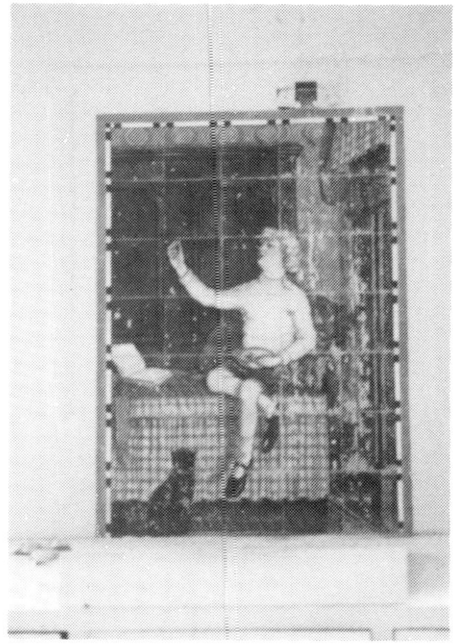

Little Jack Horner.

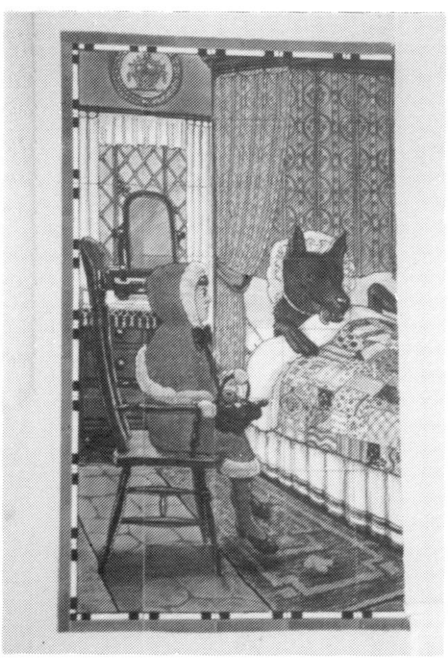

Little Red Riding Hood.

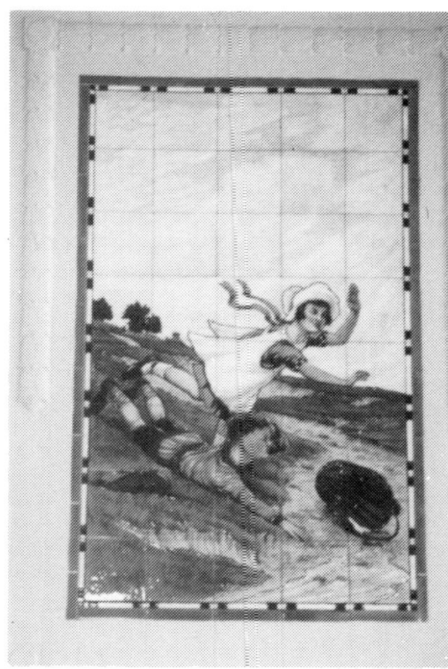

Jack and Jill.

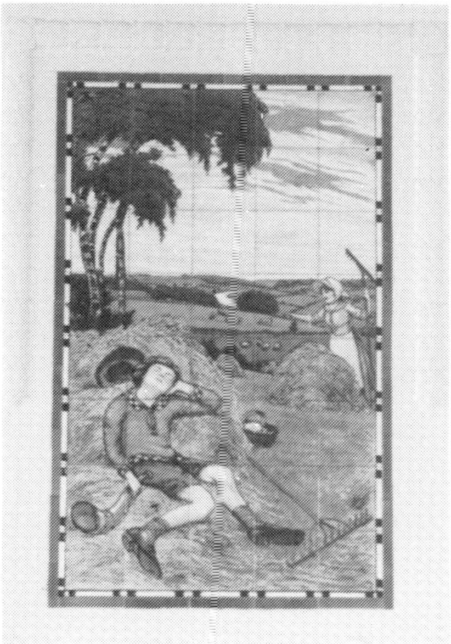

Little Boy Blue.

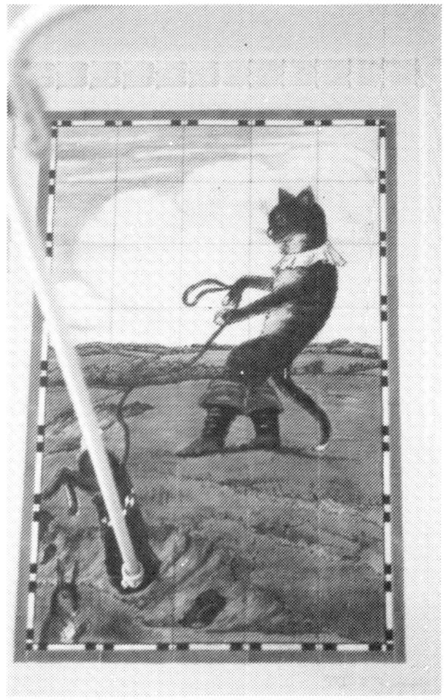

Puss in Boots.

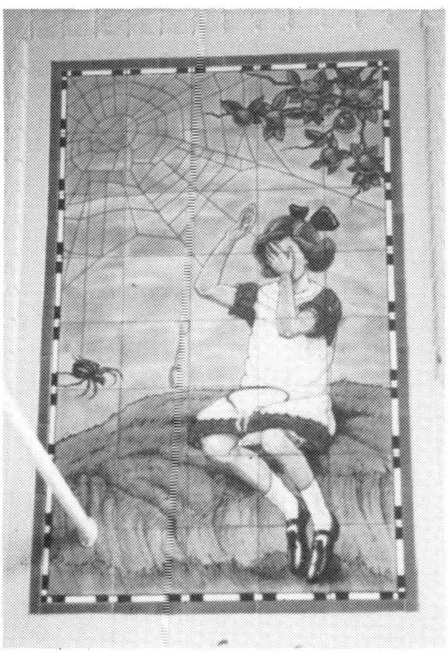

Little Miss Muffet.

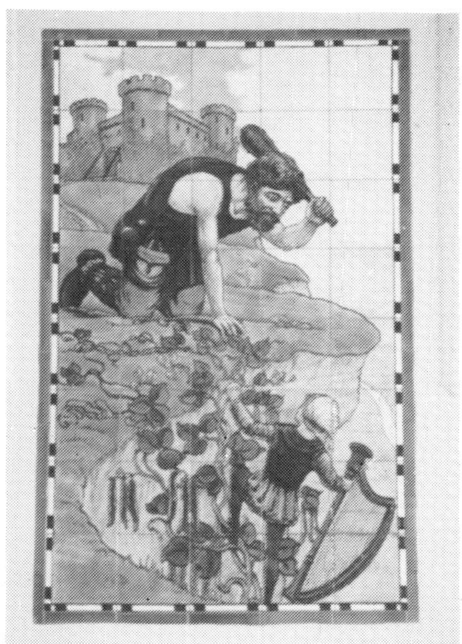

Jack and the Beanstalk.

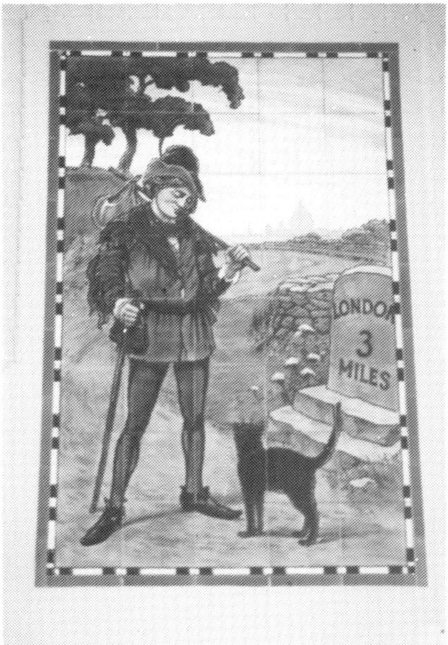

Dick Whittington.

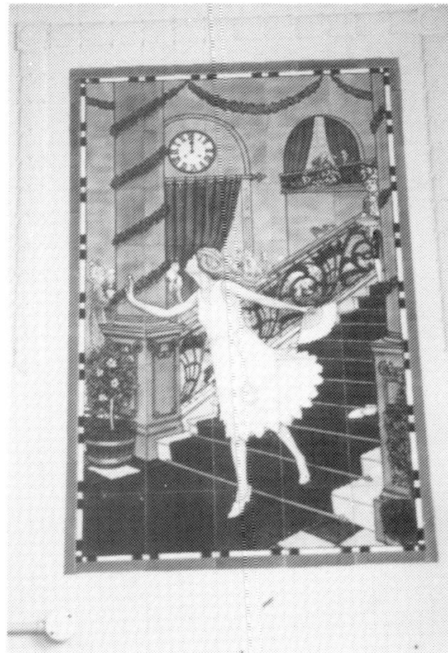

Cinderella.

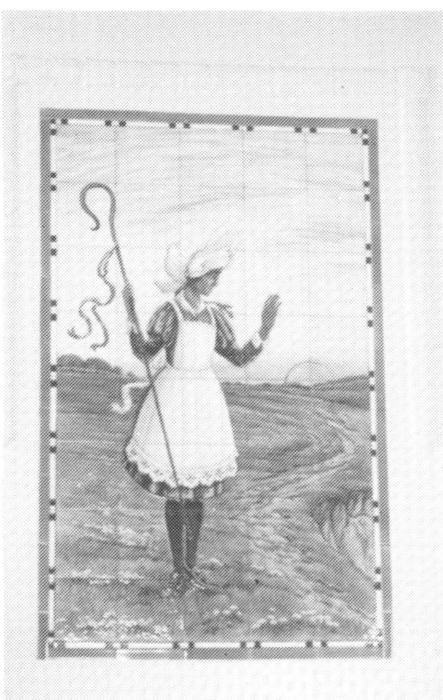

Little Bo Peep.

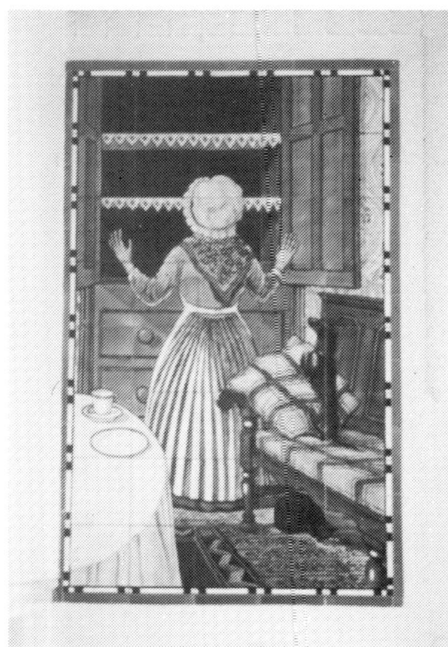

Old Mother Hubbard.

Mr. Robert M. Corbet died at his home in Dublin in September 1980 at the age of 83 years. Mr. Corbet was consultant obstetrician and gynaecologist at Preston Royal Infirmary from 1948 until he retired from the N.H.S. in 1962 at the age of 65 years to take a post as medical officer with the Canadian armed forces in Germany and carried on working until returning to Ireland in 1975 at the age of 78 years. He made many notable contributions to the advancement of knowledge in his speciality and there will be many former patients who will feel forever indebted to him for his skill and kindness.

Mr. Charles Beard, consultant plastic surgeon, died on 27th November after a year-long illness. Later Mrs. Beard unveiled a plaque naming the burns unit theatre as the Charles Beard Theatre in memory of her husband.

The death was announced of Hilda M. Foster whose name was synonymous with the annual presentation of medals in the Preston School of Nursing. The trust fund established by Miss Foster's father, a former chairman of the Hospital Management Committee provided the income for the purchase of medals for prize day.

Miss Winifred Phillips, the deputy matron under Miss Beech in maternity, died on 28th November, 1980. Among the Infirmary's staff retiring were Mr. Bill White, a pharmacy technician for 29 years at P.R.I., Mr. Norman Sutcliffe, chief salaries and wages officer, 34 years, Dr. Brierley, consultant physician at P.R.I. and latterly at Sharoe Green Hospital and Mr. Maurice who began the plastic surgery unit in Preston two years before and was known internationally for his work on cleft palates. Mrs. Vera Molloy, 25 years in the sewing room and Mr. Alan Ward, the foreman plumber, who took early retirement because of ill health. Mr. S. Rawlinson who arrived at Preston Royal Infirmary in 1954 as a senior accountancy assistant and later in February 1975 was appointed assistant district finance officer, also retired in 1980. Mr. A. J. Howcroft was appointed consultant plastic surgeon in place of Mr. D. J. Maurice with effect from 1st October 1980.

In January 1979 a new and larger incinerator had been fitted at the Infirmary to replace the old unit which had seen better days. The new incinerator was fired by gas and the monthly consumption figures were plotted. At the end of December 1979 the works department energy team discussed ways to reduce the consumption which resulted in the fitting of new controls to the incinerator and a revision in the operation of firing the unit. The end result issued in December 1980 showed a halving of the fuel bill for the Infirmary, a cash saving of over £3,000 per annum.

'1981 will be a year of change for many people, a year of fulfilment for some and year of apprehension for others but nevertheless a year of historic importance for the Preston Health District'. This was the new year message to the staff from the district nursing officer. It could also be looked upon as the end of an era where the Royal patronage had been transferred to the Royal Preston Hospital from what was now known by some people as Preston Infirmary. It could aptly be described as a period of uncertainty with shadow district health authorities due to be appointed within the year, health authority members appointed in the autumn and new district officers appointed in the early months of 1982.

Monday January 12th 1981 saw the opening of the first department at the

Royal Preston Hospital when physiotherapy patients began arriving at 9.30 a.m. Some members of the staff were left at the Infirmary to cover the department there until out-patient clinics were eventually transferred some months in the future following which the department would be allowed to 'run down gracefully'. The medical illustration department also transferred in from the Ribbleton Hospital.

Nostalgia was much to the fore at a senior staff buffet held in the Infirmary, the staff very conscious of the fact that this would be the last occasion when the present staff of the Infirmary would be together as colleagues, some moving to the new hospital and others taking the opportunity to retire. The catering staff did a wonderful job in decorating the dining room in blue and white; there was a turkey with the old Preston and Chorley H.M.C. crest emblazoned upon it and a magnificent cake with the Preston Royal Infirmary badge in icing decorating the top. The feeling of nostalgia did not, however, spoil the enjoyment of the buffet nor prevent the staff having a wonderful evening. A farewell party was held on 10th May 1985 by members of the Infirmary's laundry staff to mark the final closing of the laundry at P.R.I., the last pieces of linen being processed on 29th May 1985, after which the work was transferred to the Whittingham Hospital laundry. The event saw the retirement of Mrs. Nellie Marsden who had started work in the laundry at the age of 14 years for a weekly wage of 7/6 (37½p) and in her 46 years had served under six laundry managers.

The growth in out-patient attendances was discussed at length as the vastly improved out-patient accommodation was already fully utilized. A suggestion was made that patients south of the Ribble, excepting Penwortham, might find it easier to attend the out-patient facility at Chorley Hospital although a considerable enlargement of the out-patient department at Chorley would be necessary for this to allow for the population of Chorley and Leyland, Bamber Bridge, Walton and Hoghton etc. It was reported that in the short period the medical records department had been based in the R.P.H. difficulties had arisen regarding staffing due to an increase of 40% in the number of out-patients seen. There were not sufficient experienced staff available to cope with what had turned out to be a mammoth task when combined with major new procedural problems associated with the centralisation of records and a master index — all this at a time when the Royal Preston Hospital was not yet fully operational.

It was in June 1981 that a requisition was passed for the purchase of disposable catering materials, paper cups, plates, serviettes etc., to be issued to all the catering departments in celebration of the Royal Wedding of their Highnesses the Prince and Princess of Wales, at a cost of £454.32. In the same month the District Management Team received a request from Daniel Thwaites & Co. Ltd., to purchase land within the boundary of the R.P.H. site on which to build a public house. This request was turned down by the D.M.T. 'as not being in the best interests of the Hospital'.

Upgrading of the Infirmary's telephone system at a cost of £7,100, to ensure that an efficient telephone service was maintained was carried out in June and at the same time the addressograph model was replaced at a cost of £621, the old model having been in service for 21 years. A further £7,000 plus V.A.T. was expended for a replacement tube for the Infirmary's E.M.I. scanner as the old x-ray tube was nearing the end of its life.

The district finance officer reported an overspending of £250,000 overall for the three months to 30th June 1981. He stated 'while it was not possible to judge the true significance of the overspending due to so many extraordinary factors currently occurring e.g. delays in the commissioning of the R.P.H. and continuing high "on costs" for Sharoe Green Hospital and the Infirmary, the high degree of expenditure in meeting short-comings and deficiencies in departments and equipment for the new hospital, a lack of progress on the agreed efficiency savings programme and also the growth in the number of patients treated at the R.P.H. and Chorley'. Later it was announced that the overspending figures of 31st July 1981 continued to rise, the figure now being £355,531. Extra revenue was requested from the Regional Hospital Authority but the district nursing officer suggested that in the event of this claim being rejected there would have to be a curtailment of recruiting of nursing staffs with the consequent reduction in beds and expenditure at the R.P.H.

In September the D.N.O. reported to the D.M.T. a shortage of nursing staffs for the operating theatres at the Royal Preston Hospital and the Infirmary and made a request that the operating lists should be reduced. The shortage of trained theatre nurses was exacerbated by the unrealistic theatre lists extending on some occasions to 7 p.m. and 9 p.m. with very late starts and long interruptions in the lists were also adding problems. A letter was sent to all the consultants and a meeting arranged of the theatre users' committee to try to iron out these problems. This situation was not helped when a further stage in the commissioning of the R.P.H. was reached in the summer of 1981 with the opening of the operating theatres and surgical wards. Four theatres were brought into use, their first case being an emergency operation.

The hospital chapel was formally dedicated in the name of St. Barnabas by the Rt. Rev. D. F. Page, Bishop of Lancaster, Rt. Rev. B. Foley, R.C. Bishop of Lancaster and the Rev. T. J. Booth, chairman of the Preston Free Church Federal Council. The name of St. Barnabas is well known to the people of Preston with the houses situated nearest to the Infirmary itself being in St. Barnabas Place. In the Infirmary's own chapel there are six stained glass windows, one for the P.R.I. nurses league, one for Florence Nightingale, one for St. John, St. Luke, St. Paul and another for St. Paul's friend and contemporary, St. Barnabas.

Wards 9, 10 and 15 opened at R.P.H. on 12th September 1981 with the transfer of urological and surgical patients and during the week-end of 26th/27th September the accident and emergency department, intensive care unit and coronary care, Brown Ward, orthopaedic, medical and West wards all transferred out of the Infirmary together with the fracture and orthopaedic out-patient clinics. Following this mass exodus, the Infirmary seemed strangely quiet and still after so many years of activity.

The quiet was soon broken, however, when the decision was taken to upgrade Albert and Alice Wards to accommodate gynaecology while Sharoe Green Hospital was being converted into a new ward block for the District's gynaecological services. Tenders were received on 5th August 1981, the cost of the upgrading exercise being £15,699.20 although the overall cost was £24,000.

Further problems were arising at R.P.H. in the eye theatre associated with the vibration of the microscopes used by the eye surgeons during operations which was causing delay in the transfer of eye patients into the new hospital.

The year 1981 was marred by a tragic death at the Royal Preston Hospital; Mr. Cliff Whewell, a shift fitter at the hospital, died on duty when steam tore open a valve on which he was working; he had joined the hospital's staff 18 months previously. A former member of the Infirmary's staff, Les Lee, died on the medical ward, having retired just 18 months before, and also Roland Beare, former chief stores clerk, and Ted Chapman, a retired porter, died during 1981. Staff throughout the Health District were shocked by the sudden death of Alice Shaw on 11th December 1981. Trained at P.R.I. and a stalwart of the nurses league; also of the District's hospital choir, she had served in many capacities, as sister on the medical ward and Green Ward and latterly as nursing officer.

Among staff retiring during 1981 were Harold Eastough, night telephonist for many years and Mr. James Moss, charge nurse in the out-patient department. Miss Violet Hitchen, sister of East Ward for many years and latterly of the surgery and out-patient clinic of the dental and maxillo-facial unit at P.R.I. retired in November 1981 after 42 years service. Dr. Robert Gibb retired on 28th May 1981 having served the Preston District for more than 30 years in the field of radiotherapy. His appointment as director of the Christie Hospital in Manchester did not break Dr. Gibb's link with Preston when he made the decision to retain the clinic held weekly in the Infirmary. Mrs. Gladys Morgan retired after 47 years at P.R.I., progressing from a young operator to laundry manageress; she had seen many changes over the years with the introduction of new and modern machinery in stark contrast to the flat irons used for ironing uniforms and goffering irons used for nurses caps when she commenced in the laundry at 7/6 (37½p) a week. Retirement came too for Mrs. Jean Hartley, the chief medical laboratory scientific officer in the laboratory's blood transfusion department for 30 years and also Sister Hayden, sister in charge of South Ward at the Infirmary after 35 years service.

The district nursing officer, Miss Doris Salisbury, was awarded the O.B.E. in the Honours List in 1981 and the appointment was announced of Mr. R. P. Jones, consultant plastic surgeon from 1st October 1981.

Dr. Cooper, consultant anaethetist since 1953, retired in 1982, also Dr. David Irwin, consultant radiologist and Dr. L. Robertson, director of the public health laboratory since its inception in 1958. Miss McGrath, known affectionately by everyone at P.R.I. as Rene, who had been associated with the nurses home for almost 35 years, retired late in 1982. Early in 1982 staff throughout the Health District were shocked and saddened by the sudden death of two members of staff, Pat Lane, a clerical officer in the catering department and Mr. W. J. C. Thomas, a most popular and talented consultant urological surgeon who died whilst on holiday.

An early taste of Christmas came to the Infirmary in December 1982 with the smell of roast turkey pervading the air. As the result of a hoax telephone call, hundreds of birds were collected from supermarkets throughout the region and taken to the N.W. Forensic Science Laboratory at Washington Hall, near Chorley, to be tested. The tests proved that the birds had not been poisoned as the hoaxer had claimed, but by this time they were unfit for human consumption and were sent to the Infirmary for destruction by burning in the

Infirmary's incinerator. Having carried out this mammoth task it was reported that engineer John Morris did not really fancy turkey for his Christmas dinner.

During alterations being carried out at Ribbleton Hospital, the builders found old magazines, toys and newspapers, including a copy of the *Preston Herald* dated December 23rd 1874. This contained an item called 'Christmas preparations' which stated:

> Christmas with its round of festivities and its universal good cheer is now rapidly approaching and a real old fashioned Christmas it promises to be. On every hand extensive preparations are being made for duly celebrating this holiday season and on whomsoever the blame may rest it will be no fault of our local tradesmen if the inhabitants of Preston are not fully provided with the concomitants popularly known as Christmas fare. On Friday evening the shops in our principal throroughfares were decked out in a most tempting manner, the enterprising proprietors vieing with each other in a most tempting display for the benefit of the public . . . Christmas too, is this year surrounded by many auspices, Trade is tolerably brisk, work is plentiful and there is nothing, we feel assured to prevent our people from living as they have been wont to live in years gone by at this festive season, on the fat of the land.

This together with a wealth of information on the cost of Christmas presents and the general way of life more than a century ago contained in the other material found, made interesting reading.

The death was announced on Christmas Eve 1982 of Miss Mary Thompson, a lady who had spent more than 50 years raising money for Preston Royal Infirmary as treasurer of the Ladies Comforts League. The League in 1983 held their A.G.M. in the Infirmary, handing over a donation of £629 for the purchase of equipment for the wards and the following year the members of the League decided to disband due to the run down of the Infirmary and also for lack of success in recruitment of members. The Health Authority formally recorded its appreciation for the services provided by the League over the past 72 years and were unanimous in expressing thanks on behalf of all patients whose stay in the Infirmary had been made that much more comfortable through the work of the League.

It was a sad reflection of the general economic situation at the opening of 1983 with the bleak financial outlook of the Preston Health Authority. This stemmed from two main issues; firstly, the insufficient funds available to operate the prestigious Royal Preston Hospital to its full capacity, and secondly by the insistence of the D.H.S.S. on 'efficiency savings' being made. It was anticipated that the Authority could be overspent by £1.5 million by March 1983 and the district treasurer summarised the position that 'when you are up to your armpits in alligators, its not much use remembering that the original task was to drain the swamp'. Later it was reported that the final overspending figure for 1982/83 was not as high a figure as was feared and it was claimed that this has been achieved by the combination of good housekeeping and a package of non-repetitive measures; however, the Authority continued to spend at a rate that was in excess of the funds available.

Chapter Eleven

Goodbye to the Infirmary 1981-1987

EARLY in 1981, with the transfer of staff throughout the Health District increasing apace, a recruitment campaign for nurses to work at the Royal Preston Hospital was launched by James Hunt, former World Champion Grand Prix driver. The campaign, which was to run for four months, used the message 'Join Preston's Winning Team' as its slogan.

Amid the discussion on the reorganisation of the National Health Service which occupied the administration in June 1981, further problems were evident at the Royal Preston Hospital. A proposal was made to transfer surgical beds to the new hospital, with emergency cases being admitted from 29th June 1981. There was also a call for an electronic barrier to be fitted in the car park at the Royal Preston Hospital for even at this early stage medical staff called urgently to the hospital to attend cases were finding it difficult to park their cars.

Far wider issues faced the District Management Team with the announcement in the summer of 1981 on the National Health Service reorganisation structure and management. Since the first reorganisation of the N.H.S. in 1974, the structure below the Department of Health had been based on Regional Health Authorities and Area Health Authorities, the boundaries of which were co-terminous with the local authorities responsible for social services and education. In a metropolitan county like Greater Manchester the A.H.A.s were co-terminous with metropolitan districts but in non-metropolitan counties such as Lancashire the A.H.A. was based on the county council and so this accounted for the fact that the six districts in Lancashire did not have their own health authorities.

The decisions announced for a further reorganisation from April 1982 meant that the Lancashire Area Health Authority would cease to exist and five of the six districts, namely Burnley, Blackpool, Blackburn, Ormskirk and Lancaster, would form their own health authorities corresponding substantially to their present catchment population. The Preston District was, however, to be divided with Chorley and South Ribble becoming a seventh Health District, much against the advice of the Lancashire Area Health Authority and the North West Regional Health Authority.

The decision came as a great surprise to all concerned in the health services for Preston and Chorley and South Ribble, the main concern being that instead of patient services receiving the benefit of reduced administrative costs, it was apparent that both the new district health authorities would have to be funded from the present allocation of funds based on population. To set up separate offices for the district administrator, district finance officer, nursing officer, community physician and consultant and general practitioner team members in the two new authorities would be relatively easy but the division of specialised departments would not be so simple. These would include nurse teaching, maternity services, special baby care units, psychiatric services, audiology, major accident and intensive care units, oral surgery and orthodontic laboratories, orthoptics and many more.

Many of the patient services based at Preston served other neighbouring districts and areas and devolution of some of these services would not be possible. These included a considerable load of pathology services, e.g. biochemistry, cytology, histopathology, neuropathology, virology and immunology and also haematology and blood transfusion. In-patients were also received in Preston from a wide area of the north west region for neurosurgery, plastic surgery, neurology, urology etc. The District Management Team stated:

> that in due course profiles of services within the spheres of the two Authorities would need to be prepared mainly by staff somewhat demoralised and heavily engaged on the strategic reorganisation of the District services occasioned by the commissioning of the prestigious Royal Preston Hospital and the running down of some Hospitals and the closure of others. It was hoped that public recognition would be given to those members of staff who were likely to carry a heavy burden in the coming years.

Later in the year the members of the new Health Authority were named, with Mr. R. E. Hodd becoming the first appointed chairman and Lostock Hall Continuation Hospital closed with the staff being transferred to other posts in Preston, Chorley and the community nursing service. The district nursing officer in October 1981 reported a call for assurance that nursing care would be available when the gynaecological services transferred into the Infirmary. There was considerable evidence that nursing staffs were being drained from the Sharoe Green and Infirmary complex to provide a complete service at the Royal Preston Hospital. The obstetric and gynaecological consultants were angry with this situation and insisted that the practice of removing nursing and ancillary personnel to the new Hospital at the expense of other departments would have to cease. They stated that they would not be prepared to transfer into the Infirmary unless an assurance was given that adequate nursing, ancillary and senior house officer cover would be provided. 'The Gynaecological Service is an existing and continuing one and should be serviced as such' they said. Such an assurance was later given by the members of the District Management Team.

A special meeting was held on the 6th October 1981 to discuss the Phase I and Phase II development of the new hospital. The phasing of the construction had been purely for financial expedience; however, certain essential disciplines for the operation of a large district general hospital were omitted, i.e. there was no pharmacy or laundry facilities included and no pathology services. It soon became evident that something needed to be done to remedy these omissions, especially in the case of emergencies. The consultant pathologists expressed the hope that the laboratory planned in Phase I at R.P.H. would be completed within 18 months and would include an emergency laboratory for urgent biochemical investigations, for until the pathology phase I was completed all emergency work would have to be carried out at the Infirmary.

The chief officers of the new Preston Health Authority due to be appointed from 1st April 1982 were Mr. John Roe, district administrator, Mr. John Whalley, district finance officer, Mr. Brian Wilson, district nursing officer and Dr. P. G. Holt the district's medical officer. The retirements were announced of Mr. Harry Hill, the district administrator of the Preston District, Mr. John Hindle, the district finance officer and Miss Doris Salisbury, the district nursing officer. Farewells came thick and fast during this period of change and further reorganisation. Miss Joan Topham, the chief medical records officer at Preston Royal Infirmary retired, having commenced her duties in September 1937 and served the Infirmary with unstinting dedication and loyalty for almost 45 years, Miss I. M. Eagles, chief clerical officer in the x-ray department at P.R.I. retired in July 1982 after 32 years service and Mr. Arthur Fallows, a skilled member of the maxillo-facial laboratory for many years, decided to retire.

The continuing loss of expertise of long serving members of staff during 1983 included Miss Joan Vernon, a stalwart of the finance department for 34 years and Mr. Cyril Simons also from the finance department, after more than 35 years service. From the supplies department, Mr. Frank Edmonson and Miss Elsa Buck and the deputy administrator of the Infirmary, Mrs. McGowan, Mrs. Lucy Dewhurst, for 26 years an orderly on Holden and Alice Wards, and Mr. Joe Ford with 37 years service in the Infirmary's boiler house. From the nursing division Miss Joyce James, sister on the children's ward for more than 35 years and Sister Winifred Mudge, theatre sister at P.R.I. and latterly at the Royal Preston Hospital in oral surgery; also Marion Smith who began her training in Preston in 1957 and served as a staff nurse on South Ward before becoming night sister in 1963. The deaths were announced of Mr. James Glennie, consultant thoracic surgeon, of Joan Field, medical secretary at P.R.I., S.G.H. and R.P.H. who died on 11th August 1983 and also of Mr. Bill White who had retired from the Infirmary's pharmacy just three years before.

This period saw the departure of so many long-serving members of the Infirmary's staff including Dr. Angus Gray who came to P.R.I. in November 1944 as resident anaesthetist and in 1950 became the Infirmary's only consultant anaesthetist, Dr. Hugh McIntyre, consultant anaesthetist in Preston since 1960, well known as an evangelist and remembered by many members of staff at the Infirmary for the part he played in the annual Lenten lunchtime services held in the Infirmary's chapel. Dr. Janet Woodruffe, consultant anaesthetist, Dr. G. Hesling consultant paediatrician in Preston for 30 years, Mr. W. H. Lonsdale, consultant surgeon, Mr. D. Vero, consultant dental surgeon and Mr. R. A. Daws, consultant neurosurgeon, also departed. Mr. J. W. Beare for 20 years a porter at P.R.I. on day and night duty and Mr. George Yelling, storesman at the Infirmary working in Stanleyfield Road before transferring with the District stores to Whittingham Hospital was forced to take early retirement through ill health after after more than 20 years service. Margaret Fadyan, a maid in the maternity department, the nurses home and latterly the sister's home retired after more than 20 years service. Mrs. M. Middleton, co-ordinator of medical secretaries and Stephanie Czaja, a member of the Infirmary's kitchen staff also retired during this period. Leaving the nursing service, Sister Doreen Parkinson who came to Preston in 1954 as a district nurse, commenced at P.R.I. in 1958 as a staff nurse in the accident and emergency department, becoming sister of that department in 1968 and Mrs. Horan who commenced in 1948 as a nursing auxiliary serving for many years as an S.R.N. and in the out-patient department from 1968 before transferring to R.P.H. in 1981. Mrs. M. L. Brooks who retired after more than 20 years service as a domestic at P.R.I. but who unfortunately died shortly afterwards on 2nd April 1984. The news was announced of the death in Ireland of Sister Hayden formerly sister of South Ward until her retirement in 1981, she died on the 8th August 1984 following a long illness and news reached Preston of Dr Vladimir Griffel who died peacefully at his home in Bloxham, Oxfordshire, on 14th November, 1983. Dr. Griffel had retired in September 1963 and those who remember the former consultant chest physician will recall his charm and quiet courtesy to the staff and his patients.

This was a time of constant change as more of the new hospital building became available for occupancy and further wards and departments were transferred into the large complex. The Infirmary continued to supply its services with Alice Ward carrying on unchanged and Albert Ward made ready to accept gynaecological patients from Sharoe Green Hospital. Neurology patients were admitted into brown and green wards and orthopaedic patients were transferred into the medical wards which were now 110 years old. The orthopaedic ward, another of the original Harris Fever Wards, was altered to become a small day ward and the ophthalmic ward, occupying the third fever ward, carried on as before. Some clinics were still being held in the Infirmary but the out-patients department which had seen constant activity, day and night for some 85 years, seemed strangely quiet and subdued.

In July 1983 the planning panel of the Preston Health Authority discussed their plans for the run down and the transfer of services out of the Infirmary. A demand for the early closure of the Infirmary to enable financial savings to be made was received from the R.H.A. in the same year but there was apprehension among staff members that the general disruption of services would affect in-patient and out-patient services, increase waiting lists and have a potential risk to patients and some doubts were expressed as to whether early closure of the Infirmary would achieve the overall savings anticipated by the R.H.A. The Health Authority at its meeting on Friday 21st October 1983 discussed among other matters the latest information on manpower cuts, the proposed closure of the Infirmary and the general financial situation They issued a statement 'that the closure of the Infirmary would mean a temporary loss of beds and other direct patient care facilities with a considerable amount of inconvenience and disruption to patients and staff alike'. The omission of the pathology department from the forward planning estimates of the R.H.A. early in 1984 was a blow to the Preston Health Authority as it meant that when the

Infirmary finally closed, or at least until the start of the 1987/88 period, pathology would have to remain on the Infirmary site in Meadow Street. This was considered unacceptable and undesirable from both a clinical and financial aspect by the Preston Authority and it was agreed that the N.W.R.H.A. should be asked to explain their reasons for omitting the scheme.

An upgrading of the reception/main entrance of the District Headquarters was completed, restoring some of the former glory of the Victorian edifice by sand blasting. Two wrought iron hand rails made by Mr. Harry Hall, the blacksmith from Whittingham Hospital, incorporating the Lancashire Rose and the Preston Lamb were added to blend with the front facade of the 19th-century building, the whole project being undertaken by the Health District's works department. Reference has been made by the Health Authority to the fact that none of the buildings of the Infirmary were listed as being of architectural or historical interest, which perhaps highlights the fact that no such application has been made for this to be achieved. There is no doubt that a case could be made for the preservation of the main Infirmary block on the grounds of historical interest for, as this volume shows, it has been in existence since 1833, pre-dating Stephenson Terrace built in 1851 which has already been listed for preservation. The Infirmary also has the distinction of having been enlarged by public donation as Preston's memorial to Queen Victoria which places it firmly as part of Preston's history if for no other reason than this.

A further milestone in the Infirmary's history was reached with the completion of a series of schemes involving an expenditure in excess of £2 million pounds providing the centralisation of maternity and gynaecological services at Sharoe Green Hospital. Two new 32-bedded wards were introduced at ground floor level incorporating the former day care unit for the use of gynaecological patients, a pleasing feature being the incorporation of the stained glass window depicting the madonna and child which had been transferred from the Infirmary's maternity hospital and placed within the entrance area of the new department. On the floor above linked with the main hospital corridor, is a 30-bedded maternity ward and also the ultrasound department which had been transferred in from its rather cramped accommodation on the top floor of the Infirmary's maternity hospital.

The former wards of the building had been substantially adapted to provide a central delivery suite with 16 delivery rooms, a 29-cot special baby care unit and a 4-bedded G.P. unit, while on the top floor a further two 30-bedded maternity wards were provided. It was anticipated that some 4,200 deliveries a year would make the unit one of the largest in the north west of England. Many improvements had also been made in the operating theatres which served the unit, with medical gas services being renewed, the air conditioning improved, new autoclaves installed and the operating lamps refurbished. The ante-natal clinic had been completely rewired and adapted to cope with the increased number of patients which would result following the closure of the Infirmary's clinics and minor improvements to the S.G.H. out-patient department would enable it to accommodate the gynaecological clinics. To service this new unit the midwifery training school was transferred into accommodation adapted for the purpose on the Sharoe Green Hospital site.

The final transfer of patients out of the Infirmary's maternity hospital took place during the week-end 1st and 2nd March 1986, finally overcoming the difficulty of operating the service on two sites and allowing the Health Authority to close the maternity hospital and wards. It also allowed for the re-development of the former maternity department at S.G.H. for use as an orthopaedic unit which when completed in March 1987 would allow the Infirmary to be finally closed for in-patient use.

It was following my suggestion that there was a need to identify and catalogue all the items of historical and monetary value within the Infirmary that a small working party was set up in the summer of 1985. At the inaugural meeting of this committee, attended by Mr. D. Woods, deputy administrator at P.R.I., Mr. A. Matthews, district building officer, Mr. F. Wright, divisional supplies department, Miss J. Knipe, Grange-Over-Sands (representing the P.R.I. League of Nurses) and Mr. J. H. Wilkinson, senior chief medical laboratory scientific officer, it was agreed that in order to itemise all items of historical, aesthetic and monetary value within and without the Infirmary's premises they would require some assistance to carry out what could prove to be a time consuming exercise.

With the help, therefore, of volunteers from the two retirement fellowships within the district (*viz.* the N.H.S. Fellowship and the N.A.L.G.O. Health Service Fellowship) a full and comprehensive inventory of all items, large and small, was completed, enabling the working party to finalise their proposals for the disposal of items of interest. Some idea of the volume of material listed is shown in Appendix A, although this is not a complete record of every item dealt with by the working party.

The final meeting took place, again in the board room at the Infirmary, on 30th July 1986, with Mr. Jim Kelly, acting deputy administrator for P.R.I. in the chair, when recommendations were made for submission to the District Management Team for the disposal of the more lucrative items found, bearing in mind the financial difficulties facing the Authority. A sale of furniture to staff and 'associated organisations' took place at the end of May which resulted in offers totalling some £8,500 and subsequent offers received for sanitary ware raised a further £1,400 and a second sale was to be arranged for October 1986.

The rush-bottomed chairs in the nurses dining room, which were more than 150 years old, having been made in 1821 were despatched to the Chester salerooms of Sotheby's for inclusion in their catalogues and they estimated that the 120 chairs if sold in lots of 8 should raise approximately £800 per set with a further 20 chairs realising £75 each.

Considerable interest was shown in the 12 nursery rhyme tiled panels and individual animal tiles in the children's ward. The cost of removing the tiles safely for disposal was estimated by the Heritage Tile Conservation as £6,700 with the cost of cleaning and remounting the panels probably a similar sum. Sotheby's however anticipated that each panel on offer, could realise between £1,500 and £2,500 each. The working party recommendation was that six panels should be sent to Sotheby's which would raise the finance for the removal of all the panels by Heritage Tiles and that the remaining panels should be disposed of as follows:

2 to be on permanent loan to the Harris Museum.

2 to be on permanent loan to the Museum of Childhood, Lancaster.

2 to be donated to the Paediatric Unit at the Royal Preston Hospital.

It was considered that this distribution would bring the panels to a wider audience in Preston, bearing in mind that 5 of the panels were originally purchased by the officers and work staff of Preston Corporation as a memorial to their colleagues who had died in the First World War. The Health Authority agreed with the recommendations of the working party. The chapel organ was assessed by Mr. Christopher Dickens, an expert on organs, who suggested that the instrument be offered for sale in a specialist journal; although he found the organ in poor condition parts of it he considered were good. It was recommended that the stained glass windows in the chapel would be preserved together with the kneelers, benches, chalices, crucifixes, bible etc. to go toward the formation of a chapel at Sharoe Green Hospital. There was one exception in that the Florence Nightingale window, it was suggested, should go to the District's Nurse Training School.

One of the main problems facing the working party was the disposal of more than 120 wall plaques commemorating donations to the Infirmary during previous administrations. It was agreed that the *Lancashire Evening Post* be approached in order to publicise the problem and perhaps generate interest from relatives of benefactors desirous of receiving their particular plaque. A few enquiries relating to certain plaques were received and eventually claimed; there were, however, a large number remaining unclaimed and it was finally decided to recommend that these would eventually have to be destroyed while the ceramic tiles would have to remain on site in the building.

The disposal of other items to the county archivist, pictures to the Harris Art Gallery and Museum, old records to the records officer at Sharoe Green Hospital and the signed photograph of H.M. The Queen from the board room and the photograph of Princess Mary, Viscountess Lascelles, were to be transferred into the new board room at District Headquarters, were other recommendations of the working party accepted by the members of the Health Authority.

Other items received scant attention, e.g. the polished wood panels lining the Infirmary's main corridor which in themselves are a substantial page in the Infirmary's history recording as they do the donations made to the Infirmary covering the period 1869-1940. There is also the panel recording the gifts and donations made to the Infirmary by Sir Charles Brown amounting to over £40,000, not an insignificant sum pre-1925; no mention is made of these items in the final report and their final resting place is not known.

My suggestion that the foundation stones, some 15 in number, should be recovered and perhaps placed into a commemorative wall with a seat included for the benefit of patients in the grounds of the Royal Preston Hospital or Sharoe Green Hospital, or that the frontispiece over the main Infirmary entrance recording the date of its erection (1833) or the main hospital gates should also be recovered and preserved in some capacity, received scant consideration. The reminder that there were perhaps 'Time Capsules' placed within the foundation stones containing items pertaining to the year of their laying raised little enthusiasm, neither did the reminder that the Infirmary had been enlarged as a memorial to Queen Victoria financed by the people of Preston.

The final recommendation regarding the disposal of the income arising from the sale of furniture and equipment etc. was that it should be utilised for:

(a) Removing the Nursery Rhyme Tiles.

(b) Removing the Stained Glass Windows.

(c) The purchase of a Display Cabinet.

(d) The repair of the Infirmary Bible.

(e) The establishment of a chapel at Sharoe Green Hospital.

Further items of historical interest were two busts which had rested on the Infirmary's main corridor for more than half a century and two oil paintings which adorned the main corridor walls. The paintings were of Dr. Moore who practised in Lune Street, Preston, and who was appointed a senior physician to the Preston Dispensary in April 1828 and in which capacity he continued to serve until his death in 1848, and of Dr. F. W. Collinson M.E. (Edin.), M.R.C.P. (Lond.), M.R.C.S. (Eng.), F.R.C.S. (Edin.), who was connected with Preston Royal Infirmary for the greater part of his professional career, for many years as senior surgeon and also as secretary of the honorary medical board. He resigned from the hon. surgical staff of the Infirmary on 30th April 1923 but he became a vice-president of the Infirmary and remained a member of the honorary consultant staff until his death in 1928. These paintings were accepted by the post graduate medical centre where it is hoped they will remain for many years to come as a reminder of the dedication of service not only of the two distinguised medical officers preserved in oils but also of the countless number of people who chose to put up with long hours, poor living conditions, stern discipline and very low pay to care for the sick.

The two busts now rest in the entrance hall of the District Headquarters building at Sharoe Green, one being that of Sir Charles Brown and the other of John Bairstow Esq. whose original gift of £20,500 to the Infirmary in 1869 had made possible the necessary improvements to set the Infirmary on course for expansion.

Epilogue

FROM the outset it has been a difficult task to know what to include in a work such as this as there are perhaps hundreds of episodes which will have remained vividly within people's memories of the Infirmary which have not been recorded here. One such episode that springs to mind which occurred in the 1950s concerns the two busts mentioned when, following a soirée in the doctors' mess at that time nicknamed 'The Vino Club', the busts disappeared. There followed days of speculation, including the digging up of the front lawn, where a 'pink elephant' made in the snow may have become the depository of the busts. Later, following threats of instant dismissal of the culprits if the busts were not returned unharmed, they finally reappeared with streamers blazoned across the main Infirmary corridor saying 'Welcome back to Bob and Jack', and were replaced on their respective plinths each covered with the pink spots of 'measles' which incidently took some removing without leaving some trace of the dye used. It was the talking point of the Infirmary for many weeks afterwards but the persons responsible for their removal were never found. Quite often over the years when the busts were removed from their plinths for cleaning by the portering staff, it was found that they were replaced on the wrong plinths; it is to be hoped that some means of marking them can be found to avoid such an occurrence in the future.

The atmosphere in the Infirmary held in people's memories arises from the people themselves, of course, and not from the buildings; but the Infirmary's homely atmosphere has not, and I fear cannot be, transferred to the Royal Preston Hospital as easily as it was to transfer the Royal patronage, it had built up over the years in an atmosphere which was totally different from today's 'big is beautiful' concept at the Royal Preston Hospital. There are many imponderables regarding the Infirmary and its final closure and disposal of the site by the Health Authority which has been going on since November 1980 in anticipation of the opening of the Royal Preston Hospital. Already most of the Infirmary and its original satellite establishments such as Deepdale Hospital, Fulwood Continuation Hospital, Lostock Hall Continuation Hospital etc. have either been thrown into disuse or disposed of altogether leaving little of the former H.M.C. properties available for use.

It was anticipated that the in-patient and other services remaining in the Infirmary would finally close during April 1987 with the commissioning of new in-patient services at Sharoe Green Hospital. The pathology laboratory would, however, remain in isolation fronting onto Meadow Street posing many further problems for the administration into the 1990s until a new pathology department is completed at the Royal Preston Hospital site, commencement of this being due to take place in October 1987. When my service commenced in the laboratory in April 1946 plans were already to hand for a new laboratory to be built, but with the advent of the N.H.S. in 1948 this was not achieved until 12 years later in 1958 and within two years a great amount of alteration was necessary to accommodate the full capacity of work being carried out at that time. Since then further expansion has been necessary to accommodate other specialities which have emerged in pathology such as viriology, neuropathology, electron microscopy, immunology and histochemistry, to name but a few, giving rise to a situation which borders on contravention of the Health and Safety at Work Act. Over the past 15 years several sets of plans have been prepared, discussed and agreed, later being revised and on each occasion reduced from the agreed original to accommodation which will not be sufficient to house the existing specialities leaving little scope for any expansion to keep pace with modern advances in pathology.

The progress of the Dispensary, the Infirmary and of health care generally in Preston over the last 178 years has, as this volume shows, been a struggle to survive in an atmosphere of financial constraint and whilst keeping abreast of the vast changes that were taking place in both medicine and surgery, together with the technological impact of many new branches of science. It is to the credit of the hospital administrators of the past that they achieved so much with so little although it must not be forgotten that they were helped in this by the dedication and devotion of innumerable people who were both poorly paid and for the most part shabbily treated. The main theme throughout, however, was that of expansion, enlarging the Infirmary and adding its satellites in order to accommodate more and more patients with a service that was second to none, and all this being accomplished by public subscription from the people of Preston and its surrounding district, the magnificent help given by the Workpeople's Fund and the benevolence of Sir Charles Brown.

Today we talk in millions of pounds and quite glibly record that the Preston Health District was recently stated to be overspent by £3 million; the administrators of 1869 found the £20,500 given by John Bairstow Esq. a fortune beyond their wildest dreams at a time when most of the population of Britain had no conception of what a million pounds was and yet today we see a service which is contracting into less accommodation than before and the Health District is forced into utilising the mushrooming area of private nursing homes to accommodate its elderly patients, together with many other problems of a similar nature.

The story of Preston's Royal Infirmary and that of health care generally in Preston cannot be completed at the time of writing for it still continues to operate in the capacity for which it was erected more than 150 years ago, healing the sick of Preston, albeit to a much lesser degree than in days gone by, although if the resources were available there is no doubt it could still continue to operate to the benefit of the town for many years yet to come.

With my own retirement from the Infirmary's laboratory staff after almost 40 years it must be left to some other agency, perhaps, to finish this historical account and trace the furtherance of health care in Preston in the years to come.

Appendix A

PRESTON ROYAL INFIRMARY

An Inventory of Attractive Portable Items
(Including small items of Historical Interest)

STRONG ROOM
1 'Courant' letter opener.
1 small printer's block, bearing the old Infirmary crest.
1 silver cup. Preston & Chorley H.M.C. - Ladies Singles Tennis Competition.
1 certificate of appreciation date 14th September 1947, Royal British Legion Poppy Appeal.
1 Certificate of Patronage from H.M. King George VI dated 13th August 1937.
1 programme of the visit of H.R.H. The Princess Mary dated 8th August 1929.
1 copy of 'Hospital Year Book' 1947.
1 small brass bell with wooden handle.
1 large brass bell with wooden handle.
1 gavel and block (wood).
1 cut glass vase, Whittle's Jewellers Ltd., 111 Fishergate Preston.
1 large bible containing the names of House Surgeons from 18th October 1869 to 5th August 1947.
1 'Alex Foster' Gold Medal awarded to the most efficient nurse of the year at Preston Royal Infirmary.
1 silver bowl inscribed P.R.I. M.H.
1 silver tray with three feet, presented to Mr. Wm. Tuson, October 1848.
1 presentation set of trowel and mallet which were used at the laying of the foundation stone of the new Maternity Hospital on 12th July 1934.
1 photograph of Preston Royal Infirmary circa 1925.

WALL PLAQUES, BRASS or BRONZE

The 'Hatch' cot 1943.
The 'Helena Mary Simpson' cot 1942.
The 'Croston and District Ambulance' cot 1948.
The 'Keighley' cot.

WALL PLAQUES, BRASS or BRONZE *Continued*

The 'North of Preston Flower Club' cot.
1 invitation and programme for the Preston Guild Merchant 1922.
1 invitation and programme for the Preston Guild Merchant 1952.
1 dinner invitation to attend the retirement of Mr. G. H. Warburton Steel circe March 1958.
1 invitation to a dinner held by the P.R.I. board of management, 28th June 1948.
1 invitation to the official opening of the new department of pathology and Public Health Laboratory, Meadow Street, on 11th December 1958.
1 programme of the ceremony at the opening of the medical wards on 24th January 1938.
1 invitiation to the official opening of the rehabilitation dept., 9th March 1946.
1 invitation to the opening of the new casualty dept. at Chorley District Hospital on 20th December 1957.
1 invitation to the opening of the Preston post-graduate medical centre on 25th March 1969.
1 programme to the opening of the new Maternity Hospital on 4th September 1936.
1 programme for the opening of Lostock Hall Continuation Hospital new extension on 26th June 1930.
1 programme for the opening of 'The Willows' Convalescent Hospital on 11th October 1928.
1 silver communion cup inscribed with a cross.
1 silver coloured communion cup.
1 silver coloured bowl (marked on base, W. Germany).
1 silver coloured cork screw.
1 silver communion wafer box (inscribed with cross and circle).
2 brass candle holders.
1 large silver communion cup (inscribed in memory of my parents Stephen Michael and Margaret Alice Healy) dated 1973.
1 polished wooden casket, fitted with lock and inscribed 'Presented by the members of the St. Ignatius' Altar Society' and containing two small candle holders, one wooden cross and a photograph of Sister Jeannie Gibson.
1 standard lamp.
1 communion set and casket comprising one silver wine cup and tray and one silver wine jug. The casket engraved W.C.H. 1930.
1 auriscope.
1 patella hammer.
1 stormoguide presented by Mr. Lawrence Cartwright.
1 box of sutures, some of which are gold plated.
1 craniotome.
1 very old gastroscope in a wooden box.
1 set of urethral dilators in a wooden box.
1 framed notice of 'Fire Explosion Hazard' 55/44.
1 large cylindrical swab jar.
1 gold metal catheter.
2 G.U. old catalogues.
1 picture of Princess Mary, signed and dated 6th August 1925.
1 aerial view of Preston Royal Infirmary dated June 1927.

WALL PLAQUES, BRASS or BRONZE *Continued*

1 Minute Book from 3rd May 1883-17th February 1906.
1 Minute Book from 25th April 1938-31st December 1945.
1 Minute Book from 2nd December 1949-16th January 1956.
1 bound volume of Year Book 1921-1925.
1 bound volume of Year Book 1931-1935.
1 bound volume of Year Book 1936-1940.
1 bound volume of Year Book 1941-1948.

PHOTOGRAPHS

1 nursing group dated 1902 - Arthur Winter, Preston.
1 nursing group at opening of the nurses home - Arthur Winter, Preston.

PICTURES IN FRAMES

1 Alex Foster, chairman 1924-1937.
1 David Irwin J.P., chairman 1895-1899.
1 Robert Charles Brown M.A., presented by the Preston Medico-Ethical Society circe 1912.
1 William P. Park J.P., chairman 1899-1918.
1 Robert Charles Brown M.A., photo by Geo. Devey, Preston 1903.
1 Vandyke Puix 'D. Harvey' print, published in May 1794, Laurie & Whittle, 53 Fleet Street, London.
1 Allison Davies C.B.E., J.P., member, board of management 1937-1946 and chairman from 1946-1948.
1 Sir William Ascroft D.L., J.P., chairman 1937-1946, hon. solicitor, trustee member of board of management 1906-1946, vice-president 1947.
1 Edmund Bailey J.P., chairman 1894-1895.
1 C. R. Jacson J.P., chairman 1869-1894.
1 Alderman J. C. Hamilton J.P., chairman 1918-1924.

ALBUMS

1 opening of the new Maternity Hospital by the Countess of Derby, 4th September 1936.
2 laying of foundation stone of new Maternity Hospital by the Rt. Worshipful the Mayor, Alderman Mrs. M. A. Pimblett J.P., on 12th July 1934.
2 visit of H.R.H. The Princess Mary, Viscountess Lascelles, 8th August 1929.
1 visit of H.R.H. The Princess Mary, Viscountess Lascelles, 6th August 1925.

BOOKS ETC.

Attendance Books for Committee Members 1959/1969 and 1970/1974.
Year Books, Light Department, year ending 31st December 1922.
31st December 1928.
31st. December 1931.
31st December 1932.
2 New Testaments presented by Mrs. Weight and her pupils from Ribble Bank School, Christmas 1867.
1 Museum of St. Louis Hospital, Paris 1897.
1 atlas of Venereal Diseases, Maclaren 1886.

BOOKS ETC. Continued

2 Atlas of Clinical Medicine, Dr. Byron Bramwell Vol. 1 (1892) Vol. 2 (1893).
1 Brackenbury Library Catalogue.
1 Record of Books Borrowed and Returned 1906-1961.
1 Illustrations of Dissections, Ellis and Ford, 1867.
1 Sibson's Medical Anatomy.
1 Atlas of Diseases of the Skin, H. Radcliffe Crocker, 2 Vols, 1896.
1 folder containing information regarding the 'Centenary of Preston Royal Infirmary' dated 1st January 1970.
1 sealed cardboard box containing old unidentified photographs and newspaper cuttings.

THE MAIN CORRIDOR OF THE INFIRMARY

4 large polished wood panels recording names of benefactors 1869-1948.
8 leaded light windows - two bearing the Infirmary crest.
1 main entrance door with glass panel engraved with the Infirmary's crest.
4 brass door handles.
1 staircase to Board Room with carved crests on the Newel posts.
1 painting of Thomas Moore of Preston, surgeon, died 17th April 1848.
1 painting of Frederick William Collinson, 1887-1923.
(These paintings were accepted by the post-graduate medical centre).
1 bust of Sir Robert Charles Brown M.A. 1869-1925.
1 bust of John Bairstow, 1869.
(These busts were transferred to the District Headquarters building).
1 plaque to commemorate long and devoted service of Mr. John Tierney.
1 plaque in recognition of the devoted service of all staff, dated 1948.
1 Guild plaque 'Preston & Chorley Hospital Management Committee'.

THE EXTERNAL SURVEY SHOWED:

Main double entrance gates and adjacent pedestrian entrance gates, with wrought ironwork features to the top of the four gate pillars.

THE MATERNITY DEPARTMENT

Left of the main entrance doors - a foundation stone laid by the Mayor of Preston, Alderman Mrs. M. A. Pimblett J.P., dated 12th July 1934.
Right of the main entrance doors - a stone commemorating the opening by the Countess of Derby on 4th September 1936.
Over the main door at high level, a stone denoting the date of opening - 1936.

THE NURSES HOME

Stone denoting extension - W. W. Galloway Esq., J.P., opened by the Mayor, Alderman W. E. Morris on 29th January 1940.
On Deepdale Road side of the building a commemorative stone to the 60th year of the reign of Queen Victoria - A.D. 1897.

THE INFIRMARY'S MAIN ENTRANCE

On the front aspect above the front door, a stone feature of the Coat of Arms and designation 'ROYAL INFIRMARY', also the date in Roman numerals - 1833.

REHABILITATION DEPARTMENT (Internal)

A small metal plaque recording the opening by George Tomlinson M.P. 9th March 1946.

BROWN, GREEN AND CHILDREN'S WARDS

Foundation stone denoting laying by H.R.H. The Princess Mary, Viscountess Lascelles on 6th August 1925.
stone commemorating opening by H.R.H. The Princess Mary, Viscountess Lascelles on 8th August 1929.

X-RAY DEPARTMENT (Stanleyfield Road)

Foundation stone laid by Alderman J. C. Hamilton J.P., August 1921.
Cast iron spout heads dated 1922.

MAIN OPERATING THEATRE

A commemorative stone on the gable end - 'The gift of Dr. R. C. Brown, 1900'.

THE FEVER WARDS (Medical, Orthopaedic and Ophthalmology)

Three wards each with a gable end inscription:—

1. The gift of
2. E. R. Harris
3. 1875 (in Roman numerals).

THE NURSES TRAINING SCHOOL

A glass panel in the entrance door with crest and lettering 'Preliminary Training School'.

THE NURSES DINING ROOM

Foundation stone laid by Henry Astley-Bell J.P., Guild Mayor 8th September 1922.

THE BOARD ROOM

1 signed photograph of H.M. Queen Elizabeth II, Patron of P.R.I. 1962.
1 wooden cupboard with three doors and sloping top.
1 Smith's quartz wall clock.
1 black ink-well and pen holder.
21 Board Room chairs, red leather upholstery seat and back, with casters.
1 chairman's chair, red leather upholstered seat and back, with arms.
1 solid wood table, polished, with four ornate legs, measuring 12′×6′ constructed in two pieces.
1 solid wooden table, 9′×6′ with a raised central dais and four legs. (It was decided that all these items would be transferred into the new Board Room at the District Headquarters building).

THE INFIRMARY CHAPEL

8 stained glass windows.
1st right - St. Barnabas, dedicated to Wm. Allison Davies J.P., chairman H.M.C.
2nd right - St. John, dedicated to Wm. Henry Pimblett 1887-1937.
3rd right - St. Paul, dedicated to F. R. Collinson, senior surgeon and vice-president of P.R.I.

THE INFIRMARY CHAPEL *Continued*

4th right - coloured glass window, plaque to pupil midwife Janet Preston.
1st left - Madonna holding bible, dedicated to Miss Ronson and Miss Rice by members of the Preston Royal Infirmary League of Nurses. (The bible bears the P.R.I. crest).
2nd left - St. Luke, dedicated to Alexander Foster, chairman of the H.M.C.
3rd left - Florence Nightingale window, dedicated to William Galloway, member of the H.M.C. and benefactor of P.R.I.
4th left - coloured glass window.
14 wooden pews, with red leather type seats.
1 wood and brass crucifix.
1 organ and pipes.
1 piano.
1 brass candle snuffer.
1 arched entrance in wood with coloured glass.
1 brass door handle.
1 wooden reredos.
1 wooden lectern.
1 steel flower holder.
2 wooden kneelers.
1 wooden altar.
1 wooden, glass topped, 'Book of Rememberance' display case.
1 wooden flower stand.
1 wooden piano screen.
38 home made fabric kneelers.
1 wall plaque 'In rememberance of James Tomlinson J.P.'.
6 brass window plaques, movable.
2 ladder backed chairs with rush seats.
1 small wooden table with a glass top.
1 small wooden cross.

CHILDREN'S WARD AND STAIRCASE

12 large nursery rhyme pictures in ceramic tiles.
30 single ceramic tiles of animals and birds and other picture tiles, possibly boxed in on fireplaces.
1 picture in copper bronze and also a carved wooden plaque both dedicated to the memory of Alderman Thomas Parkinson, a member of the H.M.C. whose donation of £10,000 covered the cost of the new children's ward in 1929.
20 brass door knobs/handles.
6 brass escutcheons.
4 brass door plates.
1 brass door bell.
1 stained glass window bearing the crest of 'The Royal Infirmary, Preston'.
2 wooden arched door casings.
1 curved wooden bannister rail.
In the wards and corridors of the Infirmary and the Maternity Hospital more than 120 plaques were listed recording endowments of beds and cots over a period ranging from 1893 to 1975.

Bibliographical Note

Appendix B

Records held at Preston Royal Infirmary in the 1970s

BOARDROOM CUPBOARD	
Infirmary Committee Minutes	1865-1866
Finance Committee Minutes	1870-1887
Building Committee Minutes	1868-1870
Report of Board of Management	1869
Ladies Committee Minutes	1925
Annual Meeting, Subscribers and Donors Minutes	1933-1947
Workpeople's Fund; Executive Committee Minutes	1937-1948
The Infirmary Rules	1911
Correspondence regarding legacies	1930s
Correspondence regarding Maternity Services	1937
Register of Government Emergency Stocks	1939
Subscribers' Book	1936-1949
Statement of Accounts	1948
Lancs. Voluntary Hospitals Committee Correspondence	1936-1938
British Hospital Assoc. (North-West) Minutes	1941-1947
Lancashire Council Council; Div. Health Services	1948
Report on the British Health Services (Survey by P.E.P. - Political & Economic Planning)	1937
SECTOR ADMINISTRATOR'S OFFICE	
Preston Royal Infirmary Annual Reports (bound)	1869-1921
	1926-1930
Preston Royal Infirmary Annual Reports (loose)	1871-1898
	1901-1905
	1907-1924
	1926-1927
	1945
Preston Royal Infirmary Rules	1911
Mills & Workshops Committee Annual Reports (bound)	1884-1913
(loose)	1914

MEDICAL RECORDS DEPARTMENT (basement 1)

E.M.S. Admission/Discharge Book	1939-1949
General Operations Register (10 Volumes)	1917-1941/1943-1959/1964-1970
E.N.T. Operations Register (6 Volumes)	1944-1971
Out-patient Minor Operations	1943-1953
Urological Theatre Register	1954-1956
Small Theatre Operations Register	1955-1973
Orthopaedic Operations	1956-1967
E.N.T. Waiting Lists (6 Volumes)	1954-1968

MEDICAL RECORDS DEPARTMENT (basement 2)

Weekly Statistics (6 Volumes)	1934-1954
Day Books (4 Volumes)	1947-1950
Ward Registers (47 Volumes)	1939-1957
Lostock Hall: Register of Patients (4 Volumes)	1947-1960

RECORDS HELD AT PRESTON PUBLIC LIBRARY

Preston Dispensary - 25th Annual Report	1834
Preston Royal Infirmary: Annual Reports	1928-1946
Reports on Infectious Diseases Wards	c1870
Numbers, Cost and Residence of Patients	1934
Bazaar Programme	1866
Souvenir	1925
Effort Committee: Rag-Mag	1929
Programme of opening of Maternity Hospital	1936
Catalogue of the Brackenbury Library	1895
Rev. J. Clay: Report on Preston's Sanitary condition	1844
Preston Sanitary Assoc. discussion on high death rate	1885
Dr. Charles Brown: 'Sixty Four Years a Doctor'	1922
C. Gardner: The Care of the sick poor of Preston in the Nineteenth Century (Thesis)	1967
Preston Health Committee Minutes	1900-1901

Statistical Tables

Appendix C

TABLE 1 — IN-PATIENT STATISTICS, 1948-51

	1948	*1949*	*1950*	*1951*
Total bed complement	401	401	401	401
No. of beds temporarily unavailabe on 31 Dec.	—	—	—	27
Average daily no. of beds occupied over year	322	334	329	306
Highest daily occupancy in year	368	379	365	339
Lowest daily occupancy in year	228	223	216	220
No. of patients discharged (including deaths) during year:				
General Medicine		1,313	1,371	1,234
General Surgery		2,831	2,951	2,777
Private Pay Beds		506	491	548
Unclassified		—	—	21
Genito-urinary		666	839	863
Gynaecology		864	924	859
Obstetrics		1,159	1,227	1,077
Paediatrics		—	—	—
E.N.T.		869	1,163	1,096
Ophthalmology		413	440	499
Orthopaedic		526	683	749
TOTALS	8,558	9,147	10,089	10,027

TABLE 2 — OUT-PATIENT STATISTICS, 1949-51

	1949		*1950*		*1951*	
Attendances	*New Out-patients*	*Total Attended*	*New Out-patients*	*Total Attended*	*New Out-patients*	*Total Attended*
Consultative Clinics						
General Medicine	2,235	7,015	2,458	6,103	2,734	5,913
General Surgery	4,466	8,056	4,162	8,368	3,902	8,306
Gynaecology	1,099	2,455	1,238	2,555	1,147	2,395
Obstetrics	1,136	9,810	1,342	11,275	1,998	10,892
Psychiatry	370	2,510	484	2,706	429	3,144
Dentistry	488	523	508	508	560	866
Dermatology	1,358	4,984	1,388	4,096	1,151	3,545
Ear, Nose & Throat	2,151	16,650	3,055	19,398	3,210	16,945
Ophthalmology	1,908	7,446	2,001	7,409	1,809	7,195
Radiotherapy	1,106	9,435	1,121	9,176	869	9,472
Orthopaedics	3,298	15,663	3,467	13,967	3,606	13,234
V.D.	477	5,837	449	5,324	453	4,525
Genito-urinary	572	2,300	635	1,922	664	1,936
Pathology	1,972	3,077	2,102	3,549	2,243	3,427
Thoracic Surgery	14	18	35	50	16	42
Plastic Surgery	—	—	—	—	9	11
TOTALS	22,650	95,779	24,445	96,406	24,800	91,848

TABLE 3 — ATTENDANCES, 1949-51

	1949		*1950*		*1851*	
	New Out-patients	*Total Attended*	*New Out-patients*	*Total Attended*	*New Out-patients*	*Total Attended*
Out-patient Treatment Clinics						
Radiological	15,582	15,582	15,216	15,216	15,632	15,632
Light	1,055	62,574	1,177	58,335	846	53,203
Physiotherapy	5,113	31,826	6,503	37,849	6,098	35,055
Rehabilitation	697	16,628	840	16,910	999	23,972
Orthoptics	124	4,664	92	3,337	102	3,251
Hearing Aids	1,949	5,087	2,548	11,534	2,594	13,686
Speech Therapy	14	170	17	212	5	250
Accidents & Casualties	18,260	70,318	21,007	70,100	19,738	66,829
Treatment Totals	42,794	206,849	47,400	213,493	46,014	211,878
GRAND TOTALS	65,444	302,628	71,845	309,899	70,814	303,726

TABLE 4 — STAFFING AT PRESTON ROYAL INFIRMARY, 1960-74

Year	*Nurses*	*Medical Officers*	*Admin. & Clerical*	*Prof. & Technical*	*Catering*	*Laundry*	*TOTAL Staff*
1960	298	22	53	70	42	27	716
1961	301	22	55	79	49	29	708
1962	313	29	56	79	54	29	735
1963	315	24	61	80	54	30	785·5
1964	325	22	65	77	52	29	776
1965	318	25	67	84	53	33	801
1966	358	22	67	77	55	35	819
1967	367	23	69	92	54	35	845
1968	387	22	68	94	52	33	861
1969	401	27	68	103	52	31	883
1970	466	25	78	107	52	34	968
1971	499	25	75	114	48	32	997
1972	536	26	75	116	53	36	1,084
1973	569	29	82	128	48	34	1,092
1974	573	30	89	128	49	32	1,114

TABLE 5 — PRESTON ROYAL INFIRMARY STATISTICS, 1960-74

Year	*Bed Complement*	*Average Occupancy*	*Available Staffed Beds*	*Length of Stay in Days*	*Out-Patients Attendances*
1960	409	318			143,090
1961	410	310			145,378
1962	413	296			143,749
1963	413	296			145,589
1964	413	288			147,405
1965	413	275			151,140
1966	424	277	75%	7.8	149,440
1967	424	279	71%	8.6	145,007
1968	424	281	73%	8,4	144,230
1969	416	277	71%	8.3	144,651
1970	413	270	70%	8.6	142,331
1971	413	273	73%	8.3	143,002
1972	413	306	78%	8.4	151,657
1973	413	301	75%	8.0	151,490
1974	413	271	75%	7.9	149,794

TABLE 6 — OUT-PATIENTS ATTENDING PRESTON ROYAL INFIRMARY, APRIL/JUNE 1975

Speciality	*No. of Clinics held*	*No. of new attendances*	*Total attendances*
General medicine	55	179	957
Surgical	39	517	1,867
Urology	34	235	1,232
Paediatrics	100	165	1,399
Gynaecology	43	190	986
Orthopaedics	122	1,184	4,525
Neuro Surgery	12	27	203
Neurology	12	38	321
Dermatology	42	224	517
E.N.T.	68	495	3,157
Radiotherapy	13	123	702
Dental	71	167	702
Orthodontics	40	88	723
Obstetrics	102	461	2,763
V.D.	51	316	824

Index

A

B

C

D

E

F

G

H

I

J

K

L

M

N

O

P

Q

R

X

Y